Although descriptions of the syndrome date back to the seventeenth century, akathisia has long seemed an orphan within neuropsychiatry, lacking until recently the serious attention it deserves. This book reviews the diverse published material on akathisia and related disorders, including restless legs syndrome, other forms of motor restlessness, and neuroleptic-induced dysphoria, and provides a comprehensive account of these important but insufficiently researched syndromes.

A historical overview of the underlying concepts sets the scene for a detailed exposition of current knowledge. The main focus is on drug-induced akathisia and its various subtypes, each of which is discussed in terms of the author's own criteria as well as those of other investigators. Dr Sachdev examines the relationship of drug-induced akathisia to the restlessness caused by other neurological disorders and presents a new synthesis of the underlying pathophysiological mechanisms. What constitutes akathisia is an important clinical and research question, and the author provides arguments for new operational criteria for the research diagnosis of drug-induced akathisia. Strategies for the measurement of akathisia are discussed, as are treatment approaches, and a fascinating appendix contains a translation of Haskovec's original account of the syndrome.

This is the first extended review of scientific and clinical aspects of akathisia and restlessness, and also suggests directions for their future investigation. It will be much valued by psychiatrists, neurologists and other physicians seeking a better understanding of these disabling syndromes.

AKATHISIA AND RESTLESS LEGS

AKATHISIA AND RESTLESS LEGS

PERMINDER SACHDEV

University of New South Wales
The Prince Henry Hospital

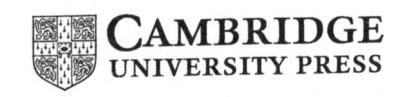

CAMBRIDGE UNIVERSITY PRESS

Cambridge, New York, Melbourne, Madrid, Cape Town, Singapore, São Paulo

Cambridge University Press
The Edinburgh Building, Cambridge CB2 2RU, UK

Published in the United States of America by Cambridge University Press, New York

www.cambridge.org
Information on this title: www.cambridge.org/9780521444262

First published 1995
This digitally printed first paperback version 2006

A catalogue record for this publication is available from the British Library

Library of Congress Cataloguing in Publication data

Sachdev, Perminder.
Akathisia and restless legs / Perminder Sachdev.
p. cm.
Includes bibliographical references and index.
ISBN 0-521-44426-8 (hardback)
1. Tardive dyskinesia. I. Title.
[DNLM: 1. Psychomotor Agitation. 2. Restless Legs.   WM 197 S121a
1995]
RC394.T37S23 1995
616.8'3 – dc20
DNLM/DLC
for Library of Congress   94-40259
                                                                          CIP

ISBN-13 978-0-521-44426-2 hardback
ISBN-10 0-521-44426-8 hardback

ISBN-13 978-0-521-03148-6 paperback
ISBN-10 0-521-03148-6 paperback

To Jagdeep, Sonal and Nupur

Contents

Foreword

In this era of rapidly proliferating scientific articles and texts, it is often difficult to identify and assimilate those publications which are truly useful addi-
tions to our knowledge base. Perminder Sachdev's scholarly and thorough
review of akathisia and restless legs provides an extremely valuable synopsis
of current information on this syndrome, and in fact represents a 'coming of
age' of akathisia.

Akathisia has come to be associated with neuroleptic drug treatment; however, restless legs syndrome (also referred to as Ekbom's syndrome) as well
as the akathisia seen in both postencephalitic and idiopathic parkinsonism
may have some important common symptoms and pathophysiological features. Therefore, it is very helpful to have all of these syndromes discussed in
one text. This volume thoroughly reviews the concept of restlessness, as well
as its manifestations in a variety of clinical and nonclinical contexts. It also
includes a compendium of instruments and techniques for assessing akathisia
and restlessness.

A detailed discussion of the definition, assessment and diagnosis of drug-
induced akathisia is provided and operational criteria for use in clinical
research are proposed. Although neuroleptic-induced akathisia can produce a
considerable degree of subjective dysphoria, the latter may apparently also
occur independently of akathisia and is generally referred to as neuroleptic-
induced dysphoria. Despite the paucity of data, the author reviews current
knowledge and potential research implications of such dysphoria.

The epidemiology of akathisia has not been studied extensively, and the
same conceptual and methodological problems that challenge differential
diagnosis of the syndrome also preclude any firm conclusions regarding its
incidence and prevalence. The existing database on this issue is thoroughly
reviewed and critiqued, providing an important stepping-stone for further
progress in this area. As new and potentially novel or superior antipsychotic

medications are introduced, it will become increasingly important to have well-developed methods for establishing the relative risk for syndromes such as akathisia associated with different drugs.

The treatment of akathisia, systematically discussed in this volume, takes on additional significance in light of the literature on the effects of akathisia on patient compliance with drug regimes, subjective well-being and suicidal and aggressive behaviour.

The relationship between acute akathisia and syndromes of chronic movement disorders such as tardive dyskinesia is crucial, both from a public health standpoint and heuristically. In addition, the potential existence of a syndrome labeled 'tardive akathisia' is an important issue in this context. Though there is still much controversy and need for further research, Sachdev suggests that the weight of the evidence supports the notion that tardive akathisia and tardive dyskinesia are separate syndromes, albeit with considerable overlap.

Perhaps the most challenging aspect of the text is the thorough review of hypotheses and data relating to pathophysiology. As with many clinical effects of antipsychotic medications, the implications for improving our understanding of neuropharmacological mechanisms of medication effects are extremely important, as are the implications for the prevention and treatment of adverse effects.

This volume contains important discussions of a number of other relevant areas, and the sum of all the parts amounts to a prodigious compilation and synthesis of data gathered from diverse fields. It will serve as an extremely valuable resource to clinicians and researchers alike.

JOHN M. KANE, MD

Acknowledgements

Numerous individuals have directly or indirectly contributed to the development of the ideas and the writing of this book. My interest in psychiatric research found able mentors in Narendra N. Wig, MD, during my New Delhi years and Gordon B. Parker, MD, PhD, in Sydney, and their influence is prevalent throughout these pages. Professor Parker was a collaborator in my first research project on akathisia. I have followed John M. Kane's research with great fascination for more than a decade and felt honoured when he agreed to write a foreword. Of the many colleagues who have critically read my papers in the past, three deserve special mention: Henry Brodaty, MD, Robert Finlay-Jones, MD, PhD, and Kit-Yun Chee, FRANZCP. Professor Finlay-Jones also deserves my gratitude for pointing out many grammatical and stylistic errors, discerned with the keen eye of a former journal editor. My research interest in akathisia was sparked by the writings of Theodore Van Putten, MD, and Thomas R. E. Barnes, MD, and if I have one hope regarding this book, it is that it will be considered to have built on and furthered their work. Dr Van Putten (1938–1993) is unfortunately no longer with us to provide criticism or approval. Dr A. E. Lang and Dr R. E. Burke were kind enough to provide preprint copies of their papers.

My research into akathisia has been ably assisted by Celia Loneragan and Jane Kruk, both exemplary research associates. They are co-authors of a number of my papers cited in this book. I am also grateful to Ms Kruk for her extensive reviews of the literature, which made my task so much easier. I have periodically sought statistical advice from the following colleagues: Dusan Hadzi-Pavlovic, Alexandra Walker, Kaarin Anstey, Anthony Kuk and Wayne Hall, and I am extremely grateful for their assistance. Ms Walker kindly agreed to translate Haskovec's paper from the French, and the translated version is presented in Appendix A.

My clinical investigations were aided by the permission granted by many colleagues to study their patients. In particular, I express my thanks to the following physicians: Marie-Paul Austin, Neil Buhrich, Stan Catts, Charles Doutney, Frank Hume, Philip Mitchell, Richard Perkins, Patrick Toohey, Kay Wilhelm and Andrew Wilson. Doutney, Hume and Toohey were collaborators in the study of tardive akathisia. The nursing staff at the Prince Henry and Prince of Wales Hospitals, as well as the community centres of the Eastern Sydney Area Health Service, were extremely helpful in the investigations. Special thanks are owed to Sister Anna Misamer and Sister Anne McKinnon for their patience and care. Sister Misamer's knowledge of German took me through some papers that would otherwise have been inaccessible.

A manuscript does not take shape without the painstaking efforts of secretaries, and I acknowledge my debt to Doreen Hanlon, who took up this challenge as 'my book' and quickly mastered the bibliography to the extent that Dr Van Putten's entries soon became a string of numbers she could recite. Without her efforts, many more publisher's deadlines would have gone by. She was assisted in this task by Dorothy Janssen and Mary Burgess.

Throughout the writing of this book, which took much longer than I had initially anticipated, Richard Barling, MD, and Laura Wise of Cambridge University Press were extremely helpful, encouraging and, above all, tolerant. The illustrations for the book were prepared by the Medical Illustration Unit of the University of New South Wales.

My research into akathisia has been supported largely by the National Health and Medical Research Council of Australia. Additional financial support was provided by the Ramaciotti Foundations, the Rebecca L. Cooper Foundation and the Coast Centenary Research Fund.

I dedicate this book to my wife, Jagdeep, and two daughters, Sonal and Nupur. Jagdeep has been a companion, friend and colleague for eight years and has provided the emotional nurture without which the task would have been impossible. Sonal and Nupur provided the joie de vivre that made the long evenings of writing bearable. To them, and my parents, I will be eternally in debt.

The author is extremely grateful to the following publishers and scientific bodies for their kind permission to duplicate previously published material: *Biological Psychiatry* and the Society for Biological Psychiatry for Appendix B; *British Journal of Psychiatry* and the Royal College of Psychiatrists, London, for Appendic C; *Psychopharmacology Bulletin* and the National Institute of Mental Health for Appendix D; the Movement Disorders Society for Figure 7.1 and Table 7.4; *Journal of Neurology, Neurosurgery and Psychiatry* and the British Medical Association for Table 7.3; Marcel Dekker, New York, for Figure 12.1; Penguin Books for the quotation from *Roget's Thesaurus* (p. 18); and Oxford University Press for quotations on pages 188 and 210.

Abbreviations

AA	acute akathisia
AC	adenyl cyclase
ACh	acetylcholine
ADHD	attention-deficit hyperactivity disorder
βA	β-adrenergic
BBB	blood–brain barrier
CA	chronic akathisia
CNS	central nervous system
CSF	cerebrospinal fluid
CT	computerized tomography
DA	dopamine
5,6DHT	5,6-dihydroxytryptamine
DIA	drug-induced akathisia
DIP	drug-induced parkinsonism
DWA	diskinesias while awake
ECG	electrocardiogram
ECT	electroconvulsive therapy
EEG	electroencephalogram
EL	encephalitis lethargica
EMG	electromyogram
EPSE	extrapyramidal side-effects
GABA	γ-aminobutyric acid
Glu	glutamate
GPe	globus pallidus externa
GPi	globus pallidus interna
HC	home cage
5HT	5-hydroxytryptamine (serotonin)
5HTP	5-hydroxytryptophan
ID	iron deficiency

LT	limb-truncal
MHPG	3-methoxy-4-hydroxyphenyl glycol
MI	movement index
MLMR	mesencephalic locomotor region
MSH	melanocyte-stimulating hormone
NCV	nerve conduction velocity
NDef	neuroleptic-induced defecation
NE	norepinephrine
NIA	neuroleptic-induced akathisia
NID	neuroleptic-induced dysphoria
NIP	neuroleptic-induced parkinsonism
NM	nocturnal myoclonus
NMDA	N-methyl D-aspartate
NREM	non–rapid eye movement sleep
OBLF	oral–buccal–lingual–facial
OCD	obsessive-compulsive disorder
OF	open field
pCPA	p-chlorophenylalanine
PD	Parkinson's disease
PET	positron emission tomography
PLMS	periodic leg movements in sleep
PLMT	painful legs and moving toes
POMS	profile of mood states
PPD	postpsychotic depression
REM	rapid eye movement
RLS	restless legs syndrome
ROC	receiver operating characteristic
SCN	suprachiasmic nucleus
SMA	supplementary motor area
SN	substantia nigra
SNr	substantia nigra pars reticulata
SP	supersensitivity psychosis
SRI	serotonin-reuptake inhibitor
STN	subthalamic nucleus
TA	tardive akathisia
TCA	tricyclic antidepressant
TD	tardive dyskinesia
TDt	tardive dystonia
TDys	tardive dysmentia
VTA	ventral tegmental area
WA	withdrawal akathisia

PART I
Introduction

1

Akathisia: development of the concept

Akathisia, a stepchild of movement disorders and an orphan of psychiatry, is beginning to receive the serious attention and clarification it deserves.

Stephen Stahl (1985)

The term *akathisia* is of Greek derivation and, translated literally into English, means 'not to sit'. It was first used by Lad Haskovec (1902) (see Appendix A) to describe two patients with restlessness and an inability to sit still. Descriptions of a syndrome resembling akathisia can, however, be traced to much earlier than the beginning of the twentieth century. The first documented description has been attributed to the British physician and anatomist Thomas Willis[1] (1621–1675), better known for his careful studies of the nervous system. The first edition of his *London Practice of Physik* was published in 1685, but Critchley (1955) quoted from his second edition, printed in 1695, as follows: 'Wherefore to some, when being a Bed they betake themselves to sleep, presently in the Arms and Leggs, Leapings and Contractions of the Tendons, and so great a Restlessness and Tossings of their Members ensue, that the diseased are no more able to sleep, than if they were in a Place of the greatest Torture' (p. 101).

The earliest nineteenth-century account resembling akathisia has been attributed to Wittmaack (1861), who referred to the syndrome as *anxietas*

---

[1] Thomas Willis introduced the experimental approach to the study of the nervous system, thus placing the brain and the nervous system on a modern footing. Willis has a number of firsts to his credit: descriptions of the hexagonal circle of arteries at the base of the brain (which gave him eponymic fame when it became known as the 'Circle of Willis'), the eleventh cranial nerve, myasthenia gravis and puerperal fever. He won great renown as a physician, researcher and teacher and, as the Sedleian Professor of Natural History, had a number of gifted pupils, among whom were Robert Hook, the inventive physicist and microscopist; John Locke, the physician-philosopher; Richard Lower and Edmund King, who performed the first blood transfusion in a human; Thomas Millington, later physician to the king; and Christopher Wren (Feindel, 1970).

tibiarum and gave a one-page account of 'die von den alteren Aerzten so genannte Anxietas tibiarum' (p. 459). It is apparent from Wittmaack's writings that earlier accounts of anxietas tibiarum existed, but Ekbom (1960) reportedly could not definitely trace them. During this period in history, the phenomenon was construed as a symptom of hysteria and, therefore, psychogenic in origin.

A late-nineteenth-century description by George Beard (1880) of what to him was 'one of the myriad results of spinal irritation' is again close to the later descriptions of akathisia. This phenomenon was broadly included under the syndrome of 'neurasthenia': 'Fidgetiness and nervousness, inability to keep still – a sensation that amounts to pain – is sometimes unspeakably distressing. When the legs feel this way, the sufferer must get up and walk or run, even though he be debilitated and is made worse by severe exercise' (pp. 41–42).

Early in the twentieth century, Haskovec (1902) described two patients with restlessness and an inability to sit (see Appendix A for a translation of Haskovec's paper). One 40-year-old man was described as follows: 'When he was required to stay seated, he rose up and down quickly and involuntary, sitting down again and repeating his behaviour. The movements impressed one as being automatic, involuntary and compulsive, and the patient also considered them this way.' The other patient, a 54-year-old man, had the following problem: 'When he was seated, he rose up and down compulsively and violently. . . . He needed to hold on to the table to stop himself from rising up involuntarily' (p. 128). Consistent with the concepts that preceded him, Haskovec's diagnoses were 'hysteria' in the first case and 'neurasthenia' in the other. Akathisia in one patient was associated with clonic movements of the diaphragm and spasm of the larynx which 'he could partially stop when one told him to keep still, to speak slowly and to breathe calmly' (p. 197). Even though the syndrome now had a distinctive name and a detailed description, and was distinguished from the restlessness associated with anxiety, depression or psychosis, it continued to be seen as psychogenic in its aetiology. Haskovec distinguished it from chorea, which was accepted as a neurological disorder.

Akathisia continued to be regarded as a nonorganic psychiatric disorder for the next two decades. Raymond and Janet (*Nouv Iconogr. de la Salpetriere*, 1902; cited in Bing, 1923) described a case which was considered to be an expression of a so-called professional abulia. While sitting, which had become for him a symbol of his profession as a goldworker, the patient was overcome by a tormented feeling of fear which eventually forced him to jump up. Beduschi (*Rivista di Patol nerv e ment*, 1904; cited in Bing, 1923) referred to an intense fear of sitting (kathisophobia). Oppenheim[2] (1923), in his book entitled *Lehrbuch der Nervenkrankheiten,* wrote: 'An unusual kind of subjective dysruption of sensations as the restlessness in the legs, it can become a tormenting problem that may continue for years and decades, and be passed on genetically, i.e. become familial. In Oppenheim's observations, psychological factors played a major role' (p. 1774).

Sicard's[3] 1923 description of a patient is reminiscent of Haskovec's account of an inability to remain seated, but he attributed it to upper-body pain. He reviewed Haskovec's cases and came to the conclusion that one patient suffered from epidemic encephalitis and the other from tic or myoclonus. He also described a series of three patients with the symptoms of forced walking (tasikinesia), diplopia and somnolence, which he diagnosed as epidemic encephalitis lethargica. The term *tasikinesia* was thus introduced. Sicard had come to the conclusion that this was part of an organic disorder, and he distinguished it from similar symptoms seen in mania, anxiety and phobia, dementia praecox, depression and certain epileptic states. Sicard (*Revue Neurologique,* 28:672) gave this description of the syndrome:

People thus affected are ceaselessly agitated, in perpetual need of movement, not being able to stay still, getting up from one seat to sit down in another, and walking up and down ceaselessly in the area of the apartment where they find themselves. A sort of anxiety siezes them, gripping them as soon as they are seated, and forcing them to leave the chairs they have chosen. They don't know rest in the seated position. They are calmer and more stable in the recumbent position.

Bing (1923) described akathisia in association with the parkinsonian syndrome related to epidemic encephalitis. In his reference to one of Haskovec's cases, he wrote:

If this case had caught our attention today (instead of Spring 1897), we would surely have made a diagnosis of the myoclonic form of epidemic encephalitis . . . we shall not attempt to hypothesise too far in this area and only stress that in our current standing of knowledge, Haskovec's patient without doubt had suffered from an acute organic brain disturbance favouring the corpus striatum. (p. 168)

---

[2] Hermann Oppenheim (1858–1919) is remembered for his description of amyotonia congenita (now called 'Oppenheim's disease') and for providing the term *dystonia musculorum deformans* (also called 'Oppenheim–Ziehen's disease'). He was an expert diagnostician, and it was on the basis of his diagnosis that the first surgical removal of a brain tumour was performed by Koehler. His treatise went to seven German editions and was translated into many European languages (Weil, 1970).

[3] Jean Athanse Sicard (1872–1929), a Parisian neurologist, is best remembered for his introduction, with his pupil Jacques Forestier, of radio-opaque iodized oil (lipiodil). He gained eponymic fame for his description of a case of traumatic injury of the neck in which the ninth, tenth, eleventh and twelfth cranial nerves were damaged (Bucy, 1970).

He agreed with Wilson that 'the symptoms . . . fall openly under the under-standing of the release phenomena . . . because it is the result of the pathologi-cal release of automatically working mesencephalic centres from the inhibit-ing apparatus of the higher centres' (p. 169). In a later treatise, Bing (1939) distinguished this syndrome from the restlessness of Parkinson's disease (PD), which he considered to be secondary to the discomfort of muscular rigidity.

With the descriptions of Sicard and Bing, akathisia came to be seen as sometimes being a symptom of idiopathic or postencephalitic parkinsonism. An influential statement in this direction was that of Kinnier Wilson[4] (1940), who wrote that even though Haskovec used the term *akathisia* for cases of 'hysterical or psychopathic nature', it could be applied to parkinsonian patients. He described patients with a mild form of the disorder who, while evidencing bradykinesia generally, tended to move their feet and legs. Others had a 'paradoxical' inability to sit even though immobilized by their illness. He felt that this was 'no doubt because they feel the cramping effect of fixed posture and have to move and stretch their limbs at intervals'. It is, therefore, not clear whether akathisia was recognized as a distinct symptom of parkin-sonism or essentially a secondary symptom with its basis in rigidity. This issue has remained unresolved until recently.

Brief descriptions of the syndrome continued to be published in the early 1940s. Mussio-Fournier and Rawak (1940) published a case of 'hyperkinesis of the lower extremities caused by paresthesias appearing during rest' associ-ated with pruritus and urticaria. This patient had a strong family history of the same disorder. Allison (1943) described 'leg jitters', which he reported to be a common problem. The paper by Ekbom (1944) was the first detailed account of the syndrome, which he denoted as 'irritable legs' and later the restless legs syndrome (RLS) (Ekbom, 1945), based on his own experience of many cases. He described the most characteristic symptom of this disorder as 'creeping or crawling sensations most frequently localised to the lower leg'. He clearly distinguished these sensations from acroparaesthesiae in that they were pre-sent not in the skin 'but deep inside, in the muscles or "bones" '. The peculiar feature of the sensations was that they appeared only when the limbs were at

---

[4] Samuel Alexander Kinnier Wilson (1878–1937) was one of the group of brilliant neurologists at the National Hospital, which included Gowers, Hughlings Jackson, Bastian and Horsley. He is best remembered for his 'progressive lenticular degeneration: a familial nervous disease associated with cirrhosis of the liver', which came to be known as Wilson's disease. He made a number of contributions to the study of what he called the 'extrapyramidal system', and his two-volume textbook *Neurology* (London: Arnold, 1940) was a landmark publication (Haymaker, 1970).

rest and they were relieved by movement. They were almost invariably present in the evening and at night. Some patients described pain rather than creeping sensations. The neurological examination was otherwise normal. Ekbom went on to describe further cases, as well as perform epidemiological studies, to suggest that RLS was a common disorder in otherwise healthy people, was equally common in both sexes, could start at any age and was often familial (Ekbom, 1945, 1946a,b, 1950, 1960). He reported that if mild cases were included, the disorder was present in 5% of otherwise normal individuals (Ekbom, 1960), and the prevalence might be as high as 11% in pregnant women and 24% in those with iron deficiency (serum iron less than 60 µg/dl). He recognized as other causes poliomyelitis and other infectious diseases, avitaminosis, diabetes, lengthy exposure of the legs to cold and the intake of neuroleptic drugs. He discussed the various treatment options and remarked that 'it should be remembered that promethazine makes the symptoms worse' (Ekbom, 1960). Ekbom recognized that a number of cases of RLS were dismissed as being 'psychogenic' or 'nervous' and that many patients 'are ashamed to talk about their discomforts to other persons', but he firmly believed that the disorder was organic. It is interesting, however, that he did not use the term *akathisia* or make any reference to Haskovec's papers in his reports. His inclusion of neuroleptics as a cause and an exacerbating factor for RLS suggests that a clear distinction between RLS and drug-induced akathisia had not emerged.

Even after the publication of Ekbom's 1944 and 1945 papers describing RLS, doubt existed about its distinct status. Purdon-Martin (1946) attributed the symptom of restlessness to acroparaesthesiae, and Masland (1947) to myokymia. Other papers were published which supported Ekbom's descriptions and some extended them. Nordlander (1953, 1954) reported restless legs in anaemic patients. Ask-Upmark and Meurling (1955) reported its presence as a late effect of gastrectomy. Subsequently, basing his claim on the anecdotal presence of postural dependence of symptoms, Ask-Upmark (1959) attributed the disorder to vascular congestion of the spinal cord. French interest in this syndrome was significant, as demonstrated by the Bonduelle and Jolivet (1953) paper and the Tolivet thesis (cited in Ekbom, 1960). In the French literature, it was referred to as *impatience musculaire*.

By the 1960s, RLS was firmly established as a neurological disorder, albeit of unknown aetiology. Grinker and Sahs (1966, p. 336) devoted a short paragraph to it, and Brain and Walton (1969, pp. 881–882) described it under the 'miscellaneous disorders of muscle', while suggesting that chlorpromazine was of great help in some patients.

Restless legs and the neuroleptic era

The first discussion of drug-induced akathisia is credited to Sigwald et al (1947), who reported that a patient with PD had developed restlessness when treated with the phenothiazine drug promethazine. After antipsychotic drugs became generally available, a number of reports of akathisia appeared in the literature, with descriptions of patients being restless, being unable to sit, marching like soldiers, etc. The similarity with the akathisia syndrome of the preneuroleptic era was recognized from the beginning, and reference was often made to the Haskovec papers. The term *akathisia* was not used consistently, however, to describe the drug effects. Barsa and Kline (1956), in referring to the effects of reserpine in psychosis, spoke of 'turbulent reactions' involving psychic excitation and motor stimulation. Sarwer-Foner and Ogle (1956) described 'paradoxical reactions'. Freyhan (1958) was one of the early authors to refer consistently to the 'akathisia syndrome' and provide a lucid description: 'If akathisia is mild, patients complain of a feeling of inner unrest, of pulling or drawing sensations in the extremities but chiefly in the legs. Once akathisia is fully developed, patients pace back and forth and can neither sit down to read or play or sleep. In severe cases, patients appear continuously agitated' (p. 198).

From its earliest descriptions, the 'paradoxical' nature of akathisia was apparent to clinicians and investigators alike; ie, drugs that were generally recognized to produce a calming effect on psychotically disturbed individuals themselves produced 'nervousness' and restlessness. The early European authors referred to it as an extrapyramidal phenomenon; its association with drug-induced parkinsonism was recognized; it was noted to be dose-related and occurring soon after the introduction of phenothiazines and related drugs; and it was known to be reversible (Deniker, 1960; Denham and Carrick, 1961). Some investigators, however, construed such symptoms as psychological responses to the physiological effects of drugs. The *American Illustrated Medical Dictionary* (Dorland, 1951) described akathisia as a 'psychosis marked by morbid fear of sitting down and resulting inability to sit still'. Lang's *German–English Medical Dictionary* (Meyers, 1951) described it as stemming from a 'neurotic inability to remain seated'. Sarwer-Foner and Ogle (1956) argued that the 'holding down' effect of the phenothiazines created feelings of increased passivity, fears of impaired bodily function and changes in bodily image, thereby resulting in enhanced anxiety and even an exacerbation of psychosis. According to them, some patients saw the administration of the drug as an assault or seduction, or otherwise resisted the abandonment of the symptoms because of the secondary gain. Sarwer-Foner (1960b) elaborated on these paradoxical behavioural reactions (listing nine categories of patients who were particularly vulnerable to drug side-effects) but accepted that a proportion of restlesness was caused by akathisia, which was a 'neurologically determined' reaction. The nature of the arguments proposed by Sarwer-Foner is suggested by the following quotation:

Drugs with powerful pharmacological effects are interpreted by some of these patients as decreasing their ability to control their own bodies. Some patients with such problems interpret the side effects as markedly threatening. These side effects suggest bodily impairment, and bring closer to the surface their fears of retribution for 'sins' and guilt in terms of bodily disease, as though it is expressed in a living tableau before their very eyes. (p. 314)

Akathisia therefore was described as either psychogenic or organic in origin, with different authors favouring different explanations. Hodge (1959) clearly described akathisia as part of the 'parkinsonian syndrome', which generally referred to the akinetic-hypertonic reaction, whereas Winkelman (1961) emphasized the similarity in the restlessness seen as a consequence of neuroleptic medication, PD or a psychoneurosis. In spite of the few interesting papers examining the psychological and psychodynamic meaning of the akathisic reaction, consensus was emerging in the early 1960s that akathisia was an extrapyramidal side-effect of neuroleptic medication. It was demonstrated that akathisia could occur in psychiatrically normal individuals when treated with neuroleptic drugs (Hollister et al, 1960). It was also suggested that akathisia could be distinguished from anxiety (Hodge, 1959; Freedman and De Jong, 1961) and that patients who developed akathisia could not be distinguished from those who did not on the basis of preexisting psychiatric or personality factors (Freedman and De Jong, 1961). The four major classes of drugs used in the 1950s and 1960s to treat psychosis (rauwolfia alkaloids, phenothiazines, thioxanthenes and butyrophenones) shared the propensity to induce akathisia as well as other neurological side-effects.

Akathisia and the efficacy of antipsychotic drugs

The prominence of extrapyramidal symptoms of antipsychotic drugs prompted a number of early investigators to consider the presence of such symptoms to be essential for achieving therapeutic effects. Two seemingly opposing concepts emerged: one group favoured the need to increase drug dosage to produce parkinsonian effects, while the other favoured the use of low dosages to avoid them and recommended the use of medication to eliminate or reduce the parkinsonian effects. The Paris school – Delay, Deniker, Green and Madaret – essentially belonged to the first group. Delay favoured the use of the term *neuroleptics* (literally, 'that which takes the neuron') to describe these drugs, and Delay and Deniker (1961) noted that the psychic excitation and dystonic reactions of the drugs (the 'excitomotor syndrome') were essential for therapeutic purposes. The synthesis of butyrophenones by Janssen in 1956 and the subsequent demonstration of their clinical profiles reaffirmed the conviction. The Leige school – Divry, Bobon, Collard, Nols, Pinchard, and Damaret – supported this viewpoint. In their report of the clinical trial of triperidol, Divry et al (1960) concluded that the manifestation of major or acute (mainly dystonia) or minor or subacute (impatience musculaire, akathisia, tasikinesia) 'neurodysleptic' excitatory reactions was of special value in the treatment of withdrawn or amotivated schizophrenics. Morosini (1967) from Italy supported this view. These investigators therefore considered the dramatic neurodysleptic manifestations to be a necessary phase in the path to improvement and were not alarmed if anxiety and panic accompanied these reactions.

The position taken by a number of Anglo-American investigators was somewhat different. Freyhan (1959) initially indicated that 'compounds which failed to elicit extrapyramidal symptoms showed the least favorable therapeutic results'. On detailed examination of his data, he modified his position, stating that drugs with higher potency (ie, with greater capacity to produce extrapyramidal side-effects) were more efficacious in mania but not in schizophrenia (Freyhan, 1961). Furthermore, the introduction of antiparkinsonian agents, while ameliorating the parkinsonism, did not antagonize the antipsychotic effect (Freyhan, 1961). Goldman, like Freyhan, changed his position after a review of 4,030 case records and concluded that 'good antipsychotic activity is available without the production of parkinsonism in most patients' (Goldman, 1958, 1961). The introduction of thioridazine, which was as efficacious as chlorpromazine but produced far fewer extrapyramidal side-effects (EPSE), supported this contention. A number of other studies followed that examined the relationship between clinical efficacy and the tendency to produce EPSE: Kam and Kasper (1959), Hollister et al (1960), Cole and Clyde (1961), Simpson et al (1964) and Bishop et al (1965), among others. These studies supported the position that 'gross EPSE bear no relation to drug response. Hence, the practice of deliberately increasing dosage to produce EPSE is unwarranted' (Bishop et al, 1965). It is unfortunate that these authors did not describe subtypes of EPSE, and it is not possible to say what their positions were with regard to akathisia.

The positions taken by Haase (1961) and Brune et al (1962) were somewhat intermediate. Haase found that clinical efficacy was apparent only when fine-motor abnormalities (eg, handwriting) were apparent, but when 'coarse'

EPSE (severe akinesia, rigidity, akathisia and dystonia) occurred, the patients did not respond. He therefore advocated the use of 'fine handwriting measures', although his data did not directly suggest that. Brune et al (1962) supported Haase's contention. This position was still different from that of Divry et al, who advocated the development of neurodysleptic symptoms such as akathisia and dystonia. It must be emphasized that the conclusions were based on different observations. For example, in the Brune et al (1962) study, the early development of anxiety or panic was seen as a negative development, but Divry et al (1960) did not place emphasis on the early developments and waited for the final outcome.

A synthesis of these contrasting positions was attempted with the suggestion that even though EPSE per se may not be necessary for the effectiveness of a drug, certain side-effects may be helpful in certain kinds of patients. The excited and assaultive patient might be helped by drugs that produce akinesia, and the inert, withdrawn patient by drugs that caused neurodysleptic excitation (Ayd, 1965). Clinicians recognized, however, that this did not work in practice and some patients reacted adversely to these effects (Chien and DiMascio, 1967). The adverse reactions continued to be considered to be psychological responses to the side-effects, much in the vein of Sarwer-Foner's (1960a,b) suggestions discussed earlier. It was not until the mid-1970s, with the influential writings of Van Putten and colleagues (Van Putten, 1974, 1975; Van Putten et al, 1974), that it started being appreciated that akathisia could have a prominent mental component that could resemble an exacerbation of schizophrenia.

In subsequent years, a number of studies have examined the relationships between neuroleptic drug doses, their plasma levels and their efficacy and propensity to produce side-effects (eg, Baldessarini et al, 1988; Rifkin et al, 1991). Most investigators now accept that it is not necessary to produce EPSE to obtain beneficial effects from neuroleptic drugs. The literature also suggests that there is a significant positive relationship between neuroleptic blood levels and EPSE, including akathisia, but the relationship is not necessarily linear (Van Putten et al, 1991). The major studies that have contributed to the development of the concepts of akathisia and restless legs syndrome are listed in Table 1.1.

The multifaceted nature of drug-induced akathisia

As akathisia became better recognized in the clinic and accepted as a common side-effect, it was apparent that its manifestations could be varied. We have already discussed some of the literature referring to the 'paradoxical' reac-

Table 1.1. *Landmark studies in the development of the concepts of akathisia and restless legs syndrome*

Contribution	Reference
First documented description	Willis (1685)
'Anxietas tibiarum'	Wittmaack (1861)
Introduction of the term *akathisia*	Haskovec (1902)
Association with parkinsonism	Bing (1923)
'Tasikinesia'	Sicard (1923)
Description of RLS	Ekbom (1944)
Description of drug-induced akathisia	Sigwald et al (1947)
'Paradoxical reactions' to neuroleptics	Sarwer-Foner and Ogle (1956)
Consistent use of *akathisia* for drug-induced syndrome	Freyhan (1958)
Further description of RLS and association with iron deficiency, uraemia, etc	Ekbom (1960)
'Persistent muscular restlessness'	Kruse (1960a,b)
Prevalence figures for akathisia	Ayd (1961)
Association of RLS with nocturnal myoclonus	Lugaresi et al (1965)
Multifaceted nature of akathisia	Van Putten (1975)
Clinical characteristics of akathisia	Braude et al (1983)
Use of propranolol for the treatment of akathisia	Lipinski et al (1983)
Subtypes of akathisia	Barnes and Braude (1985)
Clinical characteristics of TA	Burke et al (1987)
Description of akathisia of PD	Lang and Johnson (1987)
L-Dopa treatment of RLS	Akpinar (1987)
A rating scale for akathisia	Barnes (1989)
Diagnostic criteria for akathisia	Sachdev (1994a)

tions to neuroleptics, with many anecdotes of an exacerbation of psychosis resulting from the drugs. In a series of 80 patients treated with phenothiazines, Van Putten et al (1974) reported 9 who developed an exacerbation of psychosis. All had an associated subtle akathisia, and the exacerbations remarkably reversed with the parenteral administration of biperiden, an anticholinergic agent. These exacerbations were viewed as 'extrapyramidal equivalents'. Van Putten (1975) went on to describe 'the many faces of akathisia'. Akathisia was described as being associated with strong affects of fright, terror, anger or rage, anxiety and vague somatic complaints. It could lead to decompensation of various forms. In one patient, it was even experienced as a sexual torment. Violence was reported as a manifestation (Keckich, 1978), including homicide (Schulte, 1985). Other authors reported suicidal behaviour in response to, or associated with, akathisia (Shear et al, 1983; Drake and Ehrlich, 1985). The varied nature of the presentations further emphasized the fact that akathisia was an underrecognized side-effect, which, even when subtle, could have significant effects on the management of the patient. It was also appreciated that the manifestation of akathisia was primarily subjective, which was a major cause of noncompliance with the medication regime in schizophrenic patients (Van Putten, 1974).

As the understanding of the multiple symptoms of akathisia improved, it became clear that there were two aspects to akathisia: a *subjective,* or psychological or cognitive, component, and an *objective,* or motor, component. Recent research has highlighted this distinction, but any consensus as to whether akathisia is a mental disorder or a motor disorder or both has been slow to emerge (Kendler, 1976; Barnes and Braude, 1985; Stahl, 1985; Editorial, 1986). The characteristic features of akathisia are not generally accepted by all researchers. It is not certain how patients with objective manifestations in the absence of any subjective complaint should be diagnosed. Dysphoric reactions to neuroleptic drugs have been reported in the absence of akathisia, either in response to the other side-effects of the drugs or as a psychological response to the fact of being, or having to be, medicated. Even when the diagnosis of akathisia is well accepted, the clinician is called on to make a number of judgements: Are these normal restless movements, dyskinesias or some other abnormality? Should the movements be described as voluntary or involuntary? Is the patient distressed, and if so, is the distress due to akathisia or anxiety, depression, agitation, exacerbation of psychosis or some other psychiatric cause? Clear guidelines to answer these questions have only recently begun to emerge.

Akathisia, acute, chronic and tardive

Much of the preceding discussion referred to akathisia that develops soon after the introduction of neuroleptic drugs, the so-called acute akathisia (AA). It has for some time been recognized that akathisia may develop as a delayed side-effect in patients on long-term medication, either while drugs are being continued or soon after they are withdrawn. This is analogous to tardive dyskinesia (TD) and has been referred to as 'tardive akathisia' (TA). There is frequent reference to this syndrome in the earlier literature, although the term *tardive akathisia* is of relatively recent origin (Braude et al, 1983). Uhrbrand and Faurbye (1960), in their description of patients with irreversible orolingual dyskinesia, described 'rocking and torsionary body movements and incessant tripping and shuffling movements so that the patient cannot stand still'. They did not indicate whether these were irreversible as well. Kruse (1960a) described three patients with 'persistent muscular restlessness' who had severe motor restlessness and an inability to sit still along with subjective restlessness, and for whom the symptoms persisted for 3–18 months after neuroleptic withdrawal. Similar patients were described by a number of other authors (Hunter et al, 1964; Pryce and Edwards, 1966; Schmidt and Jarcho, 1966; Kennedy et al, 1971). Crane (1973), who can be credited with popularizing the syndrome of TD in the United States, included the description of 'shifting weight from foot to foot' (which later was considered to be one of the characteristic features of akathisia) as a feature of TD.

While it was accepted that many patients with TD had features suggestive of akathisia, it was only in the mid-1970s that researchers began to focus on the akathisic component of this syndrome and to describe patients who did not have the classical choreoathetoid movements of TD, yet exhibited persistent akathisia of late onset. Forrest and Fahn (1979) used the term *tardive dysphrenia and subjective akathisia* for patients with a combination of dyskinesia and akathisia. Kidger et al (1980) described three subsyndromes of TD, one of which included movements of trunk, arms, hands and legs that could be described as restless or fidgety movements, but lacked the subjective component of akathisia. The concept of TA gradually gained wider usage, and the publication of the Barnes and Braude (1985) paper, along with a leading article by Stahl (1985), provided a much-needed impetus. The distinction between AA and TA became well established.

But some controversies remained. Not all authors agreed that it was useful to subdivide the tardive syndromes into TD, TA and others (eg, tardive Tourette's syndrome, tardive dystonia, tardive myoclonus, tardive dysmentia), and a debate between the 'lumpers' and 'splitters' ensued (Stahl, 1985). Recent work (Burke et al, 1987, 1989; Sachdev and Chee, 1990; Sachdev and Loneragan, 1993a,c) suggests that TA may have pharmacological and treatment-response differences from TD which argue for its separate delineation. The overlap between the syndromes, however, makes for difficult research decisions. The relationship between AA and TA remains uncertain. Is TA the same as chronic akathisia? Do some patients with AA develop chronic akathisia if they continue on the medication, and should they then be diagnosed as having TA? A term, *acute persistent akathisia,* has been used (Barnes & Braude, 1985) which sits uneasily between AA and TA. Does this term presuppose that AA is of short duration and self-limiting? What is the status of withdrawal akathisia in relation to TA? Many of these questions are only beginning to be addressed (Sachdev, 1994a).

Another term that has added to the heterogeneity of the concepts is *pseudoakathisia.* It has been suggested in the literature as a term for the manifestations of TD that may be mistaken for akathisia (Munetz and Cornes,

1982) or the objective manifestations of akathisia in the absence of the subjective component (Barnes and Braude, 1985). The term, however, begs the question: is it or is it not akathisia? If it is akathisia in which the patient either has developed tolerance of the subjective distress or has significant apathy and lack of insight to not be concerned by it, then it is, in fact, true akathisia. If it is not akathisia, but restlessness or chorea masquerading as akathisia, then it cannot be considered a subtype of akathisia. The term therefore adds little to the understanding of the syndrome it purports to describe. It is reminiscent of some of the problems with the term *pseudodementia,* which, in spite of its demonstrated limitations (Sachdev et al, 1990), persists in the literature, if only to be severely criticized each time it is brought up. I have recently (Sachdev, 1994a) proposed a typology for akathisia which attempts to settle some of the confusion with regard to terminology.

The akathisia of Parkinson's disease

Loneragan and I (Sachdev and Loneragan, 1991a) have already referred to the early writings of Sicard and Bing concerning the association of akathisia with PD and have previously termed it *Bing–Sicard akathisia.* An earlier historical description is that by Trousseau of Napoleon III's chamberlain, who, owing to his PD, was obliged to rise from his seat every 5 minutes and walk about, even in the presence of Napoleon himself (Bing 1939). Charcot referred to the 'cruel restlessness' suffered by some of his parkinsonian patients. Gowers spoke of the 'extreme restlessness . . . which necessitates . . . every few minutes some slight change of pressure' (cited in Sacks, 1983, p. 10). Many investigators, however, continued to regard the restlessness seen in PD patients as being due to muscular discomfort caused by rigidity and bradykinesia (Wilson, 1940). Restlessness in PD has also been attributed to tremor, dyskinesia (such that movement decreased the dyskinesia), sensory symptoms or psychiatric problems (anxiety or depression) (Lang and Johnson, 1987). Many neurologists have always accepted that there were two sides to parkinsonism, which one of Sacks' (1983) patients referred to as 'the goad and the halter' and Sacks himself called 'Parkinsonism-on-the-boil, Parkinsonism in its expansile and explosive aspect' (p. 10).

Descriptions of postencephalitic parkinsonism, as opposed to idiopathic parkinsonism, included symptoms resembling akathisia as prominent features of the disorder. Indeed, the explosive and obstructive aspects of the disorder were much more severe than the idiopathic syndrome, and patients were often described as engaging in violent movements and frenzies (Jelliffe, 1932). Patients could move from states of 'frozen' catatonia to profound restlessness, often associated with bizarre perceptions, thoughts and emotions. Sacks (1983) provided some excellent descriptions in his book *Awakenings*. Not only was restlessness a feature of 'epidemic encephalitis' and the states that followed, but many patients developed it after being treated with L-dopa. One of Sacks' patients was described as follows:

I found her intensely agitated and akathisic, constantly kicking and crossing her legs, banging her hands, and uttering sudden high-pitched screams. . . . A constraint caused intense frustration, and heightened her agitation and frenzy: thus if one tried to prevent her kicking her legs, an unbearable tension developed which sought discharge in pounding of the arms. (p. 94)

A recent study in which PD patients were examined specifically for the presence of restlessness revealed it to be a common symptom, usually unexplained by other motor, sensory or psychiatric aspects of the disease (Lang and Johnson, 1987). This study has to be replicated, but the idea that akathisia may be a not uncommon feature of PD is becoming generally accepted. The association of akathisia with drug-induced parkinsonism has also received attention, with some authors suggesting that there may be two subtypes of drug-induced akathisia, one being associated with parkinsonism and having a different pharmacological profile (Braude et al, 1983). This aspect remains open to further investigation.

Restless legs syndrome and akathisia

In spite of its origin in the pre–neuroleptic era, the major association of akathisia with neuroleptic drugs has led to the term *akathisia* becoming largely synonymous with drug-induced akathisia. The syndrome of RLS, also referred to as Ekbom's syndrome, is the preferred term for the idiopathic disorder which has remained in the territory of neurology. While there is some overlap of symptoms, the two syndromes can be distinguished on a number of features, which will be discussed later. The similarities are not to be completely forgotten, however, and findings in one disorder have periodically led to the testing of similar hypotheses in the other. The possible aetiological role of iron deficiency and the treatment potential of β-adrenergic antagonists are two such examples. The further development of the concept of RLS will be discussed in Chapter 12.

Conclusion

The concept of akathisia has a long and interesting history, resulting in a diversity of meanings that the term has come to represent. The clinical importance of at least two disorders that it has been used to describe – drug-induced akathisia and RLS – is beyond dispute. Yet akathisia has remained the Cinderella of psychiatric research until recently (Stahl, 1985). This book is an attempt to synthesize the current information on this syndrome and remedy its neglect.

2

The anatomy of restlessness

Restlessness: aimless activity, pottering, desultoriness, inattention, unquiet, fidgets, fidgetiness, agitation, fever, fret, frenzy, eagerness, enthusiasm, ardour, abandon, warm feeling, vigour, energy, dynamism, aggressiveness, militancy, enterprise, initiative, push, drive, ego, pep, vigorousness, watchfulness, vigilance, carefulness, wakefulness, sleeplessness, insomnia.

Roget's Thesaurus (1983)

To place akathisia and RLS in perspective, it would be helpful to review the usage of the term *restlessness* in neuropsychiatry in general. The term has been applied in a variety of clinical states, often without a precise definition. It has also been used to describe some aspects of normal behaviour. A number of related terms have additionally been used – akathisia, agitation, fidgetiness, hyperactivity, jitteriness – to describe phenomena that resemble, or overlap with, restlessness. They share the common theme of *aimless motor activity that is poorly organized and represents a state of physical or mental unease.* The clinical application of various terms related to restlessness has been imprecise and often idiosyncratic. Some terms have dominated descriptions in certain contexts; yet without accompanying definitions, their use is limited. For example, in the context of melancholic depression, *agitation* has been the preferred term (Lewis, 1934; Nelson and Charney, 1981), even though a distinction from restlessness or hyperactivity is not always clarified. The term *jitteriness* has been used to describe restlessness induced by tricyclic drugs (Pohl et al, 1988), but its phenomenological distinction from restlessness due to other drugs has not been examined. Akathisia is often used synonymously with neuroleptic-induced restlessness; yet the term was introduced well before the first neuroleptic drugs became available (Haskovec, 1902). In this chapter, we will examine the various forms of restlessness that have been described in the neuropsychiatric literature in order to assess the merits of the diverse terminology and look for common ground in the descriptions.

The term *restlessness* has also been used to describe a not uncommon behaviour in psychiatrically normal individuals. In this context, restlessness may be a particular state a person is in, or it may represent a personality trait. When used to connote a state, references such as the following are common: 'He is feeling restless in his current job and wishes to move'; 'Ever since his wife died, he has been restless'; 'The set-back has made him restless'; 'He is restless and in search of something'. On the other hand, a person may be described as being generally 'restless'. The dictionary meaning of this word is 'finding or affording no rest; uneasy, agitated, constantly in motion, fidgeting etc.' (*Concise Oxford Dictionary,* 1983). The connotation may be positive when enthusiasm, vigour, ardour, initiative and enterprise are involved and the individual is tirelessly reaching or searching for a goal. 'Youth' is sometimes described as 'being restless', implying that at this stage in life, individuals are often reaching out and searching for status, position, purpose or role. As long as it remains within the limits considered acceptable by society, restlessness is treated without apprehension and even encouraged. If the restless energy is dissipated without a target being kept in sight or conflicts being eventually resolved, thus leading to little productivity or growth, the description of restlessness takes on a negative connotation. Such restlessness is seen as a weakness of character.

Another word commonly used in lay parlance is *restive.* While it has the same implications as *restless* in terms of overt behaviour, *restive* implies resistance. Children can be restless from boredom, but can be restive only if someone is trying to make them do something they do not want to do. Like restlessness, fidgetiness, self-manipulation of body and nervous habits have been construed as personality variables (Mehrabian and Friedman, 1986). Because our emphasis here is clinical, we will not discuss the personality dimension of restlessness in any detail.

The aetiology and prevalence of restlessness

In the clinical setting, restlessness can be caused by psychological factors or organic and nonorganic psychiatric disorders, and the list in Table 2.1 is not exhaustive. Observations of medically ill patients highlight a number of personal and environmental factors that can produce or promote a state of restlessness. Pain, frustration, irritation, tension and discomfort are well recognized in this context. Pain and discomfort are known to promote restlessness and even delirium in postoperative patients (Layne and Yudofsky, 1971; Lipowski, 1990). Further suggestion that psychosocial stress plays a role in promoting restlessness comes from the study of the causes of delirium

Table 2.1. *Neuropsychiatric causes of restlessness*

Organic disorders
Drug-induced restlessness (cf. akathisia or RLS) (see Table 2.2 for a list of drugs)
Drug withdrawal syndromes (see Table 2.2)
Delirium
Dementia
Head injury
Hypoglycaemia
RLS and related syndromes (see Chapter 12 for differential diagnosis of RLS)
Peripheral neuropathy
Peripheral vascular disease
Myelopathy

Nonorganic psychiatric disorders
Affective disorders
Psychotic disorders
Anxiety disorders
Childhood disorders
    ADHD
    Conduct disorder
    Autism

(Lipowski, 1990), although the empirical evidence remains tentative. Social isolation, sleep loss, relocation to an unfamiliar environment and fatigue have been implicated as stresses that can lead to hyperarousal and restlessness, and in some cases facilitate the onset of delirium (Kral, 1962).

More convincing research evidence comes from studies investigating fidgetiness in both healthy and ill individuals. A number of studies have examined the behaviour of normal individuals in certain experimental situations to observe the effects of boredom or frustration. Krout (1954a,b) reported that when subjects were placed in conflict situations, they had an increase in nervous gestures. Jones (1943a) frustrated the efforts of subjects to solve arithmetic problems by prohibiting the use of writing implements, counting on fingers or counting aloud, and observed more restless movements. In another study, the same author (Jones, 1943b) made the subjects drink 10 glasses of water over a 2-hour period without permitting them the use of bathroom facilities. The subjects in this uncomfortable situation had a significant increase in restless movements, especially of the legs. Other investigators have used delays in reinforcement of behaviours or imposed unnecessarily long waiting periods to induce frustration and observe its effect on behaviour. Kachanoff et al (1973) increased the time interval before schizophrenic patients, previously on a fixed-interval schedule, now received pennies as reinforcement. These patients paced and increased their water consumption. Wallace and Singer (1975) performed a similar study in normal university students, comparing two reinforcement schedules, one with a 60-second, the other a 5-second interval. The students with the longer interval showed increased movements such as pacing, stretching, eating, rocking, grooming and digital movements. Other investigators enforced unnecessarily long waiting periods when subjects solved mazes (Wallace and Singer, 1976), gambled (Clarke et al, 1977) or played backgammon (Fallon et al, 1979), and all reported increased fidgety and restless movements as well as behaviours such as eating, drinking and grooming that were incidental to the focus of the activity. In conclusion, empirical evidence supports the relationship between fidgetiness and states of anxiety, frustration, distress or boredom. It can be argued that if the motor activity of the subjects had not been constrained by the experimental situations, they would have demonstrated restlessness as well (Mehrabian and Friedman, 1986).

These studies also found that the psychological stresses were more likely to provoke restlessness in individuals who had a 'fidgeting tendency', thus linking it to a trait of personality. Mehrabian and Freedman (1986) systematically examined the relationship of fidgeting (defined as engaging in manipulations of one's own body parts or other objects) with personality traits and found that fidgety persons were also more anxious and hostile. The authors also provided evidence linking fidgetiness with restlessness and a tendency to engage in activities (eg, cigarette smoking, consuming alcohol, eating, day-dreaming) that were extraneous to the task at hand, and suggested that fidgetiness was an overflow of the tendency toward motor overactivity and thus represented a form of restlessness. It can therefore be argued that the authors provided indirect evidence to link restlessness with overarousal (manifest as anxiety and hostility) as a personality dimension.

Nonorganic psychiatric disorders

Affective disorders

Motor disturbance is a characteristic feature of affective illness, and restlessness is seen in both depression and mania, although the two are qualitatively different. The restlessness of depression is generally described as 'psychomotor agitation'. Many clinicians consider the presence of agitation as supporting a diagnosis of endogenous depression or melancholia, and regard 'agitated depression' as a distinct subtype with a characteristic presentation and differential treatment response. Others consider the motor activity as a feature of all depressive states, with the intensity of the disturbance commensurate with that of the mood state (Parker and Brotchie, 1992). Still others consider it the outward expression of anxiety in the setting of depression (Hamilton, 1989). It is described more commonly in women than men.

The restless overactivity of mania is qualitatively different from depressive agitation, even though Kraepelin (1921) considered the two to be similar, and Henderson and Gillespie (1956) considered the latter a 'mixed affective state'. The restlessness of mania may at first appear goal-directed and purposive, but as the disorder becomes more severe, increasing disorganization sets in.

Psychotic disorders

Restlessness can be a feature of any of the major nonorganic psychoses but has been classically associated with catatonic schizophrenia. The motor abnormalities were recognized to be intermittent, variable and often dramatic by investigators as early as Kraepelin (1911) and Bleuler (1911). The motor restlessness may be generalized and persistent or interspersed with prolonged bursts of energy that are often chaotic, disorganized and even frenzied. The motor abnormality may be construed as an essential, even a core, feature of the schizophrenic disturbance, or as being either secondary to the distress and frustration caused by the illness or the response of the patient to delusions or hallucinations. While motor excitement may be a more general disturbance in schizophrenia, many specific motor abnormalities have been described and comprehensively reviewed (Taylor, 1990). The term *catatonia* generally refers to a cluster of these motor symptoms, and it is important to recognize that in addition to schizophrenia, it may result from a number of organic mental disorders.

Anxiety disorders

An anxious person may experience trembling, twitching and shakiness as well as become restless both physically and mentally. The motor hyperactivity is typically associated with autonomic arousal and vigilance, as well as a subjective experience of unrealistic anxiety and worry. In an acute anxiety or panic episode, the individual is often pacing restlessly, moving arms and legs aimlessly and complaining loudly of inner turmoil. Activity may become totally disorganized.

Childhood disorders

The prototypical childhood disorder with restlessness is attention-deficit hyperactivity disorder (ADHD), in which nonpurposive motor activity is prominent in the preschool and elementary school years, and generally becomes less obvious with increasing age (Schachar et al, 1981). Adults with ADHD in childhood may continue to be fidgety and restless (Weiss and Hechtman, 1986). The additional presence of inattention and impulsivity characterize the disorder. A remarkable diversity of terms has been used to describe it: minimal brain damage, minimal brain dysfunction, hyperkinetic child, hyperkinetic impulse disorder, developmental hyperactivity, etc. Rutter et al (1970) found that one-third of the boys in their study of 10- to 12-year-old children on the Isle of Wight were described as restless by their mothers, and half of that proportion were so described by their teachers. The diagnosis of ADHD was, however, given in only 0.1% of cases. The epidemiological data in this field are confounded by lack of consensus definitions and the subjectivity in the measures applied. Prevalence rates as high as 5% have been stated for U.S. cities (Stewart et al, 1966; Schuckit et al, 1978). Lambert et al (1978) performed a comprehensive prevalence study in San Francisco, using parents, teachers and physicians to identify 'hyperactive' children. They found that 5% of children were considered to be hyperactive by at least one defining system and 1.2% by all three. It is generally accepted that boys are five to nine times more likely to be diagnosed as being 'hyperactive' than girls (Weiss and Hechtman, 1979).

If the restlessness is characterized by reckless behaviour, low frustration tolerance, irritability and temper tantrums and is associated with behaviours that break basic rules or violate the rights of others, *conduct disorder* is diagnosed. Schachar et al (1981) reported that 3% of boys in a semirural area had this problem. Rutter et al (1975) reported that the rates in an inner-city area were twice as high. In a child psychiatry clinic, 75% of boys and 50% of girls referred for aggressive conduct disorder were also hyperactive (Stewart et al, 1981).

Hyperkinetic and restless behaviour is also seen in association with autism. Rutter et al (1967) reported that 24 of a series of 50 autistic children were hyperkinetic when first assessed in a psychiatric clinic at the mean age of 6 years. This hyperactivity decreased with age.

Organic disorders

Drug-induced restlessness

Some of the drugs that produce motor restlessness in therapeutic or nontoxic doses are listed in Table 2.2. The most important clinical syndrome in this context is that of drug-induced akathisia produced typically by dopamine antagonists and depleters, but also reported with buspirone, lithium carbonate,

Table 2.2. *Drugs that produce restlessness in nontoxic dosages (including drugs that cause akathisia)*

Dopamine antagonists, eg, phenothiazines, butyrophenones, thioxanthenes,
   benzamides, dibenzoxazepines, dihydroindoles and other antipsychotic and
   antiemetic drugs
Dopamine depleters, eg, tetrabenazine, reserpine, α-methyldopa.
Heterocyclic antidepressants, eg, amoxapine, imipramine
Serotonin reuptake inhibitors, eg, fluoxetine, fluvoxamine
Serotonin antagonists, eg, methysergide
Calcium channel antagonists, eg, diltiazem, cinnarizine, flunarizine
Mood-stabilizing drugs, eg, lithium carbonate
Central stimulant drugs, eg, amphetamine, cocaine, caffeine
Arylcyclohexylamines, eg, phencyclidine
Antimuscarinic drugs, eg, atropine, scopolamine
Withdrawal from the following: opioids, alcohol and sedative-hypnotics,
   heterocyclic antidepressants, monoamine oxidase inhibitors, nicotine

---

Note: Often, both akathisia and general restlessness due to the same causes have been reported in the literature. Doses that produce altered consciousness (delirium) are not included as evidence.

calcium channel antagonists, etc. (Sachdev and Loneragan, 1991a). Tricyclic antidepressants have been reported to cause restlessness in panic disorder patients, a syndrome that has been referred to as 'jitteriness' (Beasley et al, 1993). Some tricyclic drugs (eg, amoxapine) have an intrinsic dopamine antagonist property which may explain tricyclic-induced akathisia, but akathisia has also been reported in patients treated with tricyclics and oestrogen (Krishnan et al, 1984). Serotonin reuptake inhibitors, of which the prototypical drug is fluoxetine, have been reported to cause agitation and restlessness in some patients (Beasley et al, 1992). Increased motor activity is an important feature of the 'serotonin syndrome' (which includes salivation, piloerection, hyperthermia, tremor, stereotypic behaviour and seizures) in animals (Hwang and Van Woert, 1980). Psychomotor agitation is a feature of central stimulant drug use (amphetamines, cocaine and related drugs), which is usually associated with hypervigilance, euphoria and sympathetic overactivity (Gawin and Ellinwood, 1988). While maladaptive behaviours are a feature of hallucinogen use, purposeless motor activity is more likely to occur as part of an acute syndrome, or 'bad trip'. Phencyclidine and related arylcyclohexylamines produce a variety of maladaptive behaviours that include psychomotor agitation as well as assaultativeness and impulsivity (Clouet, 1986). Restlessness produced by excessive use of caffeine has been underrecognized and is likely to be associated with nervousness, excitement, insomnia, gastrointestinal disturbance and sympathetic overactivity (Jaffe, 1989). Restlessness has been reported as an effect of antimuscarinic drugs such as atropine and scopolamine in the absence of delirium (Newhouse et al, 1988).

Drug withdrawal syndromes

Alcohol and sedative-hypnotic withdrawal may result in a delirium in which hyperactivity is a prominent feature. There are some drugs whose abrupt cessation will lead to a syndrome with restlessness as a major feature in the absence of delirium. Withdrawal from heterocyclic antidepressants, neuroleptics and monoamine oxidase inhibitors may produce restlessness (Dilsaver, 1990). Withdrawal from nicotine in dependent individuals results in anxiety, irritability and restlessness that may last for some weeks (West et al, 1989). Opioid withdrawal may produce restlessness due to either nonpurposive non-goal-directed behaviour or activity (complaints, pleas, manipulations) directed at getting the drug (Jaffe, 1989). This restlessness may persist in sleep (so-called yen sleep).

Delirium

Some patients with delirium manifest psychomotor hyperactivity, tending to move constantly in a purposeless fashion, respond excessively to stimuli, shout and resist restraint. This is usually associated with hyperalertness and autonomic arousal and has been termed the hyperactive-hyperalert variant of delirium (Lipowski, 1990). The prototypical disorder is delirium tremens, but in general the motor hyperactivity of delirium is not specific to any particular aetiology. Some patients manifest hyper- and hypoactivity at different times. Delirium tends to be hypoactive in certain metabolic encephalopathies, after infarction in the right middle cerebral artery territory and in the elderly (Blass and Plum, 1983).

The term *terminal restlessness* has been used in geriatric medicine for the behaviour of some patients with advanced malignancy or other end-stage illnesses. It usually describes agitated delirium in a dying patient (Burke et al, 1991), indicating central nervous irritability, as evidenced by the presence of multifocal myoclonic jerks or convulsions, and does not refer to restlessness due to pain or discomfort.

Dementia

Agitated behaviours in the elderly, especially those with dementia, have received considerable attention, particularly as they pose problems for management in nursing homes and other care facilities. The behaviours described are general restlessness, pacing, aimless wandering, repeated requests for attention, complaining, screaming, biting, fighting and cursing (Cohen-Mansfield et al, 1989). The behaviour is inappropriate either qualitatively (abusive or aggressive toward self or others) or quantitatively, socially inappropriate, not explained by the needs of the individual and not due to any of the other causes listed earlier, in particular delirium. Unfortunately, most of the literature is anecdotal or deals with pharmacological management, with few attempts at understanding the aetiology. A study that examined personality change in Alzheimer's disease patients reported purposeless hyperactivity in nearly 30% of subjects (Bozzola et al, 1992). Agitation was reported in 25 out of 35 patients with Alzheimer's disease in one study involving hospital outpatients, the majority exhibiting agitation in the morning (Gallagher-Thompson et al, 1992). Hamel et al (1990) reported that 57.2% of their patients with dementia demonstrated aggressive behaviours. Merriam et al (1988) reported agitation in 61% of their Alzheimer's disease patients. Wandering has been reported in 5% (Teri et al, 1989) to 19% (Burns et al, 1990) to 26% of patients (Teri et al, 1988) in different studies. Sinha et al (1992), in a study of 45 patients with primary degenerative dementia, reported the following inappropriate behaviours: hoarding (49%), attention-seeking behaviour (42%), hostility/aggression (35%), uncooperativeness (35%), wandering (29%), noncompliance (27%), disruption of others' activities (22%), destruction of property (8%) and sexually inappropriate behaviour (4%). The prevalence is reported to increase with the severity of dementia in some studies (Teri et al, 1989). However, Cohen-Mansfield (1986) reported that within the demented group, the agitated group did not differ from the nonagitated in age, cognitive level or waking up at night.

Studies of elderly residents of nursing homes that have not specified the medical status of their subjects have also reported the high frequency of restless behaviours. Cohen-Mansfield et al (1989) examined 408 residents aged 70–99 years (male 92, female 316) of a large suburban nursing home, and found that 93% manifested one or more agitated behaviours at least once a week during at least one nursing shift.

Head injury

Many patients have been described as going through stages of agitation and restlessness as they recover from head injury (Corrigan and Mysiw, 1988), such that some clinicians have described it as part of the natural recovery process (Denny-Brown, 1945). Levin and Grossman (1978) observed agitated or restless behaviour in 34%, Corrigan and Mysiw (1988) in 55% and Reyes et al (1981) in 50% of patients. It is likely that the high rates reported in these studies reflect the fact that patients were in tertiary referral centres, and restlessness that was due to delirium was not distinguished from restlessness in clear consciousness. In a careful prospective study, Brooke et al (1992) reported agitation in only 11% of 100 consecutive admissions due to closed head injury, with restlessness lasting less than 1 week in the majority of cases.

Hypoglycaemia

Restlessness, along with sweating, tremor, hunger and lack of concentration, is a major symptom of hypoglycaemia and was reported in 44% of episodes in one study (Egger et al, 1991). The symptoms often progress to confusion and frank delirium. Aggressiveness occurs infrequently, being reported in 3% of all reports (Egger et al, 1991).

Restless legs syndrome

The epidemiology and pathophysiology of RLS is discussed at some length in Chapter 12. Two large surveys (Ekbom, 1960; Strang, 1967) reported the prevalence to be 5% and 2.5% of the population, respectively. It is commonly associated with myoclonic jerks and periodic movements in sleep. The many factors of possible importance in the aetiology of RLS will be discussed later.

Other disorders

The clinical picture of uncomfortable sensations in the legs leading to restlessness may result from sensory or sensorimotor neuropathy, myelopathy or peripheral vascular disease. There are a number of disorders in which a neuropathy cannot be established with conventional electrodiagnostic studies, yet the symptoms plague the patient (Spillane et al, 1971). The diagnostic possibilities in such cases include metabolic-endocrine disorders, autoimmune illnesses, infections, drug toxicity, deficiency disorders, systemic malignancies and genetic disorders, and the details are discussed in Chapter 12.

Clinical manifestations

The characteristic feature of restlessness is motor activity that is purposeless, non-goal-directed, repetitive and poorly organized. Individuals may pace about, move their arms and hands constantly, wring their hands, grimace and furrow the brow, move their legs and torso while sitting, rock, rub their bodies, attend to various stimuli in the environment, and groan or produce other inappropriate verbalizations. The activity most often occurs in clear consciousness and, indeed, in a state of increased, albeit ill-sustained, alertness. However, the patient may be confused, and delirium is not unusual. When restlessness is mild, the individual may sometimes incorporate it in increasingly 'busy' and seemingly appropriate activity, as with an agitated housewife engaged in relentless cleaning of the floor or a hypomanic businessman promoting his business (Jaspers, 1963). The activity reflects a mental state of inner tension and distress, and restlessness may sometimes be experienced subjectively without its overt expression. Jaspers (1963) called it a 'state of inward excitement' (p. 113) which was usually linked with anxiety but may occur on its own. It may arise as a feeling that 'one has to do something', 'one has not finished something' or 'one has to come into the clear about something' (p. 114) and in severe cases may be experienced as heightened tension and even 'oppression'. There are therefore two aspects of restlessness: a *motor or objective component* and a *mental or subjective component*. Clinical experience suggests that it is possible to have the subjective component without objective restlessness. On the other hand, since subjective distress is difficult to assess, many investigators assess only the observational component. While this may be a useful research strategy, attempts to diminish or abolish agitated behaviour without regard to the distress or its cause may be counterproductive. The motor component of restlessness is typically considered to be under voluntary control. The subject usually recognizes this as such and is able to modify its expression or suppress it totally for varying periods. There is, however, a compelling need to move, and suppression of movement results in mounting distress.

The many terms that have been used to describe phenomena that overlap with, or are included in, the concept of restlessness are given in Table 2.3 along with suggested definitions. The published literature does not clearly attempt to distinguish agitation, fidgetiness, hyperactivity or jitteriness from restlessness. Many authors have used agitation and restlessness to reflect different degrees of abnormality on the same dimension. Others have used agitation in certain specific contexts, in particular when related to depression and dementia. Hyperactivity has been typically described in the context of ADHD. We will examine some of the commonly used terms.

Psychomotor agitation of depression

In the context of depression, Kraepelin (1921) described agitation as 'anxious restlessness ... [patients may] beg for forgiveness, entreat for mercy, kneel,

Table 2.3. *Some definitions of restlessness-related terms in the literature*

Restless: Finding or affording no rest; uneasy, agitated; constantly in motion, fidgeting, etc (*Concise Oxford Dictionary,* 1983)

Restive: Implies resistance; children can be restless from boredom but can be restive only if someone is trying to make them do what they do not want to do (Fowler, 1983)

Restlessness: State or trait of excessive and inappropriate motor activity usually associated with mental and/or physical unease

Fidgetiness: (1) Bodily uneasiness causing a person to seek relief in spasmodic movements (*Concise Oxford Dictionary,* 1983); (2) manipulation of one's own body parts or other objects, such actions being peripheral or nonessential to central ongoing events or tasks (Haskovec, 1902)

Hyperactivity: Excessive motor activity that is poorly organized and differs from the norm for one's age in both quality and quantity (DSM-III-R)

Agitation: (1) Excessive motor activity associated with a feeling of inner tension; usually nonproductive and repetitious; when agitation is severe, may be accompanied by shouting and loud complaining (DSM-III-R); (2) inappropriate verbal, vocal or motor activity judged by an outside observer not to result directly from the needs or confusion of the individual (Jaspers, 1963)

Terminal restlessness: Agitated delirium in a dying patient, frequently associated with impaired consciousness and multifocal myoclonus (Blass and Plum, 1983)

Jitteriness: Troublesome side-effect of TCAs in the treatment of panic disorder characterized by restlessness, trouble sitting still, insomnia and increased energy and anxiety (Nelson and Charney, 1981)

---

pray, pluck at their clothes, arrange their hair, rub their hands restlessly, give utterance to inarticulate cries' (p. 87). Lewis (1934) described agitation as 'the outward expression of mental unrest, which may, however, be expressed only in words . . . the inner unrest is the constant thing, the motor unrest is variable'. Not all investigators consider agitation to be an outward expression of inner anxiety. Some consider it to be a primary feature of melancholia and, when considered along with retardation, may even be a core feature of the disorder (Parker et al, 1990). While agitation may seem antithetical to retardation, the two may coexist, with patients alternating between agitation and retardation or manifesting some features of retardation, such as reduced facial responsiveness and poverty of speech, at the same time as they demonstrate increased and purposeless motor activity. In studies that have examined the loading of 'agitation' on the 'endogeneity' factor of depression, the results have been conflicting. Some earlier studies (eg, Hordern, 1965; Rosenthal and Klerman, 1966; Rosenthal and Gudeman, 1967) demonstrated a significant positive loading for endogeneity, while others reported a weak relationship (Hamilton and White, 1959; Kiloh and Garside, 1963; Carney et al, 1965) and even a negative loading (Mendels and Cochrane, 1968). These differences were partly explained on the basis of the relationship of agitation to sex, with studies that included only women showing a clear positive loading of agitation on the endogeneity factor (Mendels and Cochrane, 1968). More recent studies have reemphasized agitation as a discriminant between endogenous and reactive depressions. Feinberg and Carroll (1982) found it to be an important discriminant, with a correlation of .40 with the discriminant function separating endogenous from nonendogenous depressions. Parker et al (1990) reported agitation in 47% of endogenous and 43% of nonendogenous depressives in a sample of 202 patients. Agitation also appears to have a relationship with age, although research evidence does not always support this.

The agitated depressive patient usually fidgets a great deal, shifting position continually in the chair or playing with cigarettes, handbag or the fingers. In the early stages, patients are usually aware of this restlessness and may try to compensate for it. They may try to control their agitation by gripping something or holding on firmly to the arms of the chair. In such cases, the motor activity in the arms and the body may cease, but it often becomes apparent in the form of restless legs and feet. In the more severe cases, the agitation may be the most outstanding symptom. Patients may be unable to sit down, tend to pace up and down or rock backwards and forwards, and tear at their hands, face and hair. When unable to sit at all, the patient may present a picture of extreme anguish (Hamilton, 1989).

Agitation in dementia

A number of studies have examined agitated behaviour in elderly individuals residing in nursing homes or in the community. A large proportion of these patients suffer from dementia, although the aetiology of restlessness and agitation in these cases is usually multiply determined. Unfortunately, most studies have focused on the pharmacological management of agitation, and detailed behavioural descriptions are few (Cohen-Mansfield and Billig, 1986). Studies of agitation in dementia have included a range of unacceptable behaviours under the term *agitated behaviours* (Cohen-Mansfield and Billig, 1986; Sinha et al 1992). These include hostility, aggression, destructiveness, disruption of others' activities, uncooperativeness, noncompliance, attention-seeking, sexual inappropriateness, wandering, hoarding and self-injury. This broad conceptualization may be misleading since the different behaviours included may have diverse aetiologies, may not be always associated with subjective distress and may necessitate different interventions.

Cohen-Mansfield and Billig (1986) operationally defined agitation in the elderly as (i) inappropriate verbal, vocal or motor activity that is not judged by an outside observer to result directly from the needs or confusion of the agitated individual; and (ii) *always* socially inappropriate, because (a) it is abusive or aggressive or (b) it is performed at an inappropriate frequency or (c) it is in conflict with the social standards for the specific situation. In a preliminary study of 66 cognitively impaired elderly nursing home residents, Cohen-Mansfield (1986) used this definition of agitation to describe a range of inappropriate behaviours. Broadly, these behaviours could be subgrouped as being aggressive or nonaggressive, and the author found that the various behaviours were strongly interrelated, with nonaggressive behaviours such as pacing and constant requesting for attention occurring more frequently. The same author and her colleagues (Cohen-Mansfield et al, 1989) performed a further study of 408 nursing home residents in the age range 70–99 years using a nurses' rating questionnaire (the Cohen-Mansfield Agitation Inventory; Cohen-Mansfield, 1986), which included 29 behaviours considered to be part of agitation. Over the three nursing shifts, the residents exhibited a mean of 9.3 behaviours at least once a week. The most frequently manifested behaviours were general restlessness, pacing, complaining, repetitive sentences or questions, negativism, constant requests for attention and cursing or verbal aggression. An attempt at factor analysis of the behaviours by these authors is worth examining. They obtained four factors for agitation in the elderly.

Factor 1. Aggressive behaviour: hitting, kicking, pushing, scratching, tearing things, cursing or verbal aggression, grabbing (biting, spitting)

Factor 2. Physically nonaggressive behaviour: pacing, inappropriate robing or disrobing, repetitive sentences or questions, trying to get to a different place, handling things inappropriately, general restlessness, repetitive mannerisms

Factor 3. Verbally agitated behaviour: complaining, constant requests for attention, negativism, repetitive sentences or questions, screaming

Factor 4. Hiding/hoarding behaviour (daytime only)

The first three factors were stable for time of day, suggesting that these behaviours were highly related across nursing shifts.

An unexpected finding of the Cohen-Mansfield et al (1989) study was that the agitated behaviours were overall worse in the daytime. This is contrary to the literature supporting a 'sundowning' phenomenon in elderly individuals with cognitive impairment. Evans (1987) reported that restlessness and verbal agitation increased in the late afternoon for 11 out of 89 (12.3%) elderly nursing home residents. A closer examination of the Cohen-Mansfield et al data suggests that a proportion of their patients (14%) had more agitation during the evening shift, although there was a subgroup of 17% that was worse dur-

ing the day. In another study, Gallagher-Thomson et al (1992) reported sundowning behaviours in 11 out of 35 Alzheimer's disease subjects and found
that these were related to increased perceived stress in the caregivers.

Restlessness of attention-deficit hyperactivity disorder

Descriptions of hyperactivity in children go back to ancient literature, but it
was not until the nineteenth century that an attempt was made to characterize
it as a disorder. Ireland (1877) described a group of 'mad idiots' who were
restless and hyperactive, making them prone to violent outbursts and destructiveness. To quote one of his descriptions,

> ... a boy of seven or eight years of whom his parents were very anxious to get rid, and
> no wonder. He tried to seize and tear everything that met his eye in my office and
> gnawed the marble chimney piece with his teeth. He would rush out of his father's
> house and into those of his neighbours, breaking and destroying everything he could
> get hold of. (p. 274)

The behavioural manifestations of ADHD depend on the age and stage of
development of the individual. Infants may manifest feeding difficulties, poor
sleep, 'colic' and excessive crying. Toddlers are often described as children
'who never walked but ran' and are difficult to contain in their cribs or seats.
Two-year-olds are 'into everything', unable to stick to any form of play, 'driven' from one object or situation to the next, prone to accidents and 'fearless'.
By the age of 3 or 4, impulsivity, lack of concentration and poor frustration
tolerance become more apparent. Disciplinary problems come to the fore, and
interpersonal and scholastic difficulties become obvious. Disciplining is usually unsuccessful. The child touches everything, breaks things and sparks off
other children. If constrained in one place, the child is fidgety. Thorley (1984)
performed a factor analysis on the clinical symptoms in 73 children assessed
at the Bethlehem and Maudsley Hospitals in London and obtained four factors, which he labelled conduct disturbance, disturbance of relationships,
emotionality and developmental immaturity. The hyperactivity decreases
after the teenage years, although poor concentration and impulsivity may persist in many cases. However, adults with this disorder may continue to show a
number of features of hyperactivity, as well as other emotional and behavioural problems (Borland and Heckman, 1976).

Fidgeting or fidgetiness

The term *fidgeting* has usually been defined as 'manipulations of one's own
body parts or other objects, such actions being peripheral or nonessential to
central ongoing events or tasks' (Mehrabian and Friedman, 1986; LaBan et al,

Table 2.4. *Behaviours included in a questionnaire measuring a fidgeting tendency*

Rubbing one's neck, legs, scalp, forehead, eyes, arms, fingers
Pinching one's cheek; blowing or puffing
Playing with something in one's hand; jiggling pen when not working with it
Closing eyes tight and then opening them
Making clucking or smacking noises; sucking on tongue; clicking teeth
Scrunching shoulders; stretching out arms
Bending paper cups or crushing aluminum cans after drinking their contents; playing with straw when drinking
Pressing hands/fingers against each other; lacing fingers together; tapping or drumming on things
Scratching oneself frequently; fondling or playing with clothes
Moving restlessly when seated; moving torso when seated; tapping foot
Swinging legs back and forth when they are unsupported
Biting one's lip on purpose; sucking on lips or cheeks; rolling tongue in mouth; biting cheek
Putting nonedible objects in the mouth
Ripping napkins, wrappers, etc into little pieces
Playing with hangnail or picking a scab, making it worse
Shifting weight from one leg to another when standing

Source: Mehrabian and Freidman (1986), 40-item questionnaire.

1990). Behaviours such as rubbing body parts, playing with objects in the hands, scratching oneself, making clucking or smacking noises, swinging legs back and forth, biting or sucking objects, etc are described as part of fidgeting. Table 2.4 lists the behaviours included by Mehrabian and Friedman (1986) in their questionnaire measuring a fidgeting tendency. A factor analysis of these items yielded two factors: localized self-stimulation (rubbing fingers and hands, biting the lip, pulling on the ear, etc) and object manipulation (picking at loose threads in furniture or clothes, moving ring around finger, etc). A second study by the same authors also yielded two factors, being interpreted as localized self-stimulation and restless gross body movements and object manipulation. The two factors correlated with each other at .64 and .60, respectively, in the two studies. Interestingly, when gender bias was removed from the items, there was no sex difference in fidgetiness in the sample of undergraduate students who participated in this study.

Like restlessness, fidgeting has been treated as a state (transitory behavioural) or a trait (stable behavioural pattern) variable. Studies that have attempted to correlate these behaviours with personality variables – such as Eysenck's extraversion or neuroticism scale (Williams, 1973), the Woodrow–Mathews measure of emotional stability (Mathews, 1923) and the manifest anxiety scale (Tyron, 1968; Ballinger, 1970; Deardoff et al, 1974;

Walker and Ziskind, 1977) – have, however, been generally negative, with some exceptions (Vernallis, 1955; Mehrabian and Friedman, 1986). More often, fidgeting has been reported as a state-dependent behaviour induced by discomfort, tension, frustration or irritation. It has been reported to correlate positively with tendencies to engage in extraneous activities such as eating, cigarette smoking, consuming alcohol, day-dreaming, restlessness and insomnia (Mehrabian and Friedman, 1986).

Some of these behaviours – such as nail biting, thumb twiddling, nonnutritive sucking and self-scratching – have also been called 'nervous habits' (Olson, 1929; Jones, 1943a,b; Williams, 1973). Much of the research on these behaviours has been in children and adolescents. Even though there is an implicit acceptance that these behaviours are related to emotionality or tension, the studies that have examined the relationship between nervous habits and personality variables have found an inconsistent relationship (Seham and Boardman, 1934; Koch, 1935; Krout, 1954a,b; Tyron, 1968; Williams, 1973). Williams (1973) argued that the lack of a linear relationship of nervous habits with either extraversion or neuroticism on the Eysenck Personality Inventory (Eysenck and Eysenck, 1964) was possibly due to idiosyncratic variability in the behaviours being studied, making their measurement less than ideal. Vernallis (1955) focussed on one behaviour (teeth grinding) and found a significant relationship with anxiety. Mehrabian and Williams (1969), on the other hand, suggested that the behaviours may be differentially related to anxiety and neuroticism, with some becoming more apparent during periods of relaxation and social interaction, which may explain the inconsistencies in the literature. One may conclude from these studies that while some nervous habits, when present in excess, may indicate anxiety and neuroticism, many commonly observed behaviours do not show this relationship with any consistency.

The jitteriness syndrome

This syndrome was reported in some patients with panic disorder who were treated with tricyclic antidepressants (TCAs) (Zitrin et al, 1978, 1980; Pohl et al, 1988) and comprised restlessness, trouble sitting still, 'shakiness inside', insomnia, increased energy and an increase in anxiety. It usually occurred in the first week of treatment (Pohl et al, 1988) and, in some patients, a dose as small as 10 mg imipramine was sufficient to cause it. Zitrin et al (1980) reported it in 20% of agoraphobic women treated initially with a 25-mg/day dosage of imipramine. Pohl et al (1988), in a systematic study of the phenomenon, reported it in 49 of 158 panic disorder patients, usually developing at dosages less than 75 mg/day and occurring more frequently with desipramine. Interestingly, patients with bulimia nervosa and major depression who were treated with the same medication did not develop the syndrome, leading to the suggestion by the authors that it was specific to panic disorder.

In addition to restlessness and a subjective feeling of jitteriness, the subjects experience increased anxiety which may amount to a panic. Insomnia, irritability and an amphetamine-like 'speeding' response may occur. Patients complain that the medicine has made them worse. The symptoms often wear off in a few hours to a day. The occurrence of this side-effect usually results in a slower increase in medication dose, such that the Pohl et al study patients who developed jitteriness had a poorer response in the early stages. Age, sex and duration of illness did not appear to relate to the development of the side-effect (Pohl et al, 1988), but patient history did. Some preliminary evidence suggests that iron deficiency, as reflected in a low serum iron status, may predispose one to the development of jitteriness (Yeragani et al, 1992). A proportion of patients develop the side-effect when switched to a monoamine oxidase inhibitor like phenelzine. Anecdotal reports suggest that jitteriness responds to benzodiazepines (Klein et al, 1980) and phenothiazines (Pohl et al, 1986).

Jitteriness is considered to result from increased noradrenergic activity produced by TCAs (Pohl et al, 1988). That it (i) is an acute effect, (ii) tends to occur in panic disorder patients who have a baseline of increased noradrenergic activity and (iii) is most common with desipramine, which is a potent noradrenergic reuptake inhibitor, supports this hypothesis. It is phenomenologically different from drug-induced akathisia, and the suggestion that it responds to benzodiazepines and phenothiazines argues for a different pharmacological profile.

The clinical features of drug-induced akathisia are discussed in Chapters 6 and 7 and those of RLS in Chapter 12.

Operational definition of restlessness: a proposal

The diversity of the definitions in the published literature suggests that no consensus exists regarding the precise definition of the term *restlessness*. We consider this to be a serious deficiency and suggest that a consistent definition be applied to all disorders in which restlessness is thought to manifest. We propose the following definition:

1. The following should *always* be present:
    a. excessive and/or inappropriate motor activity, which is recognized as voluntary and can at least be partially suppressed for various periods of time

  b. repetitious and nonproductive activity which either leads to difficulties
     for the individual, those immediately around him or her or his or her
     caregivers, or leads to the individual being judged socially unacceptable
  c. an associated mental or subjective distress either reported by the indi-
     vidual or inferred from the behaviour
2. One or more of the following may *sometimes* be present:
  a. excessive or inappropriate verbal activity
  b. aggressive or violent behaviour
  c. self-manipulating or self-harming behaviours

Pathophysiology

The functional neuroanatomy and the neurochemical basis of restlessness are
both poorly understood. Leads are provided by our partial understanding of
some of the disorders involved, the possible mechanisms of drug-related
restlessness and the existence of animal models of hyperactivity. A discussion
of possible pathomechanisms and a model are presented in Chapter 10. The
model was developed for akathisia, but we feel that it can be applied to
restlessness due to any cause. The key elements of the model are the following:

1. The neuronal circuits involved in the pathogenesis of restlessness have
   complex afferent and efferent connections with large parts of the neo-
   cortex.
2. The key elements are cortical–subcortical neuronal loops that involve
   dopamine (DA), glutamic acid (Glu), γ-aminobutyric acid (GABA) and
   other neurotransmitters.
3. Motor activity is increased if subcortical structures are disinhibited, possibly through a number of different processes that involve distinct pathways
   leading to the same goal.
4. The primary disturbance will often determine what additional behavioural
   disturbance is produced, since restlessness is never present in isolation.
5. The involvement of dorsal vs ventral circuits will determine whether
   motor or affective disturbances predominate.
6. Certain drugs can nonspecifically reduce restlessness without addressing the cause or the primary disturbance, simply by altering the output
   pathways.
7. Because higher cortical centres retain some control, restless behaviour can
   be inhibited with effort for short periods. The movements are recognized
   as being intentional.

Measurement

Restlessness and related syndromes have been measured in research studies by means of rating scales designed either to assess syndromes of which restlessness or agitation are symptoms or to address specifically one of the restlessness-related syndromes such as fidgetiness or agitation. We will briefly summarize the psychometric properties of some of the scales that have been used and that have some demonstrated reliability and/or validity in the literature. Restlessness has also been quantified by means of electromechanical devices, especially in animals. These measurement methods will be discussed at length in Chapter 9. Summary characteristics of the scales are as follows:

1. General
   a. Behavioural Observation Schedule (Atakan and Cooper, 1989). Type: Symptom/behaviour scale. Subject area: Psychological and behavioural impairments in patients suffering from functional psychotic disorders. Administration: Rated during the course of normal clinical interview. Time axis: Present. Item selection: Based on the Psychological Impairments Rating Schedule (Jablensky, 1978). Revised edition contains more precise definitions, reducing overlap between items and additional items regarding other commonly observed aspects of behaviour. Number of items: 97. Item definitions: Behaviours rated on 3-point scale of frequency or severity, depending on the individual item; overall impression rated on 5-point scale of severity for each category. Psychometric validity: Face validity high. Reliability: Interrater reliability high. Comments: Recognized by WHO; however, more validity and reliability studies are required, as is a manual for the scale.
2. Fidgeting
   a. Fidgeting Tendency Questionnaire (Mehrabian and Friedman, 1986). Type: Behavioural scale. Subject area: Fidgeting tendency. Administration: Self-rating. Item selection: Descriptions of fidgeting behaviour drawn from the literature. Number of items: 40. Item definitions: Rated on a 9-point scale of agreement with the item (-4 = *very strong disagreement*, 0 = *neither agreement or disagreement*, $+4$ = *very strong disagreement*). Psychometric validity: Factor analysis revealed two factors – 'localized self-stimulation' and 'restless gross body movements and object manipulation'. Response bias minimized by both positively and negatively worded items. Reliability: Cronbach's alpha significant.
   b. Social Behaviour Schedule (Wykes and Sturt, 1986). Type: Behaviour/symptom scale. Subject area: Assessment of the nature of difficul-

ties likely to occur in patients who are dependent on psychiatric services. Administration: Rated by staff member. Time axis: Preceding month. Item selection: Based on previous scales designed to measure behaviours in long-stay psychiatric patients. Number of items: 30; one item – 'overactivity and restlessness'. Item definitions: Behaviours rated on 5-point scale of severity or frequency, depending on the individual item. Last 5 items deal with reason for being in setting, handicaps, etc, and are coded accordingly. Psychometric validity: No data available. Reliability: Interrater, interinformant and test–retest reliability coefficients calculated and found to be high. Comments: Reliable instrument for the rating of psychiatric patients under long-term care; easy to administer though validity has not been examined.

3. Tobacco withdrawal
   a. Withdrawal Questionnaire (Hughes and Hatsukami, 1986). Type: Symptom scale. Subject area: Tobacco withdrawal. Administration: Self-rating. Time axis: Immediate present. Item selection: Based on review of the literature and previous studies. Number of items: 22; 19 self-rated; 3 physiological measures. Item definitions: Symptoms and signs rated on a 3-point scale of severity (0 = *not present;* 1, 2, 3 = *mild, moderate, severe*). Psychometric validity: Profile of Mood States (POMS) completed concurrently. Most items on this correlated with the withdrawal scale. Reliability: High interrater and intrarater reliability on most items.

4. Catatonia
   a. Modified Rogers Scale (Lund et al, 1991). Type: Symptom scale. Subject area: Catatonia. Administration: Observer rated. Time axis: Immediate present. Item selection: Modified from Rogers (1985) Scale of Motor Disorder. A greater range of catatonic phenomena were included and a more refined approach to scoring was initiated. Number of items: 36 items identified as 'marked activity' (observed behaviour) and 'overactive' (reported behaviour). Item definitions: Symptoms rated on 3-point scale of severity (0 = *absent,* 2 = *severe and/or pervasive*). Psychometric validity: Concurrent validity examined against behaviour observation schedule and found to be highly significant. Reliability: Interrater and test–retest reliability significant. Comments: A valid and reliable measure of assessing motor, volitional and behavioural disorder in schizophrenic patients.

5. Attention deficit disorder
   a. Child Behaviour Checklist (Achenbach and Edelbrook, 1983). Type: Behaviour scale. Subject area: Children's behaviour. Administration:

Parent rated. Time axis: Preceding 6 months. Item selection: Items drawn from literature. Number of items: 138; one item – 'can't sit still, restless or hyperactive'. Item definitions: Behaviours rated on a 3-point scale based on agreement with the item (0 = *not true*, 2 = *very true or often true*). Additional items cover the social functioning of the child. Psychometric validity: Construct, discriminant, concurrent and predictive validity calculated. Reliability: Test–retest and interrater reliability high; internal consistency high. Comments: Frequently used in selecting subjects for research. Very good representative norms exist.

  b. ACTeRS – the ADD-H Comprehensive Teacher Rating Scale (Lund et al, 1991). Type: Behaviour scale. Subject area: Attention-deficit disorder in primary school–aged children. Administration: Teacher ratings. Time axis: Based on teacher's overall impression of the child's behaviour. Item selection: Items from Needleman's scale (1979) selected and converted to 5-point scales and a pilot study completed. A factor analysis revealed two factors: 'attention' and 'restlessness and fidgetiness'. Four other items were added to give a total of 43 items, which were reduced to 24 after a principal-components analysis was performed. Number of items: 24; items – 'fidgety' and 'restless' rated A.M. and P.M. Item definitions: Each behaviour rated on a 5-point scale of frequency (1 = *almost never*, 5 = *almost always*). Psychometric validity: Principal-components analysis revealed 4 factors – 'attention', 'hyperactivity', 'social' and 'oppositional'. Reliability: Alpha highly significant on all factors. Comments: Has been studied for use as a clinical tool for several years; quick to complete and is useful in evaluating an individual's response to medication.

  c. Rutter Scale (Rutter, 1967). Type: Behaviour scale. Subject area: Children's behaviour. Administration: Teacher rated. Time axis: Present. Item selection: Items drawn from literature. Number of items: 26; items – 'restless' and 'squirmy' relevant. Item definitions: Items rated on 3-point scale based on agreement with the item (0 = *does not apply*, 2 = *certainly applies*). Psychometric validity: Factor analysis supported three factors. Reliability: Test–retest reliability moderate. Comments: Used in several countries; useful in longitudinal studies of child development and behaviour.

6. Agitation in depression

  a. Hamilton Depression Scale (Hamilton, 1967). Type: Symptom scale. Subject area: Depression; symptom profile and severity. Administration: Observer rated. Time axis: Preceding 3 days. Item selection: Based on clinical experience and published literature. Number of items:

17 (other versions exist); one item – 'agitation'. Item definitions: 8 items defined 0–2, and 9 items 0–4. Psychometric validity: General severity factor confirmed by factor analysis; for all items, cut-off of: 8–14 = *mild depression,* 15 or more = *moderate to severe depression;* interrater reliability high (intraclass correlation coefficient .86).

b. Zung Self-Rating Depression Scale (Zung, 1965). Type: Symptom scale. Subject area: Depression; severity of depressive states. Administration: Self-rated. Time axis: na. Item selection: Descriptors of depression drawn from literature. Number of items: 20; one item – 'I am restless and can't keep still'. Item definitions: Sentences rated on a 4-point scale of frequency (1 = *not at all or some of the time,* 4 = *most of the time*). Psychometric validity: Positively and negatively worded items included. Reliability: Split-half reliability measured. Comments: Has been used extensively in individual screening and in evaluation of change in depressive state.

c. Mental State Rating Schedule (Parker et al, 1993). Type: Symptom scale. Subject area: Depressive disorders. Administration: Interviewer ratings. Time axis: Duration of normal clinical intake interview. Item selection: Items clinically observed that appeared to describe depressed behaviour included, as well as items that had demonstrated some discriminatory capacity in previous studies. Number of items: 18; one item – 'motor agitation'. Item definitions: Symptoms rated on a 4-point scale of frequency (0 = *absent,* 1, 2, 3 = *slight, moderate, severe*). Psychometric validity: Factor analysis revealed 2 or 3 factors; 'retardation', 'agitation' and a 'noninteractive' dimension; bootstrap sampling also carried out. Reliability: Interclass coefficients high. Comments: Designed to quantify psychomotor disturbances in depressed patients.

7. Agitation in the elderly

a. Blessed Dementia Scale (Blessed et al, 1968). Type: Symptom scale. Subject area: Dementia. Administration: Observer scale – based on information from close relatives or friends. Time axis: Preceding 6 months. Item selection: Items drawn from literature. Number of items: 22; one item – 'purposeless hyperactivity'. Item definitions: Varied – first 8 items measuring everyday functioning scored on 3-point scale of severity (0, .5, 1: 1 = *total incompetence*). Changes in self-care habits (3 items) rated on a 4-point scale of severity. Changes in personality, interests, drive (11 items) scored as present or absent. Psychometric validity: Scale scores highly correlated with counts of plaques in 60 patients. Reliability: No data reported. Comments: Widely used in research on dementia; elements of this scale have been used in the formulation of other batteries.

b. GERRI – Geriatric Evaluation by Relative's Rating (Schwartz, 1983). Type: Symptom scale. Subject area: General functioning in geriatric patients. Administration: Observer scale – completed by significant other. Time axis: Preceding 14 days. Item selection: Short sentences assessing frequency of behavioural complaints drawn from literature. Number of items: 49; one item – 'appears restless and fidgety'. Item definitions: Symptoms rated on 5-point scale of frequency (1 = *almost all the time*, 5 = *almost never*, 6 = *does not apply*). Psychometric validity: Response bias decreased by the inclusion of both positively and negatively worded items. Discriminant validity assessed. Reliability: Interrater reliability and internal consistency measured. Comments: Has been translated into several languages and used in the assessment of drug therapy and therapeutic interventions; consists of three clusters – cognitive functioning, social functioning and mood.

c. MS-E – Mood Scales, Elderly (Raskin and Crook, 1988). Type: Symptom scale. Subject area: Mood disturbances in the elderly. Administration: Self-rated. Time axis: Immediate present. Item selection: Adjectives of mood selected from the literature. Number of items: 50; items – 'restless' and 'jittery' included. Item definitions: Adjectives rated on 5-point scale of severity (1 = *not at all*, 5 = *extremely*). Psychometric validity: Seven factors revealed by factor analysis. Construct validity was investigated by examining three diagnostic groups. Statistically significant differences were found between these groups using scale measurements. Reliability: Significant alpha values recorded. Comments: Has been used in drug trials with depressed inpatients. Normative data have been obtained as well as data on elderly patients with mood disorders.

d. Dementia Mood Assessment Scale (Sunderland et al, 1988). Type: Symptom scale. Subject area: Severity of depression in dementia patients. Administration: Rated by interviewer. Time axis: Immediate present. Item selection: Partly derived from the Hamilton scale, with additional items relating to the functional mood of dementia patients. Number of items: 24; one item – 'physical agitation'. Item definitions: Rated on a 7-point scale of severity (0 = *within normal limits*, 6 = *most severe*). Psychometric validity: Concurrent validity moderate; construct validity high. Reliability: Interrater reliability high. Comments: Not intended for use as a diagnostic tool; useful in longitudinal monitoring of mood in dementia.

e. Behavioural Problem Checklist (Niederehe, 1988). Type: Behaviour/ symptom scale. Subject area: Dementia. Administration: Completed by caregivers. Time axis: Coded on 5-point scale for each item (0 = *never*, 5 = *2+ years ago*). Item selection: Expanded and modified from the Memory and Behavioural Problems Checklist (Zarit et al, 1980). Also includes items from several other scales. Number of items: 52; one item 'being very restless or agitated'. Item definitions: Behaviours rated on three 5-point scales of frequency (0 = *never*, 4 = *daily*), duration (see 'time axis') and severity of reaction of caregiver (0 = *not at all*, 4 = *extremely*). Psychometric validity: Homogeneity of scaling method reveals seven symptom clusters, refined into six subgroupings. Discriminant validity investigated and found to be significant. Correlated with the Short Portable Mental Status Questionnaire (Pfeiffer, 1975) and the Hamilton Depression Scale ratings. Reliability: Cronbach's alpha high; test–retest reliability high. Comments: Has been used in several studies of caregivers of dementia patients. May possibly be used by professionals in clinical settings.

f. Cohen-Mansfield Agitation Inventory (Cohen-Mansfield, 1986). Type: Behaviour scale. Subject area: Agitated behaviours in the elderly. Administration: Nurses' ratings. Time axis: 8-hour period. Item selection: Descriptions of agitated behaviours drawn from the literature. Number of items: 29 – all relevant; one item – 'general restlessness'. Item definitions: Descriptors rated on a 7-point scale of frequency (1 = *patient never engages in behaviour*, 7 = *patient manifests behaviour several times an hour*). Psychometric validity: Factor analysis revealed 3 types of agitated behaviours from this scale. Reliability: Interrater reliability significant. Comments: Discriminates between aggressive, physically nonaggressive and verbally agitated behaviours.

Treatment

Since restlessness is a symptom, the recognition and treatment of the primary disorder are often sufficient to deal with it. The causes may be multiple, and each needs to be addressed. For example, a demented patient may be restless ostensibly because of pain after a fall and a fracture, but this may be exacerbated by large doses of analgesics or the use of sedative drugs. In many cases, however, restlessness must be treated in its own right because of its negative impact on the patient and caregivers (Reisberg et al, 1987). Restlessness can lead to exhaustion, dehydration, accidental injury, an inability to provide adequate medical care because of uncooperativeness and the disruption of ward routines. This is most apparent in patients with dementia, delirium, affective disorder or psychosis. The overall strategy has to be tailored to the disorder and the individual.

First, the various psychological, social and environmental determinants of restlessness have to be identified and rectified. Measures should be taken to provide an optimal sensory and social environment. Such an environment should provide some stimulation to the patient without being overstimulating, be reassuring, guarantee the safety of the patient as well as those caring for him or her and permit appropriate medical intervention. It is important to remember that in predisposed individuals even minor changes in the environment may lead to restlessness. Excessive noise or heat, a change of roommate, altered daily routine or staff changes may be important. The details with regard to the nursing requirements have been discussed by Lipowski (1990) in the case of delirious patients, and the same principles apply to any patient with restlessness, especially if cognitive impairment is a feature. The individual's fluid, electrolyte and nutritional needs have to be met; pain, hypoxia or other exacerbating factors must be addressed; the role of sensory loss needs to be considered; and the medical problems need to be appropriately managed. Psychodynamic factors should not be ignored: the perception of reduced autonomy, the denial of the need for a nursing home placement, conflict with a family member, etc may all exert an influence (Leibovici and Tariot, 1988).

Second, the patient may need drug therapy to reduce motor activity and subjective distress. Drugs used to treat restlessness or agitation include the neuroleptics, benzodiazepines, β-adrenergic antagonists, antidepressants, lithium and carbamazepine, and the choice of a particular drug is guided by the setting and the possible aetiology. It must be emphasized that the literature is replete with accounts of the inappropriate use of psychotropic drugs in the management of agitated behaviour, in particular in the elderly (Prien et al, 1976; Salzman and van der Kolk, 1979; Ray et al, 1980; Seifert et al, 1983) and the mentally retarded populations (Sachdev, 1991). This practice is to be deplored for the following reasons: (i) The underlying causes of restlessness may be ignored, often with disastrous results. (ii) Most psychotropic drugs have toxic effects which may either worsen the patient's state or impose added problems. A worsening of the agitation may lead to an increase in dosage of the drugs, thus starting a spiral of toxicity leading to further deterioration in the person's state (Ancill and Holliday, 1988). (iii) Drug treatment may be used as a substitute for more appropriate nursing and general medical management, as sometimes happens in institutions for the mentally ill or the mentally retarded (Sachdev, 1991).

The literature on the treatment of agitation in dementia has been reviewed by Leibovici and Tariot (1988), and that for delirium by Lipowski (1990). The large number of drugs that have been used suggests that no one drug is uniformly beneficial. The choice of drug can be guided by certain specific symptoms, but in many cases a trial-and-error approach is warranted, with the dosage of the most suitable drug then being tailored to the individual's response. Leibovici and Tariot (1988) recommend a detailed behavioural analysis to identify a 'psychobehavioural metaphor' – a subtype of agitation or restlessness – that would respond differentially to a particular drug. Patients who, along with their restlessness, show pressured speech and decreased sleep may be considered for treatment with a mood-stabilizing drug like lithium or carbamazepine. Patients who are aggressive are more likely to benefit from β-adrenergic antagonists, lithium or carbamazepine (Yudofsky et al, 1984). The coexistence of anxiety may suggest the use of benzodiazepines, and of dysphoria and irritability that of antidepressants. In the same vein, neuroleptics would be chosen if there is a suggestion of psychosis, although these drugs often tend to be used as first-line drugs for many different restless behaviours.

Neuroleptics are probably the drugs most commonly used for the management of agitation in dementia and delirium (Helms, 1985). They are certainly the drugs of choice if a psychotic disorder forms the basis of the restlessness or exists concomitantly. Published research studies ($N = 68$) involving more than 5,000 patients were reviewed by Salzman (1987), with the conclusion that antipsychotic drugs were indeed beneficial in a number of patients. If all studies were pooled, nearly 65% of patients showed a positive response. However, if only rigorous studies were considered, the results were far less impressive, suggesting that the effect may not be very powerful. The literature does not suggest that any particular drug is more effective, and the clinical practice of preferentially using sedating drugs, such as thioridazine, is not supported by empirical evidence. The choice of a particular antipsychotic drug depends on the patient's symptom profile and the presence of any associated problems. For example, a patient with parkinsonism will tolerate a high-potency neuroleptic poorly, and one with orthostatic hypotension may get worse on thioridazine. It has been suggested that patients with irritability, suspiciousness and paranoia tend to improve on neuroleptics (Risse and Barnes, 1986), so that the antiagitation effect of these drugs may be related to their antipsychotic properties. Other behaviours such as wandering, socially inappropriate behaviour and calling out are not improved by these drugs (Risse and Barnes, 1986). The antiagitation dosages of neuroleptics are much smaller than their antipsychotic dosages and are of the order of 0.25–5 mg of haloperidol per day or its equivalent (Salzman, 1987). There is some evidence from the literature that the effect is short-lived, and long-term treatment is not to be advised. The few discontinuation studies that are available suggest that agitated patients are often treated for too long (Barton and Hurst, 1966).

Benzodiazepines are quite extensively used in the treatment of agitation, and a number of studies attest to their efficacy in some patients (Risse and Barnes, 1986). It is not certain whether it is the subgroup with anxiety that responds positively. Side-effects of these drugs must be carefully considered prior to use, and sedation, ataxia and cognitive effects can sometimes make the primary disorder worse. A paradoxical increase in agitation is known to occur sometimes. These drugs should, therefore, be used for short periods and for insomnia, anxiety or mild agitation. It is preferable to use drugs with a short half-life, eg, lorazepam or oxazepam (Hyman and Arana, 1987). Ancill et al (1991) recommended the use of alprazolam because of fewer side-effects compared with lorazepam. It is also important to be aware of the problems associated with withdrawing patients from the benzodiazepines.

β-Adrenergic antagonists have been used to treat aggressive behaviour in patients with dementia (Greendyke and Kanter, 1986), head injury (Yudofsky et al, 1987), mental retardation (Ratey et al, 1986), etc. Their use for the management of restlessness or agitation in the absence of aggressiveness is limited to a few published anecdotes (Petrie and Ban, 1981). Propranolol, a lipophilic, nonselective antagonist, is the drug most commonly used, but other more selective drugs may be used with the same efficacy (Mattes, 1985; Greendyke and Kanter, 1986).

The efficacy of lithium and carbamazepine is supported by case reports of improvement in some patients, but rigorous studies are generally lacking (Williams and Goldstein, 1979; Neppe, 1982). The use of antidepressants – tricyclics and monoamine oxidase inhibitors – is similarly limited, and it is possible that the potential of these drugs has not been fully exploited (Tariot et al, 1987).

Future research

There is a definite need for strict and operational definitions of the terms used so that consistency can be achieved and study results can be compared. The application of a standard definition of *restlessness* is therefore advisable. The clinical manifestations of each of the syndromes described should then be rigorously investigated. Large epidemiological studies should include unselected or randomly selected populations. The measures of severity of restlessness should be further evaluated for their psychometric properties. Once the clinical profiles of the syndromes have been studied, the pathophysiology of the various aspects of restlessness can be investigated. The treatment studies have been few and are methodologically weak, and amends must be made in this regard. While animal models may be appropriate for investigating the different aspects of the pathophysiology of restlessness, human studies using positron emission tomography (PET) and other functional imaging would be necessary to confirm the validity of the models. Future strategies for the management of restlessness will then be based on the underlying mechanisms, thus improving on the currently available empirically derived interventions.

3

Neuroleptic-induced dysphoria

One must be crazy, either literally or figuratively, to take these drugs [neuroleptics].

Leo E. Hollister (1992)

Neuroleptic drugs are unpleasant for both normal people and many psychiatric patients, and this behavioural side-effect has been recognized from the time these drugs were first introduced. Hollister (1957) cited a study in which 80 normal individuals were given a single 50-mg dose of chlorpromazine. Twenty (25%) experienced increased fatigue, sleepiness and generally unpleasant feelings. A number of other authors have reported distressing feelings in normal people or nonpsychiatric patients in response to these drugs (Hollister, 1961; Kendler, 1976; Belmaker and Wald, 1977; Anderson et al, 1981). To quote Belmaker and Wald (1977, p. 222), who injected themselves with 5 mg haloperidol iv:

Within ten minutes a marked slowing of thinking and movement developed, along with profound inner restlessness. Neither subject could continue work, and each left work for over 36 hours. Each subject complained of a paralysis of volition, a lack of physical and psychic energy. The subjects felt unable to read, telephone or perform household tasks of their own will, but could perform these tasks if demanded to do so. There was no sleepiness or sedation; on the contrary, both subjects complained of severe anxiety.

A number of descriptions of neuroleptic-induced dysphoria (NID) in the literature suggest that only a proportion of this dysphoria is due to akathisia. It is for this reason that NID is discussed in this book separately. The general literature on this topic, in spite of being spread over three decades, is somewhat scanty and will be briefly surveyed here.

Description of the dysphoric response

The simplest generalization of this phenomenon is that individuals given the drug in the absence of clear evidence for akathisia, drowsiness, depression or

47

cognitive impairment report feeling unwell or dislike the drug for its effect on the body or the mind. The manifestations are varied and may be categorized as follows.

'The drug disagrees with me' report

It is not uncommon for patients to say that neuroleptic drugs make them 'dull', 'unable to think' or 'goofy, lazy and mummified', give them a 'permanent hangover' or put them 'in a chemical straitjacket' (Van Putten and May, 1978). As one Tourette's syndrome patient (Caine and Polinsky, 1979) described it: 'It was as if a shade suddenly came down'. Many complain of being 'drugged', being 'tired and slowed down', 'having no drive or ambition', feeling 'strange, frightened or weird' or being 'suppress[ed] . . . from having ideas' (Van Putten et al, 1984a). Patients experience a slowing of both body and mind, and a distressing lack of freedom of will. They can usually distinguish these experiences from depression and anxiety. The response can be attributed by the individual to the drug, and it is dosage-related.

Van Putten and May (1978a) measured the subjective response of 42 newly admitted schizophrenic patients to neuroleptic drugs at 4, 24 and 48 hours after a test dose of chlorpromazine (2.2 mg/kg) (which was repeated at 25 hours and, at twice the dose, at 48 hours) using a blind rater and found that 17 (40%) had a dysphoric response. Four were so distressed that they refused to take the drug again. Dysphoria was assessed on a rating scale of −11 to +11 in response to the question, 'How does the medication agree with you?' Interestingly, the remaining 25 (60%) were described as having a 'euphoric' response. (The authors later found this term inappropriate.) The same group of investigators (Van Putten et al, 1981) challenged another set of 63 newly admitted schizophrenic patients with thiothixene (0.22 mg/kg) and found that 14 (22%) had a dysphoric response. Of those remaining, 31 (49%) had a syntonic response, 12 were noncommittal and 6 were inaccessible. In yet another study (Van Putten et al, 1984c), the authors reported that 16 (25%) of 65 patients treated with thiothixene and 9 (23%) of 40 patients treated with haloperidol had a dysphoric response to the first dose of the drug. The authors concluded that there was consistent evidence that a significant minority of patients reacted adversely to the medication.

Weiden et al (1989) performed a naturalistic study in 50 consecutively admitted acutely psychotic patients and found that 13 (26%) were consistently dysphoric, with 4 refusing the readministration of drugs. Caine and Polinsky (1979) described a dysphoric response in 6 of 72 patients with Tourette's syndrome treated by them with haloperidol, but this was not a prospective study.

Noncompliance

A dysphoric response may lead to a refusal by the patient to take the offending drug. While this has always been appreciated by clinicians, a systematic study of this phenomenon was performed by Van Putten and colleagues. Van Putten et al (1981) reported that a dysphoric response was a powerful predictor of noncompliance with medication ($p < .0001$). Of the 14 patients with dysphoria, 6 vehemently refused to take a second dose of an antipsychotic, even at a much smaller dose. The remaining 8 could be persuaded to take a smaller dose (mean dose of thiothixene, 9.9 mg for this group vs 27.2 mg for the nondysphoric group), but only 4 persisted in taking the drug beyond 2 weeks. In the Van Putten et al (1984b) study, 10 (62%) out of 19 dysphoric responders did not continue thiothixene beyond 2 weeks, compared with 5 (11%) out of 49 syntonic responders ($p < .001$). The figures for the haloperidol group were 67% and 20%, respectively (ns).

There are many determinants of compliance which have to be considered by a clinician in any patient who refuses medication or is found to neglect or 'forget' to take it. The preceding studies suggest that a dysphoric response may be one potent determinant of noncompliance. Van Putten et al (1981) called it the 'sauce bearnaise phenomenon', quoting Seligman (1972, p. 8):

Sauce Bearnaise . . . used to be my favourite sauce. It now tastes awful to me. This happened several years ago, when I felt the effects of the stomach flu about 6 hours after eating filet mignon with Sauce Bearnaise. I became violently ill and spent most of the night vomiting. The next time I had Sauce Bearnaise, I couldn't bear the taste of it.

The drug refusal was attributed to 'interoceptive conditioning with a somatically based dysphoric response' by Van Putten et al (1981, p. 190).

Anxiety and derealization

A number of patients report that the drugs make them 'anxious', though they are usually able to distinguish this 'anxiety' from that associated with stress and worry. Singh and Kay (1979) considered it an important feature of dysphoria, giving it a weighting of three on their six psychopathological measures of dysphoria: depression ($\times 3$), anxiety ($\times 3$), ideas of guilt and worthlessness ($\times 2$), suspiciousness/persecution ($\times 2$), hostility ($\times 1$) and suicidal ideas and actions ($\times 1$). It is uncertain, however, whether anxiety accurately describes the subjective experience of the patients. Some patients report a feeling of depersonalization and/or derealization attributable to the medication. This has been observed by the author in two patients being treated with pimozide for Tourette's syndrome; the patients obtained some relief from the administration of benztropine and responded to a reduction of neuroleptic dosage.

Shapiro et al (1988) reported what they called 'fog states' characterized by feelings of depersonalization, paranoia and slowed mentation lasting from a few seconds to several hours in patients with Tourette's syndrome being treated with haloperidol. One patient also reported several episodes in which his thoughts were fixated on a part of his body, an object or a word. A second patient reported repetitive psychopathological fantasies.

School and work avoidance, and the neuroleptic separation anxiety syndrome

With the extensive use of neuroleptics, in particular haloperidol and pimozide, in the treatment of Tourette's syndrome, reports of an unexpected side-effect of school and work avoidance have appeared. Mikkelsen et al (1981) first drew attention to this in their report of 15 patients with Tourette's syndrome, all being treated with haloperidol at low dosages (mean 2.5 mg/day; range 1.0–7.5). These patients (mean age 19.9 ± 12.4 years), 9 of whom were less than 15 years old, experienced such symptoms as unprecedented, severe feelings of anxiety and school or work avoidance soon after the introduction of the drug (mean 8 weeks; range, 1–28). They had no past history of phobic symptoms, were all relatively successful and high functioning and did not experience akathisia, except for 1 patient who responded to antiparkinsonian treatment. All improved completely with the discontinuation of the neuroleptic drug. Some quotations from the case reports are instructive:

Case 1: 'A 42-year-old man became fearful of going to work because of "terrible anxiety about making mistakes", and he was aware of a dysphoric feeling. He was obsessed with the idea that he would be unable to manage the large number of people in his section'.

Case 2: A 12-year-old boy suddenly became afraid of going to school, 2 weeks after starting the medication. 'He was reluctant to leave home in the morning, and when he arrived in school he insisted on repeatedly telephoning home to talk with his mother. When the principal refused permission for these telephone calls, B. became acutely panicked'.

Case 10: A 35-year-old man reported, 'In the morning I found I was afraid to get out of bed. At one point it took me 4 days before I could even get out the door'.

The authors argued that these responses were phobic, emphasizing separation anxiety, and could not be explained on the basis of dysphoria or cognitive deficits induced by neuroleptics. None of the patients had a major depressive reaction, and all experienced benefit from the drug in the control of their tics. The authors speculated on the biochemical basis of this response and wondered whether these patients (15 out of a total of 90 in their sample) constituted a distinct subgroup. Other authors have also reported separation anxiety in response to haloperidol (Bruun, 1982; Shapiro and Shapiro, 1993).

A few reports of separation anxiety in response to pimozide have also been published. Shapiro (cited in Linet, 1985) observed school anxiety or avoidance in 5 of 51 patients treated with pimozide. Linet (1985) reported an 11-year-old boy who developed school phobia on each of three trials with pimozide, exhibiting the usual fantasies of being trapped in school and irreversibly separated from his parents.

Painful sensory symptoms

It is generally accepted that many patients (about 40%) with PD or postencephalitic parkinsonism report painful or other distressing sensations that cannot be attributed to gross motor or sensory pathology, the so-called primary sensory symptoms of parkinsonism (Snider et al, 1976; Koller, 1984; Goetz et al, 1986). Snider et al (1976) categorized these symptoms into paraesthesiae (burning, coldness, tingling and numbness) and pain (poorly localized painful sensations without thermal or anaesthetic characteristics and not associated with increased muscle contraction or affected by movements or pressure). The pathogenesis of these symptoms is not understood, but reduced DA function in the basal ganglia or other systems has been implicated (Snider et al, 1976; Koller, 1984; Nutt and Carter, 1984).

Sigwald and Solignac (1960) first drew attention to the presence of disagreeable or painful sensations in association with neuroleptic treatment that were similar to that in PD. A systematic but preliminary study of these phenomena was performed by Decina et al (1992), who reported that painful sensory phenomena, but not paresthesiae, were more common in neuroleptic-treated patients compared with those receiving other medication. Fourteen (23%) of 60 patients receiving neuroleptics reported experiences of spontaneous pain subjectively attributed to pharmacological treatment. The pain was described as intermittent by 10 of the 14, and characterized most commonly as 'aching' ($n = 12$). Twelve located their pain in all four limbs, 5 in the back, with the head and torso being spared. Those who had pain also suffered more often from EPSE and akathisia. On univariate and multivariate analyses, the best predictors of pain were tremor and postural imbalance rather than rigidity or bradykinesia, and akathisia was not significant. No demographic or drug-related predictors emerged. The authors expressed caution about the preliminary nature of the findings because of methodological limitations in the assessment of the sensory symptoms.

Depression

Whether neuroleptics can cause depression and, if so, what the nature of that depression is has been debated for more than two decades, and will not be discussed in any detail here. Various positions have been suggested by previous investigators.

Some authors have described a severe depression in patients emerging from psychotic states. This was first described by Mayer-Gross (1920) as postpsychotic depression (PPD), long before the introduction of neuroleptics. The topic was extensively reviewed by McGlashan and Carpenter (1976), who described a retarded depression with strong neurasthenic and schizoid components. They were uncertain about the causal role of neuroleptic drugs. They cited studies (Steinberg et al, 1967; Stern et al, 1972; Ollerenshaw, 1973) in which virtually all patients with PPD had been given phenothiazines. However, in two studies (Cohen et al, 1964; Warnes, 1968), there was no difference in the use of neuroleptics between those schizophrenics who were depressed or suicidal and those who were not. The authors concluded that it was possible that some cases of PPD were caused by neuroleptics.

Hirsch (1982) argued that since a high proportion of recently hospitalized schizophrenics suffered from depression (Johnson, 1981; Knights and Hirsch, 1981), posttreatment depression was an integral, 'revealed' aspect of the schizophrenic syndrome. Hirsch argued that the cause of depression in schizophrenics may prove to be heterogeneous, but drugs were unlikely to be a major contributor.

Some authors (eg, Galdi, 1983) have argued strongly in favour of neuroleptic-induced depression. Several studies have reported excess depression in patients treated with depot neuroleptics (De Alarcon and Carney, 1969; Johnson, 1969; Marjot, 1969; Ray, 1972; Keskiner, 1973; Hogarty et al, 1979), but methodological problems make the conclusions not totally convincing. Galdi et al (1981) argued that schizophrenics who developed neuroleptic-induced depression were genetically predisposed to affective disorder, thus arguing for a pharmacogenetic induction. The Hogarty et al (1979) data supported this, but Hirsch (1983) questioned the significance of these studies in light of many negative studies. Further, the depression in the Galdi et al study often responded to anticholinergic medication, suggesting that it may have been misdiagnosed hypokinesia.

The relationship between neuroleptic-induced akinesia and depression has also been debated. Van Putten and May (1978b) presented data to suggest that patients who developed akinesia in response to neuroleptics were more likely to report and be judged as having depression. When the authors examined the published literature, however, they did not find evidence that patients who received high doses of neuroleptics, and therefore had more akinesia, had a higher prevalence of depression. Some authors have reported that depression associated with neuroleptics responds to acetylcholine (ACh) antagonists in many cases (Galdi et al, 1981; Johnson, 1981). The question remains, however, whether the depression described in these studies is true depression or merely misdiagnosed hypokinesia. It has not been shown that depression can be reliably distinguished from hypokinesia, and 'akinetic depression' may in fact be a pseudodepression. The akinesia syndrome can arise in the absence of other EPSE (Siris, 1985) and be accompanied by blue mood (Van Putten and May, 1978a,b; Siris, 1985), thus making the distinction particularly difficult.

Singh and Kay (1979) described a dysphoric response to neuroleptics, which they characterized as a combination of anxiety, depression and accusatoriness. This response typically occurred in the 'nonparanoid, nuclear schizophrenic', was associated with an autonomic arousal and was an early response.

In conclusion, while a dysphoric response to neuroleptic drugs is not uncommon, the evidence that a depressive syndrome commonly occurs is not convincing, and in fact there is more evidence to the contrary.

Determinants of the dysphoric response

As we have discussed, the dysphoric response cannot be explained on the basis of depression. Further, the role of akathisia, drowsiness or cognitive dysfunction is excluded by definition. What then are the other possible determinants of the dysphoria? In this discussion, empirical data are often replaced by educated speculation.

Neuroleptic dosage and type

In two studies, Van Putten and colleagues used standard dosages and therefore could not examine the role of neuroleptic dosage. However, a majority of their dysphoric patients could be persuaded to take smaller doses, as mentioned previously, suggesting that dysphoria may be dose-related. This is also our clinical experience. Weiden et al (1989) also reported that dysphoric patients tended to go on to receive smaller doses of neuroleptics than the nondysphoric patients.

Van Putten and colleagues (1980, 1984c) showed that dysphoric responders to chlorpromazine, haloperidol or thiothixene did not have unusual or higher plasma levels of the drugs. There was, therefore, no obvious pharmacokinetic explanation for the individuals' responses.

The published literature does not suggest that any drugs are particularly likely to produce dysphoria, although it tends to be reported more commonly with high-potency drugs such as haloperidol. If one considers the rates reported by Van Putten for chlorpromazine, thiothixene and haloperidol, dysphoria is probably equally common with the low-potency drugs, although these rates were reported in different studies and did not reflect direct comparisons of drugs. It is likely that dysphoria associated with akinesia or severe EPSE is more common with high-potency drugs.

Other drug-related variables

Factors like previous exposure, rate of increment and the duration of neuroleptic use have been inadequately examined to make any definitive statement. It is recognized that dysphoria is generally an acute response and can start within minutes of the first dose of the drug (Belmaker and Wald, 1977), and certainly within days. In the Van Putten and May (1978a) study, there was no difference in the length of drug treatment between dysphoric and 'euphoric' responders.

EPSE: akinesia, rigidity and tremor

The relationship between dysphoria and akinesia has already been discussed, and it has been previously stated that it is unclear whether akinesia and depression coexist or are mistaken for each other, or the individual responds to the akinesia with subjective distress and dysphoria, or the real relationship is indeed a combination of these possibilities. Detre and Jarecki (1971) observed that 'suicidal ideation often develops after the patient discovers that he is too anergic to function as he did before he first fell ill and therefore assumes that he is permanently damaged' (p. 135). Patients are known to respond to rigidity or tremor with distress. One of our patients made a suicide attempt in response to a severe, generalized tremor that did not respond to antiparkinsonian medication.

The research evidence linking EPSE and dysphoria is inconclusive. Van

Putten and May (1978b) reported that out of a total of 94 patients treated with antipsychotics, 28 developed a mild akinesia, which was defined as a 'behavioral state of diminished spontaneity characterized by few gestures, unspontaneous speech, and, particularly, apathy and difficulty with initiating usual activities' (Rifkin et al, 1975, p. 672). Sixteen (57%) of the akinetic patients developed a concomitant increase in depression, but a relationship with other EPSE was not reported. In another study (Van Putten and May, 1978b), the same authors reported that 50% of the dysphoric and 17% of the euphoric patients had mild akinesia. Singh and Kay (1979) did not find an association between EPSE and NID. Reference has already been made to studies (Galdi et al, 1981; Johnson, 1981) in which ACh antagonists improved neuroleptic-induced depression, suggesting that it may be the akinesia that was being improved.

Akathisia

Akathisia is the most important cause of subjective distress in patients medicated with neuroleptics, but our definition of NID excludes it. However, not all studies of NID have been careful to distinguish it from akathisia. Van Putten et al (1984a) observed that the dysphoric response in their patients was powerfully associated with akathisia, with all dysphoric and only 16% of syntonic responders also experiencing akathisia ($p < .001$). When we later examine the clinical features of akathisia, it will become clear that it is possible to distinguish akathisia from other causes of dysphoria in these patients. We consider it important that one tries to regard NID and akathisia as separate syndromes.

Placebo response or misattribution

A proportion of the dysphoria can be considered to be a placebo response to the drugs. It must be appreciated that patients often take neuroleptics under compulsion or fear that the drugs would alter their thinking or control them in other ways and therefore have a negative expectation. They may also misattribute their illness-related distress to the medication.

Psychological factors

The importance of understanding drug side-effects in terms of the patient's personality, his or her fears and expectations, the patient's and the doctor's transferences and the setting in which the drug is prescribed was highlighted by Sarwer-Foner (1960a,b, 1961, 1963). For example, individuals who use activity as a defence against unacceptable conflicts may find the psychomotor slow-down produced by chlorpromazine threatening and may respond with anxiety and disorganization. Paranoid individuals who are constantly vigilant may poorly tolerate any drug that affects their alertness. An early study was conducted by Kornetsky and Humphries (1957), who correlated scores on the Minnesota Multiphasic Personality Inventory (MMPI) with the subjective experience and psychological task performance subsequent to the administration of secobarbital, chlorpromazine, LSD and a placebo. They reported that the higher the subject's scores on the depression and psychasthenia scales, the greater the subjective effects of these drugs. Henninger et al (1965) provided empirical support to Sarwer-Foner's observations in a normal group. Their healthy male volunteers were challenged with 200 mg chlorpromazine; the ones who were notably extroverted reacted to the drug with marked anxiety, whereas the introspective and introverted subjects became tranquil and indifferent to their surroundings. The results reported by Klerman et al (1959) were somewhat different: their type B individuals (introverted, inhibited, high on manifest anxiety) showed more hostility and depression after reserpine use than did the type A individuals (expressive of anger, extroverted).

Recent studies in patient populations do not suggest that patients who develop a dysphoric response have particular characteristics at baseline (Van Putten and May, 1978a; Singh and Kay, 1979; Van Putten et al, 1984a; Weiden et al, 1989). Nevertheless, personality and baseline psychopathology variables should be examined further in trying to understand the dysphoric response.

In summary, a number of different variables may contribute to a dysphoric response, but there is a significant component of 'individual vulnerability' that remains unexplained.

The longitudinal course of neuroleptic-induced dysphoria

Do patients with NID develop a tolerance to the dysphoric side-effect? In the Van Putten and May (1978a) study, this was not evident in the duration of the follow-up, with 88% of the dysphoric responders eventually refusing to continue chlorpromazine (vs 23% of nondysphoric responders). Singh and Kay (1979) examined their patients every 2 weeks for at least 12 weeks. The dysphoric patients had an increase in the dysphoria score in the first 2 weeks and then remained consistently dysphoric. The nondysphoric patients had a dramatic decline in their dysphoria from baseline in the first 2 weeks and then showed a more gradual but progressive decline. The preliminary evidence, therefore, is that the dysphoric response does not abate in the short to medium term. There is also a suggestion that dysphoric responders have had similar experiences in the past. The long-term course is unclear and confounded by the fact that a large number of dysphoric responders discontinue the medication, or at least reduce the dosage.

Does dysphoria predict a poor outcome?

Van Putten and May (1978a) supported the view that an early dysphoric response to chlorpromazine augured a poor prognosis for further treatment with the drug, but this could be explained on the basis of noncompliance and limitation of dosage. Singh and Kay (1979) provided further data to support the relationship with poor outcome, but for the nonparanoid and not the paranoid group of schizophrenic patients. Weiden et al (1989) added a new perspective to this issue by arguing that the dysphoric patients who did continue with the medication had a good resolution of their psychotic symptoms, with less akathisia and EPSE. Thus, if noncompliance could be disregarded, a dysphoric response proved positive for the patient.

The biochemical basis of neuroleptic-induced dysphoria: utility of an animal model

The neurobiological basis of the dysphoric response is poorly understood, and in the absence of definitive information, one can only speculate on the possible pathogenesis. Some facts must be addressed to develop one or more models: (i) All classic neuroleptics are known to produce dysphoria, and we do not know the relative risk for the different drugs. Haloperidol has most often been implicated in the nonpsychotic populations, but this may merely reflect the more common use of this drug. Neuroleptics have an effect on many neurotransmitters in the brain (Richelson, 1984), of which DA antagonism has received the greatest attention because of its correlation with antipsychotic potency (Creese et al, 1976; Seeman et al, 1976). (ii) The wide range of subjective manifestations, and the associated strong affective component, suggest that the response is of a central origin. (iii) Subjective reports of symptoms that superficially resemble NID occur in a number of disorders affecting the basal ganglia: Tourette's syndrome, PD, postencephalitic parkinsonism. DA dysfunction is arguably important in these disorders, although other neurotransmitters are also involved, and the nature of the DA change may be an increase or decrease or an imbalance in the relative actions of the drugs on different receptors. (iv) Is this kind of subjective phenomenon a consequence

of basal ganglia dysfunction? Basal ganglia are known to modify sensory perception, and electrophysiological studies indicate that they have a mainly
inhibitory influence on sensory activity (Krauthamer, 1979). There are
descending dopaminergic projections to the dorsal horn and midline thalamic
nuclei, which may be the anatomical substrates for this interaction (Bjorklund
and Skagerberg, 1979). Basal ganglia also have an interaction with the limbic
brain, which controls the affective and experiential states. How basal ganglia
dysfunction actually leads to dysphoria or sensory phenomena is, however,
unknown and worthy of exploration.

Some assistance in the study of the pathophysiology can be provided by
suitable animal models of NID. It has been known for a long time that animals are averse to neuroleptics. Berger (1972) showed that chlorpromazine
could be used as punishment in a rat model of conditioned suppression.
Hoffmeister (1975, 1977) showed that monkeys actively avoided the administration of small doses of chlorpromazine, although the effect was not as clear-
cut with haloperidol, probably because of a marked response suppression produced by the latter. Giardini (1985) showed that chlorpromazine was an
affective unconditioned stimulus in a conditioned taste-aversion paradigm,
and this response was masked by an opiate like morphine (Giardini and
Valanzano, cited in Bignami, 1991). Giardini (1985) did not find haloperidol
to have a similar effect as chlorpromazine, and he argued that it was because
of the opiate-like component of haloperidol's action, ie, because it produced
the effect when given in conjunction with naloxone.

Defecation is an index of emotionality in the rat that has been studied in
relation to neuroleptics. Originally described by Hall (1934), defecation was
considered by Broadhurst (1957) to be the 'emotionality index of choice in
the rat'. It has long been known that rats defecate excessively when in an
aroused state, such as being placed in unfamiliar or novel surroundings (Hall,
1934). In these circumstances, neuroleptics in fact reduce the level of defecation, thus acting as 'major tranquilizers' (Allain and Lechat, 1970). Russell et
al (1987a) first demonstrated that the effect of neuroleptics on emotion-
induced defecation in rats placed in a well-habituated environment is paradoxically increased. We confirmed this finding in a recent study (Sachdev et
al, 1993) in which we also showed that the dysphoric rats were not 'hyperactive' (see Chapter 10, this volume). The neuroleptic-induced defecation
(NDef) response is not due to the action of the drugs on gut DA receptors,
because a peripheral DA antagonist (domperidone), which does not cross the
blood–brain barrier at the usual doses, does not lead to the same response
(Russell et al, 1987a; Sachdev et al, 1993). It is also not a nonspecific effect
of the catalepsy induced by the neuroleptics, because morphine, which also

produced catalepsy, does not produce increased defecation in the home cage (Russell et al, 1987a). This may suggest that the NDef response in the rat is directly a result of central DA receptor antagonism. That this simple explanation was not satisfactory was demonstrated by Sanberg (1989), who reported that apomorphine, a directly acting DA agonist drug, produced a response similar to pimozide, a DA antagonist. Although this study remains to be replicated, it would suggest that the neuroleptic drug interacts with the affective state of the animal to produce a dysphoric response by some as yet poorly understood mechanism. Further studies using this and other models may help clarify the pathomechanism.

Conclusion

In this chapter, we have reviewed the relatively limited literature on the dysphoric response produced by neuroleptic drugs in some individuals. Many possible determinants of this response are recognized, but the pathophysiology is poorly understood and awaits further exploration, including the use of animal models. Meanwhile, the continuing clinical importance of this side-effect makes it necessary to investigate new drugs that are effective antipsychotics without being distressing to the very individuals they are supposed to help, so that the treatment is not worse than the illness it is supposed to treat.

PART II
Drug-induced akathisia

4

The definition of drug-induced akathisia

The greater the ignorance the greater the dogmatism.

Sir William Osler, *Montreal Medical Journal*

(Sept. 1902, p. 696)

While the importance of akathisia as a side-effect of the first-generation neuroleptics and some other drugs is now well recognized, there exists no consensus on its essential characteristics and hence its diagnostic criteria. If we are to discuss its epidemiology and pathophysiology, we must first clearly state, and agree upon, the definition of drug-induced akathisia (DIA). As no generally accepted diagnostic criteria exist, the diagnoses reported in the literature are usually based either on rating scales designed to measure the severity of akathisia (Barnes, 1989; Fleischhacker et al, 1991) or on psychiatrists' clinical opinions. The criteria for TA used by Burke et al (1989) are a rare exception. The problem of variable definitions of akathisia was highlighted by Stahl (1985) and has been reiterated by many subsequent reviewers (Burke and Kang, 1988; Adler et al, 1989b; Lees, 1990; Sachdev and Loneragan, 1991a; Lang, 1992). This chapter discusses the reasons for the difficulties encountered and outlines a proposal for the research diagnostic criteria for DIA published by Sachdev (1994a). A less detailed proposal by Lang (1994) will also be discussed. In this and the following chapters, the term *akathisia* will refer to drug-induced akathisia, and *DIA* or *neuroleptic-induced akathisia* (NIA) will be used only when the actiological importance of drugs, or specifically neuroleptics, must be highlighted.

A number of issues can be identified that have led to the confusion with regard to definition. First, while most investigators have emphasized two components of akathisia – a subjective or psychological or cognitive component and an objective or movement component – there is disagreement about the relative importance of these two aspects (Van Putten, 1975; Kendler,

1976; Barnes and Braude, 1985; Editorial, 1986). In other words, is akathisia a mental disorder or a movement disorder or both? Is the subjective report of akathisia without any observational features enough to make the diagnosis? Is it valid to diagnose akathisia in the absence of a subjective report of distress? No clear answers to these questions are available, and operational criteria have only recently been proposed. Second, no general agreement exists regarding which clinical features are specific to akathisia. Clinical judgment is called on to decide if the patient's movements are manifestations of akathisia, anxious restlessness, dyskinesia or some other abnormality, and whether the distress is akathisia or anxiety, depression, agitation, exacerbation of psychosis or has some other psychiatric cause. Third, a number of subtypes of DIA have been identified (Barnes and Braude, 1985; Sachdev and Loneragan, 1991a), which include AA, CA, TA, WA and pseudoakathisia. In addition, akathisia-like syndromes not related to drugs are well recognized: RLS (Ekbom, 1960), and akathisia of PD or other brain disorders (Lang and Johnson, 1987). Unless investigators clearly state which subtype of akathisia is being studied, communication and comparison of results become difficult. To work towards diagnostic criteria for DIA that would be acceptable to most investigators of this disorder, some resolution of the these issues is paramount.

Principles underlying the construction of a definitional scheme

Before a clear definition emerges and diagnostic criteria can be proposed, some basic principles should be set forth with regard to the essential features of akathisia.

Exposure to drugs as an essential criterion

Diagnostic criteria for DIA should certainly include drug exposure as an essential criterion. This argument may appear circular, since drugs are implicated by definition, but is necessary considering the recent literature examining the 'real' role of drugs in the aetiology of TD (Rogers, 1992). This seems less of a problem with TA since, unlike TD, a spontaneous syndrome resembling TA has not been reported (Burke et al, 1989), although here again idiopathic RLS and other syndromes may confound the diagnoses. The issue of the relationship of neuroleptic drugs and TA will be discussed in Chapter 7. Further, the existence of akathisia-like syndromes like RLS and akathisia secondary to PD or other neurological disorder makes drug exposure an important criterion for definition.

An examination of the literature suggests that a number of drugs which are not neuroleptic can cause acute DIA. The list, without being exhaustive, includes catecholamine-depleting drugs such as reserpine, tetrabenazine and α-methyldopa, buspirone, lithium carbonate, amoxapine, tricyclics when combined with oestrogen therapy, as well as calcium channel antagonists like diltiazem, flunarizine and cinnarizine (see Chapter 5 for a more detailed analysis). All of these drugs share some degree of antidopaminergic activity. Drugs acting on the serotonergic system have also been implicated in the aetiology of akathisia – serotonin-reuptake inhibitors (SRIs; Lipinski et al, 1989) and the serotonin antagonist methysergide (Bernick, 1988) – but whether SRI-induced restlessness is similar to NIA is disputed (Maany and Dhopesh, 1990). (See Chapters 5 and 10 for a more detailed analysis of the relationship between serotonin and akathisia.) At this stage of our knowledge, it is important to recognize when DIA is produced by a non-neuroleptic drug, which should then be stated in the diagnosis. Further empirical work is necessary to test this suggested distinction.

The distinctive features of akathisia

Detailed studies of the clinical features of DIA (Braude et al, 1983; Gibb and Lees, 1986a; Burke et al, 1987) have highlighted the variation in the manifestations of the disorder. From these studies and our own work (Sachdev, 1994c; Sachdev and Kruk, 1994), the following features can be identified that are very suggestive of the presence of akathisia (see Chapter 5 for details):

I. Subjective report
   A. A feeling of restlessness, inner tension or discomfort, with special reference to the lower limbs and/or
   B. A constant urge to move the legs and sometimes other parts of the body such as arms/trunk and/or
   C. Difficulty in maintaining, or inability to maintain, a posture for several minutes, such as sitting in a chair or standing in one place
II. Objective (or observational) features
   A. While sitting
      1. Semipurposful/purposeless leg/foot movements and/or
      2. Semipurposeful/purposeless hand, arm/trunk movements and/or
      3. A tendency to shift body position repeatedly in a chair and/or
      4. An inability to remain seated for several minutes, with a tendency to get up and walk/pace (the original meaning of akathisia)
   B. While standing in one spot
      1. Semipurposeful/purposeless leg/foot and/or arm/hand and/or trunk movements and/or

  2. A tendency to shift weight from foot to foot or march in one spot
     and/or
  3. An inability to stand in one spot, with a tendency to walk or pace
C. While lying
  1. Semipurposeful/purposeless leg/foot movements and/or
  2. Coarse tremor of the legs/feet and/or
  3. Myoclonic jerks of the feet and/or
  4. An inability to remain lying down

This list is by no means exhaustive but highlights the complexity of the dis-order. Furthermore, a number of uncertainties exist with regard to these characteristics.

No one feature is pathognomonic, and many features that are very sugges-tive of the diagnosis are infrequent (Braude et al, 1983). For example, Barnes and Braude (1985) considered rocking from foot to foot while standing or walking on the spot as highly characteristic and very common signs (being present in all their akathisic patients), but Gibb and Lees (1986a) found it to be present only in 26% and Burke et al. (1987) in 40% of cases. Van Putten and Marder (1986) proposed that 'the clinical sign of restless foot movements ought to become a diagnostic criterion for moderate or severe akathisia' (p. 1016). Our own data (Sachdev and Kruk, 1994) show that akathisic subjects scored significantly ($p < .01$) more on all these features than the control group of nonakathisic patients being treated with neuroleptics. On discriminant function analysis, the features that emerged as being the most significant were shifting weight from foot to foot or walking in one spot, inability to keep legs still, feelings of inner restlessness and shifting of body position in a chair, and these were present in 65.6%, 52.6%, 86.2% and 58.1% of akathisic patients, respectively. Though some akathisic patients do manifest these signs and symptoms, the data do not suggest that the features can be assigned a hierar-chy of weightings, and we suggest that each symptom or sign be given the same weight in the diagnostic schema.

The patient must usually be observed in more than one position before a diagnostic decision is reached. Movements may be observed in only one posi-tion in milder cases. Braude et al (1983) suggested examining the patient in the sitting, standing and lying positions. Our data (Sachdev, 1994c) suggest that it is appropriate to examine patients in both the sitting and standing posi-tions, and an examination in the lying position does not necessarily provide any additional information, at least in AA. Further, the movements are not constant and are usually present for only a proportion of the observation period.

Some characteristics of the aforementioned movements help distinguish them from dyskinetic movements, which is important as TD often co-occurs with TA. There is likely to be little confusion between akathisia and the oral–buccal–lingual–facial (OBLF) dyskinesia, but the limb and truncal dyskinesia of TD may be confused with akathisia. Dyskinetic movements are more stereotyped than the akathisic movements, are often asymmetrical, as well as slow and rhythmical, and the patient is unable to control the movements, although they may be modified by voluntary movement or psychological factors. Crane, Naranjo and Chase (1971) note: 'While the movements of patients with akathisia may have an extremely driven quality to them, they are in fact voluntary movements in response to the subjective discomfort'. The akathisic patient is usually able to suppress his or her abnormal movements voluntarily for at least short periods, although this may not be possible in the more severe cases. The akathisic patient reports that his or her movements are the consequence of an irresistible urge to move, with the movement temporarily and at least partially satisfying the urge. Dyskinetic movements are experienced as totally involuntary, without a subjective urge determining their manifestation. As Munetz (1986) puts it, 'One tries to determine whether the patient is restless and therefore moving (akathisia) or moving and therefore restless (dyskinesia)'. (The issue of voluntary vs involuntary status is discussed further in Chapter 6.) The akathisic movements are frequently more complex, may appear purposive (eg, face rubbing, pacing) and demonstrate an intact motor control. In our experience, if the patient can, on request, sit absolutely still for a few minutes, the movements are almost certainly akathisic rather than dyskinetic. In practice, however, the distinction can sometimes be difficult, not only because some patients are uncooperative in their examinations, but also because the subjective distress in some TA patients may be minimal or absent. TD and akathisia may also co-occur, further complicating the differential diagnosis of the movement disorder. The co-occurrence of TD, however, does not necessarily imply that the akathisia is of the tardive subtype, as acute DIA and TD can coexist.

It is at present not certain whether the patterns of movements in AA and TA are different. The published literature and our own experience suggest that the same range of movements is seen in both subtypes, although the movements of TA may be more stereotyped, ie, repeated in precisely the same manner. There is also some suggestion that axial movements may be more common in TA. We propose that for the current diagnostic criteria, any attempt to subtype akathisia on the basis of movement characteristics alone would be premature, and the same criteria should apply to both subtypes.

The symptoms are bilateral but may be asymmetrical. To our knowledge, unilateral DIA has not been reported. A report of unilateral akathisia secondary to a subthalamic abscess has, however, been published (Carrazana et al, 1989). It is possible that in a patient with a neuropathological vulnerability to akathisia, neuroleptic drugs may induce unilateral akathisia, but such a manifestation will merely serve to highlight the underlying pathology and should not be called DIA.

The certainty of diagnosis

DIA is a clinical diagnosis made in the absence of a universally accepted definition and without an external validator in the form of a biochemical or electrophysiological investigation or treatment response. It is therefore appropriate to consider the level of certainty as one variable in the diagnosis. The levels of certainty we propose are: clinically definite, probable or possible. According to our proposal, a *definite* diagnosis of akathisia should be made only if (i) both subjective and objective features are present, (ii) given that the symptoms and signs are mild (rated 1 on the scale), two of each are present, such that the sum of each of the subjective and objective item scores is 2 or more and (iii) the patient has been examined on a least two occasions, separated by a minimum of a few hours and ideally a day. If only one examination has occurred or if only one one subjective and objective feature at the mild level of severity is present (at least one of each is still necessary), a diagnosis of *probable* akathisia should be made. If characteristic subjective or objective features, but not both, are present, a diagnosis of *possible* akathisia should be made.

It must be stated that the proposal to have three levels of certainty is slightly different from our earlier proposal for two levels: definite and probable (Sachdev, 1994a). The current proposal draws on a recent analysis of some of our data. This study, which will be discussed at length in the next two chapters, involved the assessment of 100 patients admitted consecutively to a psychiatric unit and treated with neuroleptic medication for the development of akathisia. All patients were assessed with the Prince Henry Hospital (PHH) Akathisia Scale (three subjective and seven objective items; see Chapter 9 and Appendix B). A clinical diagnosis of akathisia was made in 40 subjects during the first 2 weeks of treatment, using global criteria for diagnosis. A number of other diagnostic criteria were applied to the data, as listed in Table 4.1. We examined the sensitivity and specificity of the diagnostic criteria presented in the table using receiver operating characteristic (ROC) analysis. ROC curves were constructed, using Criteria I and II for the classification into akathisia or nonakathisia on days 7 and 14 of the study. For the first analysis,

Table 4.1. *Akathisia diagnosis using different criteria*

Criterion	Comment
I. Global score ≥ 1	Overall clinical diagnosis
II. Global score ≥ 2	Definitive clinical diagnosis
III. Total score ≥ 4	Relatively strict research diagnosis
IV. Total score ≥ 5	Strict research diagnosis
V. Sum-Sub score ≥ 2 *and* Sum-Obj score ≥ 2	Definitive research diagnosis
VI. Sum-Sub score ≥ 1 *and* Sum-Obj score ≥ 1	Loose criteria; could lead to overdiagnosis
VII. Total score ≥ 2	Very loose criteria; almost certainly leads to overdiagnosis

Note: Global score is from the Prince Henry Akathisia Scale (see Appendix B). Sum-Sub is the sum of the 3 subjective items on the 10-item scale. Sum-Obj is the sum of the 7 objective items. Total is the sum of Sum-Sub and Sum-Obj.
Source: Sachdev and Kruk (1994).

the different scores on the sum of the items of the 10-item scale (Sum scores) were plotted as the individual points. These curves are presented in Fig. 4.1, and suggest that a cut-off score of 4 or 5 yielded the highest specificity and sensitivity for the diagnosis of akathisia. ROC curves were also constructed for the different criteria presented in Table 4.1, again using Criteria I and II for the classification into akathisia or nonakathisia, and these curves are presented in Fig. 4.2. Criteria III and IV yielded similar probabilities of true- or false-positive diagnoses, affirming the preceding classification. The less restrictive Criterion II was therefore considered the most appropriate criterion for diagnosis. If Criterion V, a special condition of Criterion III in which a minimum score of 2 on the sum of both the subjective and objective items was necessary, was applied, the specificity improved but at the cost of sensitivity.

On the basis of these findings, we considered the presence of at least two features at the moderate intensity level, and four at the mild level, for the diagnosis. Since both subjective and objective features were considered necessary, the cut-off score of 4 translated into 2 or more for the sums of subjective and objective item scores (Criterion V) to yield the greater specificity. The scale used for this analysis (see Appendix B for description) makes a categorical shift between the ratings of 0 and 1, with 1 denoting a definite presence of the symptom/sign, and 1, 2 or 3 then rating its severity. The suggested criteria of a total sum score of 4, or of 2 or more on each of the subjective and objective sum scores, may seem too strict. The data, however, reflect the real-

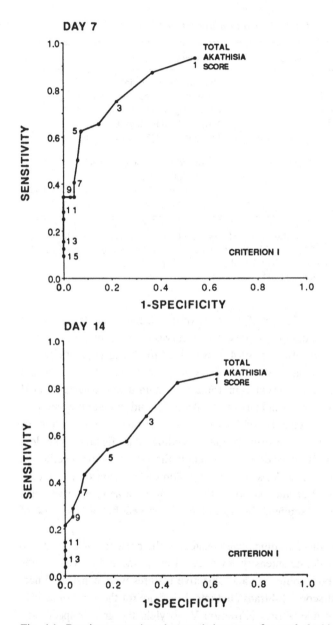

Fig. 4.1. Receiver operating characteristic curves for total akathisia scale scores on days 7 and 14. Subjects were grouped as akathisic/nonakathisic using Criterion I or II as indicated in Table 4.1. Data are drawn from the AA study (Sachdev and Kruk, 1994).

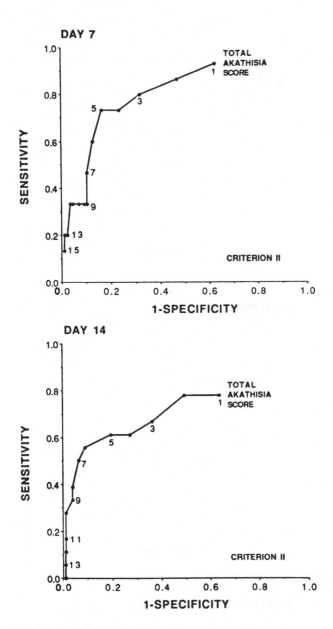

Fig. 4.1. (cont.)

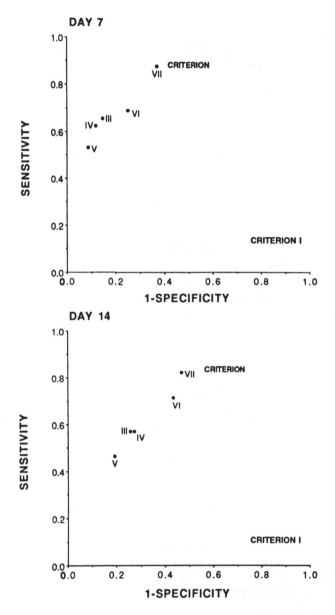

Fig. 4.2. The sensitivity and specificity of Criteria III to VII when applied to akathisia diagnosed by Criteria I and II on days 7 and 14. A description of the criteria is given in Table 4.1. Data were drawn from the AA study (Sachdev and Kruk, 1994).

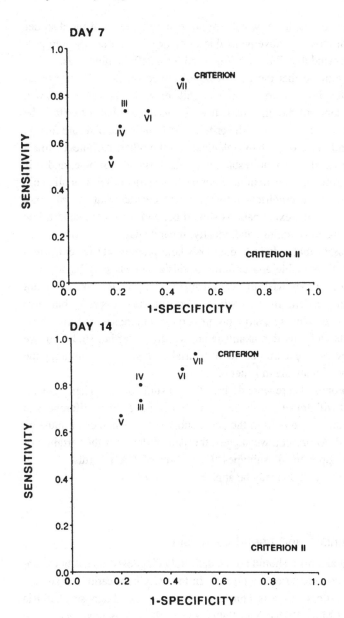

Fig. 4.2. (*cont.*)

ity of the features of akathisia, which are not pathognomonic of the disorder and overlap with those of movements due to other causes. For research purposes, we recommend that Criterion V be used for a definite diagnosis.

We also recommend that the patient be examined on two separate occasions, at least a few hours apart, before a definite diagnosis be made. This will increase the certainty of the diagnosis. It is not necessary that the criteria be equally strict on both occasions. If the criteria for definite akathisia are met on one occasion, and those of probable akathisia on the other, definite akathisia can still be diagnosed. The manifestations of akathisia are variable, and it is possible, even likely, that a patient may not meet the strict criteria on all occasions. We do not have empirical information to decide what the minimal interval between the two examinations should be, and we recommend a few hours (eg, morning and evening) and, ideally, separate days.

It is not necessary that a definite diagnosis be a prerequisite for entry into drug trials, as both probable and definite akathisia patients may be suitable. Similarly, a clinician may wish to treat a patient with probable akathisia, not only because the patient may experience considerable distress, but also because it may be possible to avert a progression to a more severe form of the disorder. Patients with possible akathisia are worthy of further study, but we recommend they not be admitted to drug trials, or studies examining the pathophysiology of akathisia in general.

The criteria proposed here were derived from a study of AA. Their applicability to TA and withdrawal akathisia (WA), which have some differences in their clinical manifestations from the acute subtype (see Chapter 7), must be further examined. At present, we suggest the same criteria for the certainty of the disorder to apply to all subtypes. Our study of CA/TA (discussed in Chapter 7) suggests that this may be appropriate (see Fig. 4.3).

Possible akathisia and pseudoakathisia

We propose that akathisia should not be definitely diagnosed unless both subjective and objective features are present. In the early publications, a subjective report of restlessness was considered sufficient to diagnose akathisia (Van Putten and May, 1978a; Van Putten et al, 1981). It is now recognized that this is too nonspecific a feature, and restlessness, as we have considered in Chapter 2, can occur for various reasons. However, clinical experience does attest to the fact that subjective akathisia in the absence of any observable features does exist, and can be clearly attributed to medication (Van

Putten and Marder, 1986). In fact, milder akathisia may manifest mainly in the subjective experience. In our study of 100 patients recently started on neuroleptic medication (AA study), 4 patients had subjective akathisia on day 7 in the absence of objective manifestations. Three of these were diagnosed to have akathisia in the second week of the study, and 2 responded to benztropine. We therefore recommend a category of possible akathisia (subjective) which acknowledges this aspect of akathisia.

The presence of the characteristic movement disorder of akathisia can occur without the subjective distress, especially in patients with TA. In AA, this is probably uncommon. In our AA study, 1 patient, on a large dose of haloperidol, had a high objective score without any reported distress. The patient was, however, acutely psychotic, hostile and uncooperative, and as his psychotic symptoms improved, his subjective distress came to the fore. In our study of 100 schizophrenic patients on long-term medication (TA/CA study), 9 patients were categorized as having objective akathisia only. Barnes and Braude (1985), in their investigation of 82 schizophrenic patients attending 'depot neuroleptic' clinics, found 10 patients with objective akathisia but not the subjective component. They called this phenomenon 'pseudoakathisia', which we propose should be referred to as 'possible akathisia (objective)'.

The term *pseudoakathisia* has had a short and problematic history. The term was introduced by Munetz and Cornes (1982) to refer to lower extremity TD, or a forme fruste of TD, that was mistaken for akathisia. The implication was that it was not akathisia, but mimicked it. Barnes and Braude (1985) applied a different meaning when they suggested it for the objective manifestations of akathisia without the subjective component. For them 'pseudoakathisia' was in fact true akathisia, but with limited manifestations. Stahl (1985) suggested that this use was inappropriate and wondered if this should not be described as a variant of TD. Furthermore, Haskovec (1902) originally suggested that the inability to sit sometimes occurred as a conversion symptom in neurotic disorders, and pseudoakathisia would perhaps be the appropriate appellation for such a presentation, although it must be exceedingly rare. We therefore are of the opinion that pseudoakathisia is an ambiguous term which should be dropped before it becomes too widely used. A parallel can be drawn with the use of the term *pseudodementia* (Kiloh, 1961; Sachdev et al, 1990; Emery and Oxman, 1992; Sachdev and Kiloh, 1994), which after three decades is now in decline as our understanding of dementia and cognitive processes has increased and it is has become generally accepted that the dementia of pseudodementia, even when due to depression, is in fact real dementia.

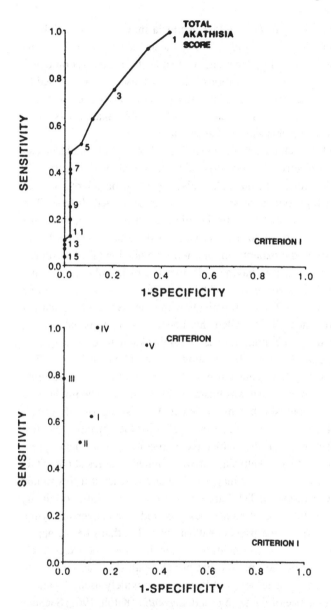

Fig. 4.3. Receiver operating characteristic curves for total akathisia scale scores and
Criteria I to V for the tardive akathisia subjects. Subjects were grouped as aka-
thisic/nonakathisic using Criterion I or II. Data were drawn from the TA/CA study
(see Chapter 5).

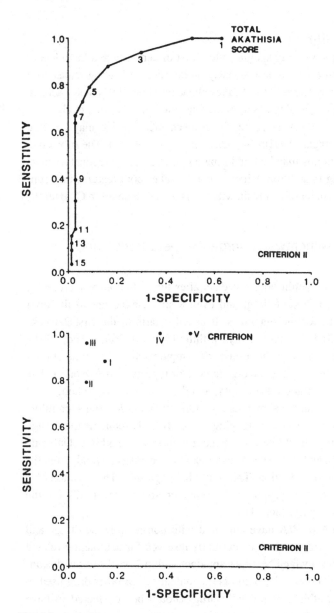

Fig. 4.3. (*cont.*)

Criteria for severity

A decision regarding severity should follow that of certainty and be independent of it. It is appropriate to base severity on the scores of rating scales such as those developed by Barnes (1989), Fleischhacker et al (1991), and Sachdev (1994c). Alternatively, analogue scales may be constructed (Adler et al, 1985; Sachdev and Chee, 1990), or some electromechanical device may be used (Sachdev and Loneragan, 1991a) (see Chapter 9, this volume). The subjective and objective symptoms may be rated separately, but most investigators have used a global rating in addition, which generally takes both features into consideration. Measurement of akathisia will be discussed in detail in Chapter 9.

Tardive onset; withdrawal emergence, persistence and chronicity

Acute DIA can start within hours or days after the initiation or increase in dosage or change in type of drug, and even a single exposure to the drug should be sufficient for the diagnosis. It usually starts in the first 2 weeks (Braude et al, 1983) and almost always within the first 6 weeks (Ayd, 1961). It would be appropriate to consider onset of symptoms after 3 months of continuous use of the drug without change in dose or type as a *tardive* onset. The choice of 3 months' duration is arbitrary, and draws on the TD (Schooler and Kane, 1982), rather than the akathisia, literature, the latter lacking such information. Onset within 6 weeks of stopping or significantly reducing the dosage of a neuroleptic drug should be considered a withdrawal akathisia (Dufresne and Wagner, 1988), and if the diagnosis of akathisia persists beyond 3 months after drug cessation or reduction, TA should be diagnosed. The duration of 3 months is similar to that proposed by Schooler and Kane (1982) for the research diagnosis of persistent TD.

No reports of TA or WA have appeared with non-neuroleptic drugs, and these diagnoses should therefore be currently reserved for neuroleptic-related side-effects. Akathisia which becomes apparent within 2 weeks of the discontinuation of an anticholinergic, β-adrenergic antagonist or other drug used in the treatment of akathisia (therapeutic drug) should be considered to have been unmasked, and classified according to its chronological relationship to the aetiological agent. This presumes that the akathisia would have manifested if the therapeutic drug had not been administered.

It is important to operationalize the use of the term *chronic* in the context of akathisia. We suggest that akathisia which continues for 3 months or longer be referred to as chronic. Chronic akathisia (CA) may, therefore, have an acute, delayed or withdrawal onset, and at present there are no empirical data to decide whether this makes any difference to its clinical manifestations.

Response to treatment

Response to a pharmacological challenge using a double-blind technique has been employed by at least one group (Van Putten and May, 1978a; Van Putten et al, 1984b) to diagnose akathisia. An ACh antagonist drug has been generally used, in particular biperidin or benztropine. Recent literature (see review in Chapter 11) suggests that such a strategy is prone to error. First, akathisia does not always respond to any one drug, and ACh antagonists are successful in treating only some patients with akathisia. Second, the response may not be the same in all subtypes of akathisia. For example, ACh may in fact worsen some patients with TA. Third, the pharmacological strategy of diagnosis leads to circular reasoning when drug treatment of akathisia is being investigated. Fourth, such a strategy is invasive and would be of limited value in clinical practice even if its validity were established. We therefore do not support this method of diagnosing akathisia. A parallel may be drawn with affective disorders. The practice of 'diagnosing' depression by response to an antidepressant drug was abandoned when it became clear that many depressives were 'resistant', and antidepressants were effective in disorders not construed as depression or equivalents.

The 'objective test' of Maltbie and Cavenar

Maltbie and Cavenar (1977) state that 'the accentuation, or recruitment, of cogwheel rigidity by the voluntary performance of alternating movements in the wrist or elbow is a useful sign in confirming the diagnosis of akathisia' (p. 37). The co-occurrence of extrapyramidal rigidity with akathisia in many patients has been reported by a number of authors (Braude et al, 1983; Van Putten et al, 1984b), but akathisia can occur in the presence of normal muscle tone, even when recruitment is used during clinical testing. Current thinking is that this represents a co-occurrence which may or may not reflect a common vulnerability, and to use the presence of rigidity as a diagnostic criterion of akathisia would be grossly in error.

Akathisia unrelated to drugs

Significant differences exist between DIA and RLS to consider them as separate disorders, even though they share some characteristics (see Chapter 12).

The akathisia seen in PD or secondary to other brain disorders, although diagnosed using the same subjective and objective criteria as DIA (Lang and Johnson, 1987), should again be classified separately (see Chapter 8). Such a classification can be supported as being aetiological, and will permit a separate examination of the pathophysiology of DIA and other akathisias. The clinical features of these other akathisias also need to be examined.

Research diagnostic criteria for DIA

Prerequisites

Based on the preceding arguments, the following three prerequisites are proposed for all diagnoses of DIA (Sachdev, 1994a):

1. A history of exposure to drugs known to cause akathisia (neuroleptic drugs can cause all subtypes; non-neuroleptic drugs can cause acute DIA and chronic DIA with acute onset)
2. Presence of characteristic subjective (Sub) and/or objective (Obj) features of DIA

   Definite: ≥2 Sum-Sub *and* ≥2 Sum-Obj features and on two occasions separated by at least a few hours

   Probable: (i) ≥2 Sum-Sub *and* ≥2 Sum-Obj features on first occasion
   (ii) 1 Sum-Sub *and* 1 Sum-Obj

   Possible: ≥2 Sum-Sub *or* ≥2 Sum-Obj features (state whether Sub or Obj)
3. Absence of other known causes of akathisia, eg, RLS, PD or subthalamic lesion, and absence of peripheral neuropathy, myelopathy or myopathy

Diagnoses

The various diagnoses to be considered, all of which should meet the preceding prerequisites, are as follows (Sachdev, 1994a):

Acute DIA

(i) The symptoms began within 6 weeks of initiation or increase in dosage, or change in type of drug; (ii) a concurrently administered therapeutic drug (see earlier) was not decreased or discontinued in the 2 weeks before onset of symptoms.

Drugs responsible may be neuroleptic or non-neuroleptic. If the symptoms continue for longer than 3 months, chronic DIA, acute onset (see later) should be diagnosed.

Tardive DIA

(i) The symptoms began at least 3 months after initiation of *neuroleptic* drug; (ii) there was no increase in dose or change in type of drug in the 6 weeks prior to onset of symptoms; (iii) a concurrently administered therapeutic drug (see earlier) was not decreased or discontinued in the 2 weeks before onset of symptoms.

Diagnose as chronic if over 3 months.

Withdrawal DIA

(i) The symptoms began within 6 weeks of discontinuing or significantly reducing the dose of a *neuroleptic* drug; (ii) the patient had received neuroleptic medication for a minimum of 3 months; (iii) a concurrently administered therapeutic drug (see earlier) was not decreased or discontinued in the 2-weeks before onset of symptoms.

If symptoms continue beyond 3 months after the last change in neuroleptic medication, a diagnosis of chronic DIA should be made.

Chronic DIA

If the symptoms of DIA persist for over 3 months, chronic DIA should be diagnosed, and an acute or tardive onset specified if possible. If the patient has not received neuroleptic drugs for the last 6 weeks, 'not currently on neuroleptics' should also be specified.

The diagnosis of chronic DIA is not strictly a separate category from the others, but we list it here as such because (i) sometimes the onset of akathisia cannot be established with certainty while its duration can, (ii) many published studies of akathisia have included patients with CA but without further specification, and (iii) it remains to be empirically established whether the subcategorization of chronic DIA has any treatment or prognostic implications.

Proposals for testing the definitional schema

We have three main goals in proposing the preceding criteria: first to bring conceptual clarity and consistency to the definitions, thereby facilitating communication between research groups and across studies; second, to stimulate research in order to establish empirically derived criteria for diagnosis and severity; third, to facilitate investigation into the aetiopathogenesis of akathisia, drug-induced or other, so that prevention or treatment based on the understanding of pathophysiology may result.

The published literature and the extant but unpublished data on DIA should be examined using the recommended definitions. New studies should be designed that use clearly delineated diagnostic criteria, incorporating the ones proposed here, so that the clinical features, longitudinal course and treatment outcome may be studied. One example would be a study set up to compare and contrast the clinical features of acute and tardive DIA. The pharmacological characteristics of the two syndromes may similarly be contrasted using drug challenges or functional imaging. Similar studies examining non-neuroleptic DIA or withdrawal DIA may test their proposed criteria.

There are some aspects of akathisia that could help validate the subtyping. For example, AA is recognized to be dose-related and to subside spontaneously when the offending drug is no longer administered (Braude et al, 1983). The relationship of akathisia with the drug over time will, therefore, be an important aspect of diagnostic validation, which can also be examined longitudinally. The validity of the diagnosis of WA can be investigated empirically if a baseline examination and follow-up are incorporated in the design of the study. The usefulness of delineating chronic DIA separately, even though it overlaps with the other categories, can be examined by determining the heterogeneity in the longitudinal course of and treatment response in such cases. Similar examples can be multiplied.

If other versions of the diagnostic criteria are arrived at by varying one or more of the preceding specifications, their predictive power when applied to a particular set of data can be used to determine their relative value. Statistical techniques, such as the receiver operator characteristics method (Hsiao et al, 1989), are available for this purpose.

Comment

In this chapter, we have provided arguments and proposed tentative operational criteria for the research diagnoses of DIA. We invite challenges to these

Table 4.2. *Diagnostic criteria for tardive akathisia employed by Burke et al (1989)*

1. Onset during or within 3 months of a DA antagonist drug
2. Persistent, ie, more than 1 month in duration
3. A subjective report indicating an aversion to remaining still
4. Increased, abnormal frequency of spontaneous movements that are frequently complex and stereotyped, and give an appearance of restlessness

Table 4.3. *Classification of chronic akathisia proposed by Lang (1994)*

Subtype	Features		Onset	Duration	Comment
	Sub	Obj			
1. Acute	+	+	Increased dosage/potency, antiparkin-sonian drug withdrawal	≤6 months	Late onset may occur
2. Acute persistent	+	+	Increased dosage/potency	>7 months	Remits with neuroleptic withdrawal
3. Probable tardive	+	+	Not as in items 1 and 2	Observed on one occasion	Note if neuroleptics are currently present or absent
4. Masked, probable tardive	+	+	Same as item 3	Masked by neuroleptics within 2 weeks	—
5. Transient tardive	+	+	On neuroleptics	<3 months	Includes 'covert akathisia' at end of depot injection period
6. Withdrawal tardive	+	+	Neuroleptic withdrawal (within 2–5 weeks)	<3 months	If >3 months, persistent TA
7. Persistent tardive	+	+	Same as item 3	>3 months	Qualified as concurrent neuroleptic, neuroleptic free or unspecified
8. Masked, persistent tardive	+	+	Offset in 3 weeks of change in neuroleptic drug	>3 months	—
9. Pseudo-akathisia	−	+	—	—	Controversial

Note: Based on the Schooler and Kane (1982) classification of TD. Sub = subjective; Obj = objective.

criteria, both from a conceptual viewpoint and based on empirical examination, so that tested and valid definitions may emerge. The proposed criteria are intended for research application and may not be suitable for many clinical situations. Furthermore, their suitability for akathisia not related to drugs is unknown.

While critically examining these criteria, investigators would be expected to make decisions regarding inclusion criteria and definitions so that their studies may proceed. We recommend that these investigations include enough data for these, and perhaps other, criteria to be applied, post hoc if necessary. Investigators should be cognizant of the possible subtypes of DIA even if these do not form the basis of the investigation. The existence of subtypes should be considered in any calculation of sample size so that data collected in these studies can be used to examine the definitional schema. It is hoped that such efforts will lead to a clearer understanding of akathisia.

Proposals for the diagnosis and classification of TA have been presented by other authors. The definition of TA used by Burke et al (1989) and the proposal by Lang (1994) are presented in Tables 4.2 and 4.3, respectively.

5

Epidemiology

Introduction

With a few exceptions, epidemiological studies of akathisia have been limited for the following reasons.

While extrapyramidal side-effects of drugs have attracted attention ever since neuroleptic drugs were introduced (Delay and Deniker, 1952; Steck, 1954), in most early investigations akathisia was lumped together with other extrapyramidal reactions. Some early authors (eg, Freyhan, 1958; Ayd, 1961) did attempt to describe akathisia separately, but it was not until the mid-1970s that akathisia received serious attention in its own right and the 1980s that incidence and prevalence estimates became available from well-conducted studies. As stated in Chapter 1, this neglect has been difficult to understand. It is possible that EPSE and TD, by virtue of their more definite clinical features, received most of the attention at the expense of akathisia. Moreover, akathisia was a paradoxical response that was inconsistent with the notion that neuroleptics produced tranquillization, resulting in some resistance to its acceptance. Especially in the United States, akathisia was until recently (Van Putten and Marder, 1986) conceptualized as a subjective response, and since AA occurs in acutely psychotic individuals, it is likely that the subjective report would be misattributed to agitation or anxiety or, even worse, ignored. On the other hand, TA is generally overshadowed by TD, or subsumed by it, especially as the two often co-occur.

Until recently, no definite diagnostic criteria for akathisia had been proposed. In many studies, a clinical diagnosis was made but the process of diagnosing was not specified (eg, Ayd, 1961; Hunter et al, 1964; Kennedy et al, 1971). Even when rating scales were used, it was often not specified whether both subjective and objective features were considered necessary for the diagnosis (eg, Levinson et al, 1990; Rifkin et al, 1991). The reliability and validity of many of the scales have not been adequately examined (see Chapter 9 for a review of the measuring instruments). One group of investigators (Van Putten et al, 1974; Van Putten, 1978) used a positive response to parenteral biperiden as the diagnostic criterion for akathisia, with interesting results. It is only relatively recently that operational diagnostic criteria have been proposed (Burke et al, 1987; Lang, 1994; Sachdev, 1994a), and it is hoped that future epidemiological studies will give due regard to these criteria in arriving at the incidence and prevalence estimates.

The majority of the published epidemiological studies do not take into consideration the various subtypes of akathisia. DIA can be subdivided, depending on the relationship between recent drug history and the onset of akathisia, into AA, TA and WA. There is the additional dimension of chronicity. The epidemiological, clinical and treatment characteristics of the different subtypes need to be examined separately, something lacking in most published studies. In some studies, where a challenge with a neuroleptic drug was part of the study design, the acuteness of the akathisia is beyond doubt. Others are more ambiguous on this point. Even when acute psychiatric inpatient admissions are the point of entry into the study, as in the Braude et al (1983) investigation, it is possible that the patient was being treated with neuroleptics, often over the long term, before the admission, and the akathisia observed was not acute. Our recent AA study attempted to redress this problem in the literature on acute akathisia. The problem with TA is even greater, since no study has been prospective and longitudinal. To establish the point of akathisia onset on retrospective enquiry, as would be necessary in a cross-sectional study of TA, is prone to serious error. The Gibb and Lees (1986a), Barnes and Braude (1985) and our own TA/CA study suffer from this limitation. Only one study has examined the incidence of WA (Dufresne and Wagner, 1988), but this was limited by the fact that subjects were not examined for akathisia at baseline prior to the withdrawal of the antipsychotic medication.

A distinction has not always been made between the incidence and prevalence of akathisia. *Incidence* is the number of new cases that appear during a specified period in a given population, whereas *prevalence* is the number of all cases (new and old) of the disease that currently exist in the population. Prevalence can be expressed as point, period or lifetime prevalence. In the investigation of akathisia, the difficulty in comparing and contrasting incidence and prevalence rates stems from the fact that the natural history of akathisia is poorly understood. It is not certain at what point AA becomes chronic, and whether this is different for CA of tardive or withdrawal onset. Barnes and Braude (1985) attempted to distinguish AA that tended to persist, and yet retained its pharmacological characteristics, from TA, and called it 'acute persistent akathisia'. While this may be a reasonable distinction to make in a longitudinal study, its validity in retrospective analyses is questionable because of the difficulty in establishing that akathisia had been continuously present since its acute onset. The published literature presents a mix of incidence and prevalence data.

The preceding limitations notwithstanding, the following types of studies that deal with the epidemiology of akathisia can be identified.

Studies in which akathisia was the primary focus of an epidemiological investigation. Examples of this are studies by Braude et al (1983), Van Putten (1975), Van Putten et al (1984b,c) and Sachdev and Kruk (1994, AA study) for AA, and by Gibb and Lees (1986), Barnes and Braude (1985) and the author (TA/CA study, unpublished) for TA or CA. The ideal design of a study to examine the incidence of akathisia is a prospective longitudinal study of patients treated with a particular neuroleptic, and controls not treated with any neuroleptic. Since neuroleptics are used to treat serious mental illness, an untreated psychiatric control group is usually not possible. Further, since akathisia is by definition a drug-induced state, a control group may indeed not be necessary provided a baseline examination has excluded subjects with akathisia-like syndromes. Because neuroleptic dosage and its increment rate are potentially important for the development of akathisia, only those studies are clinically relevant that use clinical dosages and the usual routes of administration. Single-dose challenge studies (eg, Magliozzi et al, 1985) may serve the important function of identifying risk factors for akathisia, but the incidence rates obtained from such studies have limited clinical relevance. A prospective design is essential if predisposing factors to akathisia have to be studied. Retrospective studies, such as reviewing patient charts or interviewing patients for past history of akathisia, are likely to be poor epidemiological methods for this disorder because it is often underrecognized clinically, and patients find it difficult to distinguish akathisia from restlessness due to other causes.

Studies that focused on side-effects of drugs, with akathisia being one of a number of side-effects so studied. The classic paper by Ayd (1961) is an example of such a study. The advantage of this kind of investigation is that it can place any one side-effect in the proper perspective. However, the lack of focus leads to a compromise on diagnostic rigour, and predisposing factors can often not be adequately assessed.

Studies whose primary aim was to investigate the clinical aspects of some drug, and akathisia was not altogether an incidental observation. Examples are studies designed to compare different dosages of neuroleptics (eg, Levinson et al, 1990; Van Putten et al, 1990; Rifkin et al, 1991) or to study the clinical profile of a new drug in comparison with an earlier established one (eg, Claghorn et al, 1987, and Cohen et al, 1991, for clozapine) or of a non-neuroleptic drug not generally known to produce akathisia (eg, Goff et al, 1991, for buspirone).

In this chapter, we will examine some of the epidemiological studies of akathisia, while acknowledging their limitations. Even though the studies do not always clearly identify the subtype of akathisia, this will be inferred from the data wherever possible.

Incidence and prevalence of acute akathisia

One of the earliest reports was by Freyhan (1957), who examined for EPSE all patients treated either with chlorpromazine or reserpine in his hospital over a 2-year period. While he did not use the term *akathisia,* he described patients who 'complained of inner restlessness and have at times an irresistible urge to be in motion . . . reminiscent of the hyperkinetic behaviour of encephalitic patients'. This reaction was seen in 6–8% of the reserpine-treated patients but none of the chlorpromazine-treated patients. In another study, Freyhan (1959) made explicit the term *akathisia* and said that, in his opinion, 'the various references to "paradoxical reactions" or "turbulent phases" are descriptions of the syndrome of akathisia' (p. 582). He reported slightly different prevalence rates for akathisia for different phenothiazines: trifluopromazine ($n = 25$) 12%; prochlorperazine ($n = 68$) 19.1%; trifluoperazine ($n = 65$) 12.3%; perphenazine ($n = 22$) 9.1%. However, equivalent doses were not necessarily used.

The largest survey of drug-induced EPSE was that of Frank Ayd Jr (1961), which covered 3,775 subjects (1,833 men and 1,942 women) between the ages 4 and 88 years who had been treated with one of seven phenothiazines for periods ranging from 3 months to 6 years. Akathisia, described as 'motor restlessness', was diagnosed clinically in 21.2% (cf parkinsonism in 15.4% and dyskinesia – largely acute dystonia – in 2.3%) of subjects. No rating scale was used. Akathisia was more common in women (M/F 1:2) and occurred more frequently in the age range 12 to 65 years. The onset was early, slightly before the development of EPSE, with 90% of the cases developing it in the first 72 days after initiation of drugs. The onset was earlier and at smaller dosages as the potency of the offending drug increased. The author could not explain much of the variation on demographic or drug-related variables, and individual susceptibility was considered most important.

Van Putten and his colleagues from the University of California at Los Angeles have reported a number of studies of akathisia. An earlier study (Van Putten et al, 1974) examined 80 consecutive admissions to an inpatient unit in order to study phenothiazine-induced exacerbations of psychosis. Nine (11%) patients had sudden decompensations, and all of them had akathisia, sometimes subtle and evanescent, which could be reversed by an intramuscular injection of biperiden. Twenty-three other patients had EPSE (akathisia, parkinsonism or dystonia). All 9 patients being treated with fluphenazine enanthate had akathisia. In another study by the same author (Van Putten, 1975), 110 inpatients on neuroleptics were examined. The subtype of akathisia was not specified but was presumably largely acute. Diagnosis of akathisia was based on a subjective experience of restlessness and confirmed by a double-blind response to im biperiden 5 mg. Akathisia was diagnosed in 49 (45%) patients, with the manifestations being highly variable. The majority (59%) of akathisic patients also had other EPSE. The study by Van Putten et al (1984b) is of interest because of the rigour in the methodology. Subjects were challenged with either 5 mg haloperidol (*n* = 44) or 0.22 mg/kg thiothixene (*n* = 67) and examined over the succeeding 6 hours for the development of akathisia. The haloperidol group was then maintained on 10 mg/day and the thiothixene group on 0.44 mg/kg per day and followed up over the succeeding 4 weeks. In the haloperidol group, 17 (40%) patients developed akathisia after the challenge (5 mild, 5 moderate, 3 severe, 4 very severe) and 31 (76%) by the seventh day of maintenance therapy. In the thiothixene group, 13 (20%) patients developed AA, but if the 7 who received an ACh antagonist drug for dystonia are excluded from analysis, the figure becomes 28%. Over the succeeding 4 weeks, the cumulative percentage with akathisia rose to 63%.

A few published studies have examined the development of akathisia in response to neuroleptic administration in nonpsychiatric populations. Murray et al (1977) performed a double-blind cross-over study of haloperidol in the treatment of stuttering and found that 8 out of 26 patients had poor concentration, akathisia or dystonia. Magliozzi et al (1985) administered iv or oral haloperidol to normal subjects. In the iv group 8 of 12, and in the oral group 3 of 9, subjects developed akathisia. No other risk factors were identified.

A number of studies whose primary focus was the comparison of different dosages of neuroleptic drugs have also reported on rates on akathisia. Only a few such studies will be mentioned here, selected on the basis of a clear statement on akathisia. McClelland et al (1976) conducted a double-blind 6-month trial to compare very high dosages (250 mg/week) with standard dosages (12.5 mg/week) of fluphenazine decanoate in 50 patients in the 18- to 60-year age range. By the 24th week, 22% in the high- and 9% in the standard-dosage groups had developed akathisia. No specific akathisia rating scale was used. The side-effect was mild, however, and only 1 patient in the high-dosage group needed treatment for akathisia. Van Putten et al (1990) compared 3 dosages of haloperidol (5, 10 or 20 mg/day) over 4 weeks in acute or relapsing schizophrenia and measured akathisia on a 7-point scale (May et al, personal communication). Although the incidence of akathisia was not stated, there was a significant difference between the 5- and 20-mg/day groups, with the latter tending to have more akathisia overall. Levinson et al (1990) conducted a randomized, fixed-dosage, double-blind trial of oral fluphenazine and used a modified version of the Simpson and Angus (1970) scale to include a rating for akathisia. Of the 51 patients who did not receive any antiparkinsonian drugs, 22 (43%) developed akathisia, typically after 2–3 weeks of treatment. The psychosis of those patients who developed akathisia tended to worsen. Rifkin et al (1991) conducted a randomized trial to compare 3 dosages of haloperidol ($n = 29$ in each group), again using the modified Simpson and Angus (1970) scale. Akathisia showed a nonsignificant trend towards worsening over time in the 10- and 80-mg/day groups, but the three dosages (10, 30 and 80 mg/day) did not affect the overall relative risks for akathisia. Any akathisia present was mild.

An important naturalistic study that examined the epidemiology and clinical features of AA was that by Braude and colleagues (1983). The authors systematically examined, at baseline and at least weekly intervals, 104 (30 men, 74 women) patients who were consecutively admitted to a psychiatric ward and who required antipsychotic medication. The detailed symptoms of akathisia were rated, and a diagnosis of akathisia was made in 25% of cases. The main deficiencies of this study were: (i) Many patients were not drug-free at the time of admission (the authors do not provide figures on this). However, only 1 patient was assessed to be 'restless' at admission and was excluded from the final figures. (ii) Antiparkinsonian medication was not controlled, and the authors do not state how many patients received ACh or β-adrenergic (βA) antagonists. This would certainly affect the incidence figures. (iii) Subjects were not screened for RLS, peripheral neuropathy or vascular disease, that may produce symptoms like akathisia. The results of these and other relevant studies are presented in Table 5.1.

AA study

The study of the incidence of AA that we recently performed (AA study; Sachdev and Kruk, 1994) will be described in some detail. The sample

Table 5.1. *Epidemiological studies of acute NIA*

Authors	Population	Drug(s) and route	N	Definition of akathisia	Incidence/ prevalence	Percent	Comment
Primary investigations of akathisia							
Van Putten (1975)	Psychiatric inpatients	Multiple/oral	110	Subjective and response to biperiden iv	? Incidence	45	Subtype not specified; largely AA
Jungman and Schoffling (1982)	Healthy subjects	Metoclopramide/ iv bolus	—	Subjective	Incidence	25	Single-dose (10 mg) study
Braude et al (1983)	Psychiatric inpatients	Multiple/oral	104	Subjective and objective	? Incidence	25	Systematic naturalistic study
Magliozzi et al (1985)	Healthy subjects	Haloperidol/ iv and oral	12 (iv) 9 (oral)	Not specified	Incidence	67 33	—
Van Putten, May and Marder (1984)	Healthy subjects	Haloperidol and thiothixene/iv and oral phases	44 67	Subjective	Incidence	76 63	In two phases; an initial iv challenge and then used for 4 weeks
Cohen et al (1991)	Psychiatric patients	Clozapine and standard neuroleptics	23 29	Subjective and objective	? Incidence	39 45	Baseline ratings inadequate
Safferman et al (1993)	Resistant schizophrenics	Clozapine	49	Subjective and objective	Incidence	Nil	Patients previously treated with neuroleptics and had no akathisia at baseline
Sachdev and Kruk (1994)	Psychiatric inpatients	Classical neuroleptics	100	Subjective and objective (various criteria)	Incidence	31	—[a]
Studies of neuroleptic-induced side-effects that included akathisia							
McClelland et al (1976)	Psychiatric patients	Fluphenazine decanoate: 250 mg per week vs 12.5 mg per week/im	50	Clinical diagnosis	? Incidence	22 9.7	Akathisia mild: only one patient needed treatment

Table 5.1. (cont.)

Authors	Population	Drug(s) and route	N	Definition of akathisia	Incidence/ prevalence	Percent	Comment
Murray et al (1977)	Stutterers	Haloperidol/oral	26	Clinical	? Incidence	<8	Poor concentration, akathisia and dystonia (included)
McCreadie et al (1988)	Psychiatric patients	Thioridazine vs remoxipride/oral	—	Not stated	Incidence	8 4	More seen with remoxipride
Anderson et al (1990)	Psychiatric patients	Haloperidol vs remoxipride/oral	32 39	Not stated	Incidence	68 32	—
Levinson et al (1990)	Psychiatric patients	Fluphenazine/oral	51	Rating scale	? Incidence	43	Typically after 2–3 weeks of treatment
Lindstrom et al (1990)	Psychiatric patients	Haloperidol vs remoxipride/oral	48 48	Not stated	Incidence	57 32	—
Van Putten et al (1990)	Schizophrenic patients	Haloperidol, 5 vs 10 vs 20 mg/ oral	22 + 38 + 20	Rating scale	Incidence	—	More with 20 mg
Rifkin et al (1991)	Psychiatric patients	Haloperidol, 10 vs 30 vs 80 mg	29 each group	Rating scale	Relative severity	—	Usually mild; no difference between groups
Selected studies of therapeutic drug effects, akathisia also assessed							
Freyhan (1959)	Psychiatric patients	Trifluoperazine Prochlorperazine Trifluopromazine Perphenazine/oral	65 68 25 22	Clinical diagnosis	Prevalence	12.3 19.1 12 9.1	Open study; paradoxical reactions considered to be akathisia; doses of drugs not equivalent
Ayd (1961)	Psychiatric patients	7 phenothiazines/ oral	3,775	Clinical diagnosis	Prevalence	21.2	Largest open study
Van Putten et al (1974)	Psychiatric inpatients	Multiple drugs/ oral	80	Subjective + response to biperiden iv	? Incidence	>11	Phenothiazine-induced exacerbations primarily studied

[a]See Table 5.2 for more detailed figures for different criteria.

comprised 100 patients admitted consecutively to the psychiatric units of two teaching hospitals of the University of New South Wales. All suffered from nonorganic psychotic disorders and were treated with neuroleptic medication. On admission, they had been free of a DA antagonist drug for a minimum of 2 weeks (6 weeks if a depot preparation had been used), as well as ACh or βA antagonist drugs, and other drugs known to cause or modify akathisia. Patients with PD, RLS, peripheral neuropathy, diabetes mellitus or peripheral vascular disease were excluded.

All patients were comprehensively assessed at baseline, before the initiation of neuroleptics (except in nine cases for which 'emergency' neuroleptic drugs were used), and any patients with akathisia at baseline were excluded. Subjects were started on neuroleptics on day 1 by the treating psychiatrists, who agreed to the following: (i) to not use ACh or βA antagonists prophylactically, and introduce any antiparkinsonian and antiakathisia measures only after consultation with the research team. The choice of the neuroleptic drug and the rate of its increment were determined by the treating psychiatrist as a 'clinical' decision. Polypharmacy was generally avoided. Patients who developed acute dystonia and were treated with regular ACh antagonists and manic patients treated with lithium in the first two weeks were excluded.

Baseline assessment included the administration of the PHH Scale and its global rating (Appendix B). Other rating scales administered were the Abnormal Involuntary Movements Scale (AIMS; National Institute of Mental Health, 1976), the Rating Scale for Extrapyramidal Side Effects (Simpson and Angus, 1970), the Self-Rating Depression Scale (Zung, 1965), the Spielberger State-Trait Anxiety Inventory (Spielberger et al, 1967) and the Brief Psychiatric Rating Scale (Overall and Gorham, 1962). Subjects were assessed daily with the global rating for the development of akathisia. The comprehensive assessment was repeated on days 7 and 14, or earlier if akathisia developed.

The percentage of subjects who received a global rating of 1 or more over the 2 weeks is presented in Fig. 5.1. The first cases of akathisia were usually diagnosed by day 3, and an initial peak was reached by day 6. The incidence of akathisia depended on the criteria used for the diagnosis. Both strict and loose criteria, based on the global rating, or the ratings on the PHH Scale, were applied, and the results are presented in Table 5.2.

We had realized from our examination of the baseline data that patients rated positively on many of the items of the PHH Scale even when they did not receive a clinical diagnosis of akathisia. We therefore decided on the overall clinical rating as the standard for diagnosis (Criterion I). By this criterion (ie, global rating of 1 or more), 32 patients had akathisia on days 7 and 31 (33.3%) on day 14. Of the 68 subjects not akathisic on day 7, 8 went on to

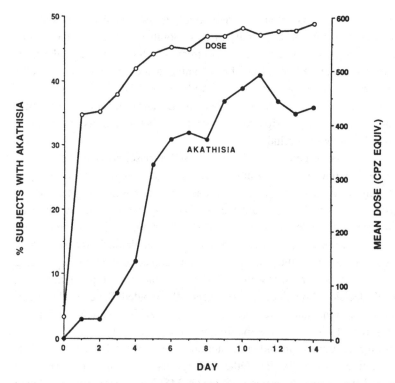

Fig. 5.1. The percentage of subjects diagnosed as having akathisia (solid circles) and the mean neuroleptic dose in milligrams of chlorpromazine (CPZ) equivalents for all subjects (open circles) over the first 2 weeks after initiation of medication in the AA study (Sachdev and Kruk, 1994).

develop akathisia in the second week, thereby giving a 2-week incidence of 40%. However, the majority of patients had only a mild disorder, which was not clinically significant and was often not noted by the treating team. Therefore, a definitive clinical diagnosis was agreed on as 'the need to intervene because of akathisia' (ie, reduction in dose or change in type of neuroleptic or introduction of antiakathisia medication). To us, this was akin to the diagnosis of moderate to severe akathisia (global rating of 2 or 3; Criterion II). By this more strict criterion, 15 subjects had akathisia on day 7 and 18 (19.8%) on day 14. Of the 85 patients not akathisic on day 7 by this criterion, 6 developed akathisia in the second week, giving an overall incidence of 21% in the first two weeks.

We used the scores on the PHH Scale items to arrive at incidence figures, as shown in Table 5.2. The sums of the three subjective and seven objective

Table 5.2. *Akathisia diagnosis using different criteria (AA study)*

Criterion	Number with akathisia		
	Day 7 (*n* = 100)	Day 14 (*n* = 91)	Total (2 weeks) (*n* = 100)
1. Global score ≥1	32	31	40
2. Global score ≥2	15	18	21
3. Total score ≥4	31	33	41
4. Total score ≥5	25	27	32
5. Sum-Sub score ≥2 *and* Sum-Obj score ≥2	23	26	31
6. Sum-Sub score ≥1 *and* Sub-Obj score ≥1	39	48	55
7. Total score ≥2	53	58	61

Note: Global score is from the Prince Henry Akathisia Scale (see text). Sum-Sub is the sum of three subjective items on the 10-item akathisia scale. Sum-Obj is the sum of two objective items on the 10-item akathisia scale. Total is the sum of Sum-Sub and Sum-Obj scores.
Source: Sachdev and Kruk (1994).

items gave the Sum-Sub and Sum-Obj scores, respectively, and the sum of all the items gave the total score. The receiver operating characteristic analysis to determine the specificity and sensitivity of the diagnostic criteria has already been presented in Chapter 4 (Figs. 4.1 and 4.2). By using the proposed research Criterion 2 (2 or more on both Sum-Sub and Sum-Obj), 31% were diagnosed as suffering from akathisia.

A limitation of the study is the restriction of the systematic follow-up to 2 weeks. Our figures may, therefore, be underestimates but are unlikely to be too far from the real figure. In the Braude et al (1983) study, 85% of the patients developed the disorder within a week of starting the medication, and nearly all by the second week. Ninety percent of Ayd's (1961) patients on depot fluphenazine developed akathisia within four days of the injection. In the oral treatment group reported by Ayd (1961), 90% of the akathisia developed in the first 73 days, with about 70% occurring in the first month. However, the author did not make it clear how the drug dosages varied in this period and what the increments were. In the Van Putten et al (1984c) study, akathisia had developed in a majority of patients by day 7. These findings support our contention that our figures do not greatly underestimate the true incidence of akathisia.

Conclusion

The diversity of the studies does not permit a confident statement to be made on the incidence and prevalence of AA. The published rates due to conventional neuroleptics vary from 8% (McCreadie et al, 1988) to as high as 76% (Van Putten et al, 1984b). To have clinical relevance, the rates should pertain to commonly used neuroleptic drugs at the dosages and rates of increment that are applied in clinical practice. The incidence rate of 31% in the AA study is relevant in this context. When at least moderate severity is considered, an incidence of 21% was reported in this study. This figure is consistent with the 21.2% prevalence figure of Ayd (1961), who reported the largest survey, although the criteria for the diagnosis of akathisia in this study were much less rigorous. The Braude et al (1983) rate of 25%, which included mild cases, is in the same range. A conservative estimate of incidence of akathisia with classical neuroleptics at clinical dosage levels is, therefore, 20–30%, but as we will discuss in the next chapter, this rate is significantly affected by treatment-related and other variables. For example, parenteral administration, potency of the drug and initial dose used, will all affect the rate of akathisia. A distinction between incidence and prevalence rates can be made in some studies, but since AA is of short duration in most of these studies, the distinction is not of great clinical import. Most investigators will agree that AA, along with parkinsonism, is one of the most common side-effects of neuroleptic drugs.

Akathisia induced by specific drugs

A number of published studies report the prevalence of akathisia in patients treated with specific drugs. A summary of these studies is presented in Tables 5.3 and 5.4. Some notable examples are discussed in the following subsections.

Akathisia related to newer antipsychotic drugs

Studies that have examined akathisia secondary to the newer antipsychotic drugs are of particular interest because of the different pharmacological profiles of these drugs and because many of these drugs are not potent dopamine D_2 receptor antagonists, unlike the conventional neuroleptics.

Clozapine is one such drug with an atypical profile, being a relatively weak D_2 antagonist, but a more potent $5HT_2$ and adrenergic α_1 antagonist, as well as a D_4 antagonist (Peroutka and Snyder, 1980; Lee and Tang, 1984; Richelson and Nelson, 1984). Clozapine is associated with a low incidence

Table 5.3. *Acute akathisia induced by specific newer neuroleptic drugs*

Drug	Prevalence (%)	Comment	Reference
Clozapine	6.7	Similar to chlorpromazine (5.3%)	Claghorn et al (1987)
	39	Usually mild	Cohen et al (1991)
	Nil	Akathisic patients ($N = 21$)	Safferman et al (1992)
	3	Product insert; $N = 842$	Sandoz Corp (1991)
Remoxipride	30	Median dose, 600 mg/day	Lund Laursen and Gerlach (1986)
	Nil	210 mg/day over 4 days	Farde et al (1988)
	81	420 mg/day over 4 days	Farde et al (1988)
	4	Comparison with thioridazine	McCreadie et al (1988)
	36	Comparison with haloperidol	Andersen et al (1990)
	32	Comparison with haloperidol	Lindstrom et al (1990)
Sulpiride	8.7	Comparison with perphenazine	Lepola et al (1989)
	44	Comparison with haloperidol	Munk-Andersen et al (1989)
	7.9	Open study	Robertson et al (1990)
Amisulpiride	21.5	Open study	Mann et al (1984)
Metoclopramide	25	Single-dose (10 mg iv) study	Jungman and Schoffling (1982)

and severity of EPSE (Claghorn et al, 1987; Kane et al, 1988). The literature with regard to akathisia is somewhat inconsistent. Much of the earlier literature suggests that clozapine produced little akathisia (Gerlach, 1991), except at the highest dosages in vulnerable patients (Casey, 1989). Claghorn et al (1987), in a double-blind comparison of clozapine with chlorpromazine, reported that, contrary to expectation, the former produced akathisia as frequently as the latter (6.7% vs 5.3%, respectively). Cohen et al (1991), in a naturalistic study, assessed 23 patients receiving clozapine for akathisia using the Chouinard et al (1980) scale for assessment and compared them with 29 control patients receiving a standard neuroleptic. Using a total score of 3 or more (maximum possible = 9) to diagnose akathisia, they found that 39% of the clozapine group and 45% of the control group had akathisia. The mean (SD) ratings for the two groups were 2.17 (1.8) and 2.41 (2.6), respectively. However, those with severe akathisia (score of 6 or more) tended to be more

Table 5.4. *Akathisia induced by non-neuroleptic drugs*

Drug	Prevalence (%)	Comment	Reference
Serotonin-reuptake inhibitors			
Fluoxetine	9.8–25	Open study (only 20 of 51 systematically examined)	Lipinski et al (1989)
	Nil	23 cases in open study	Maany and Dhopesh (1990)
	10–15	Anxiety, nervousness and insomnia	Eli-Lilly Pty Ltd (1993)
Sertraline	—	Single case report	Klee and Kronig (1993)
	—	Single case report	Settle (1993)
Serotonin antagonists			
Cyproheptadine	—	Single case report	Calmels et al (1982)
Methysergide	—	Single case report	Bernick (1988)
Buspirone	—	Single case report	Patterson (1988)
	—	Single case report	Ritchie et al (1988)
Heterocyclic antidepressants			
Tricyclics + oestrogen	—	3 cases reported	Krishnan et al (1984)
Tricyclics	—	Multiple case reports	Zubenko et al (1987)
Amoxapine	—	4 cases of agitation	Barton (1982)
	—	9 cases	Hullett and Levy (1983)
	—	3 cases	Shen (1983)
Anticonvulsants			
Carbamazepine	—	Single case with left temporal lobe injury	Schwarcz et al (1986)
	—	2 cases	Milne (1992)
Ethosuximide	—	2 cases with questionable akathisia	Ehyai et al (1978)
Calcium channel antagonists			
Diltiazem	—	Single patient	Jacobs (1983)
Flunarizine	—	5 cases	Kuzuhara et al (1989)
	—	2 cases	Chouza et al (1986)
	—	Single case	Meyboom et al (1986)
	—	Single case	Micheli et al (1987)
Cinnarizine	—	?	Gimenez-Rolden and Mateo (1991)
Mood-stabilizing drugs			
Lithium carbonate	—	Single case	Channabasavanna and Goswami (1984)
	—	Single case	Price and Zimmer (1987)

common in the control group (14%) than the clozapine group (9%). In this study, patients were not randomly allocated to different treatments, and the dosage equivalence of the treatments was not certain. The package insert for clozapine reports an akathisia rate of 3% in 842 patients (Sandoz Pharmaceutical Corporation, 1991). Safferman et al (1992) recently examined the impact of clozapine on patients with ($n = 21$) or without ($n = 49$) akathisia at baseline after a 2-week wash-out period. Patients who did not have akathisia at baseline (acute or tardive) did not develop it during the 1 year of treatment with chlozapine (mean dosage 565 mg/day). Those with akathisia, possibly a mixture of AA and TA and/or agitation, improved considerably in the first 3 weeks and then continued to improve over 3 months, even though the dosage of clozapine was increasing. This finding is in contrast with the other two studies, and the authors argued that the other studies were deficient in not assessing akathisia adequately at baseline such that they may have included TA, or the carry-over effect of acute akathisia, as being caused by clozapine. This is an important argument since most patients who are treated with clozapine have failed trials with other drugs and are usually chronically ill. The Safferman et al study, however, suffered from the limitation of a 50% drop-out rate over the year (although no patients were withdrawn because of EPSE), and the use of a modified Simpson and Angus (1970) scale for the diagnosis of akathisia, which is less than optimal for such purposes.

It is therefore difficult to give a definite rate of akathisia secondary to clozapine. The rate for the large number of patients enrolled in the Sandoz trials suggests that akathisia may be relatively uncommon, as does the Safferman et al study. The latter study also suggests that clozapine may even permit the recovery of chronic akathisia due to conventional neuroleptics. However, the conflicting evidence presented by Claghorn and associates and, especially, Cohen and associates argues for further examination of the issue.

A number of substituted benzamides have recently been introduced that are effective antipsychotics but have an atypical side-effects profile (Lund Lauersen and Gerlach, 1986; Andersen et al, 1990). Remoxipride has been investigated with regard to akathisia. Lund Lauersen and Gerlach (1986) treated 10 patients with a median dosage of 600 mg/day (range 300–1,200) and reported akathisia in 3, with a mean rating of 1.6 on the St. Hans Hospital rating scale (rating 0–6). Farde et al (1988) administered remoxipride at 2 dosage levels – 70 mg and 140 mg tid – for 4 days. The drug was well tolerated at the lower dosage, but the higher dosages resulted in akathisia in 7 of 8 subjects. McCreadie et al (1988) compared remoxipride (75–375 mg) with thioridazine (150–759 mg) in a double-blind study of acute schizophrenia. Although the method of assessment of akathisia was not stated, it was diagnosed in 8% of thioridazine patients and 4% of remoxipride patients, it being reportedly more severe for the latter. In a multicentre, double-blind comparison of remoxipride and haloperidol, akathisia was noted to be less common with the former. Lindstrom et al (1990) reported that in their study (*n* = 48 in each group), akathisia occurred in 32% of the patients receiving remoxipride and 57% of those on haloperidol (*p* < .05). Andersen et al (1990) reported a 36% incidence with remoxipride (*n* = 39) and 68% with haloperidol (*n* = 32). The method of diagnosis of akathisia was again not specified. Another drug from this group that has received increasing attention is sulpiride. Robertson et al (1990) treated 63 patients suffering from Tourette's syndrome with sulpiride in an open study and reported that 5 developed akathisia (1 of the 26 who discontinued, and 4 of 37 who continued the drug). They suggested that the drug was better tolerated on this count than the conventional neuroleptics. In a double-blind study, Lepola et al (1989) compared sulpiride with perphenazine in schizophrenia. In the sulpiride group, 2 of 23, and in the perphenazine group, 6 of 23, developed akathisia. The criteria for diagnosis were again not specified. Munk-Andersen et al (1989) compared sulpiride (median 1,600 mg/day) with haloperidol (median 12 mg/day) in a double-blind crossover study (*n* = 16) and reported akathisia in 8 haloperidol and 7 sulpiride patients. Only preliminary data on raclopride are available (Farde et al, 1988; Cookson et al, 1989); they suggest that it does frequently produce dystonia and akathisia. In an open clinical study of amisulpiride, 3 of 14 patients reportedly developed akathisia (Mann et al, 1984). Sufficient data on other substituted benzamides (eg, emonapride) are not available.

A benzamide that is not generally used as an antipsychotic is metoclopramide. This drug is important because of its extensive nonpsychiatric usage to treat severe nausea, oesophageal reflux, dyspepsia, neurogenic bladder, orthostatic hypotension, nonprolactinemic amenorrhoea, hiccoughs, etc. Numerous reports of metoclopramide-induced akathisia have been published in the literature (eg, Bui et al, 1982; Allen et al, 1985; Saller et al, 1985; Graham-Poole et al, 1986; Richards et al, 1986). The literature with regard to metoclopramide-induced movement disorders was recently reviewed by Miller and Jankovic (1989), who recorded 1,031 reported cases, 10% (*n* = 106) of which had akathisia (acute or tardive). Good incidence data are unavailable. Borenstein and Bles (1965) administered high dosages to psychiatric patients and reported EPSE in 25% but did not specify the rate of akathisia. Jungmann and Schoffling (1982) investigated the effect of an iv bolus of 10 mg metoclopramide in healthy volunteers and found that 25% 'complained of akathisia', usually within 15–30 minutes, which lasted for 3–4 hours. That this distressing side-effect is frequently unrecognized or ignored has been repeatedly highlighted (Miller and Jankovic, 1989).

Risperidone is a novel benzisoxazole derivative that shows a different side-effects profile than do the conventional antipsychotics. It is a potent D_2, $5HT_2$ and α_1 receptor antagonist (Janssen et al, 1988). A recent double-blind parallel-group trial comparing different fixed dosages of risperidone with haloperidol suggested that the former produced less akathisia (Janssen Research Foundation, 1992). This difference is currently being investigated in greater detail in a multicentre trial.

A number of drugs that, like risperidone, act on D_2 as well as other receptors, are currently being investigated for their antipsychotic properties and side-effects profiles (Gerlach, 1991). ICI 204,636 is a dibenzothiazepine with a relatively weak D_2 antagonism but a stronger blockade of the $5HT_2$ receptor. In a small clinical study, no extrapyramidal symptoms were observed (Fabre et al, 1990). Sertindole has a biochemical profile like risperidone (Skarsfeldt and Perregaard, 1990), but its clinical profile is still under investigation. Amperozide is a diphenylbutylpiperazine with an unusual biochemical profile of potent $5HT_2$ antagonism, a moderate affinity for α_1 receptors and minimal affinity for D_1, D_2 and $5HT_{1a}$ receptors. In a small clinical study (Axelsson et al, 1991), no akathisia was reported. Savoxepine is a novel tetracyclic cyanodibenzoxepinoacepine derivative with strong D_2 antagonistic properties, which are 10 times greater for the hippocampal than the striatal receptors (Bischoff et al, 1986). Additionally, it blocks D_1, $5HT_2$, α_1 and histamine H_1 receptors. In three open studies, it was found to commonly produce EPSE including akathisia (Butler and Bech, 1987; Moller et al, 1989; Wetzel et al, 1991).

Partial D_2 agonists have recently aroused interest as potential antipsychotics, and a few drugs (eg, SDZ HDC912, terguride, roxindole and B-HT 920) have been tried mostly in open clinical trials. The occurrence of EPSE, including akathisia, has been low or absent in these trials, but the data are preliminary, and more definitive studies are awaited (Gerlach, 1991). Dopamine D_1 antagonists have shown promise as potential antipsychotics in animal studies and may produce fewer or different side-effects, but clinical trials are yet to be published.

In conclusion, the preliminary evidence from the use of the newer antipsychotic drugs in relation to AA is encouraging, and further systematic work is necessary. The dosages used should be kept in mind when rates for different drugs are compared, since it is likely that newer drugs are used at relatively lower dosages.

Other drugs that reportedly produce acute akathisia

Serotonin reuptake inhibitors

Akathisia, quite indistinguishable from that caused by neuroleptics, has recently been reported to occur with serotonin reuptake inhibitors (SRIs) used in the treatment of depression and obsessive compulsive disorder. Lipinski et al (1989) reported 5 cases of fluoxetine-induced akathisia. The akathisia was rapid in onset, starting from within hours to 5 days of the initiation of the drug, was mild, manifested subjective and objective features and responded to dose reduction or treatment with propranolol. In one case, akathisia continued for more than a year while the patient was maintained on fluoxetine. Fluoxetine-induced akathisia was not associated with parkinsonism or dystonia. Interestingly, 4 of the 5 patients reported were young women with obsessive-compulsive disorder (OCD); one man had a depressive illness. The incidence of akathisia with fluoxetine is uncertain. The Lipinski et al cases were observed in a series of 51 patients so treated, but only 20 patients were systematically examined, suggesting that the incidence could be anywhere between 9.8% (5/51) and 25% (5/20). The product insert for fluoxetine describes 'anxiety, nervousness, and insomnia' in 10% to 15% of treated patients, leading to drug discontinuation in 5%. It is likely that a proportion of these suffer from akathisia.

The issue of fluoxetine-induced akathisia, in spite of this report, remains controversial. Maany and Dhopesh (1990) challenged the Lipinski et al paper, arguing that the observed side-effect was in fact not akathisia or could be attributed to neuroleptics or trazodone. They cited their own experience of treating 23 patients with fluoxetine, noting anxiety and insomnia in 1 but no cases of akathisia. The criticism was, however, adequately rebutted by the authors, and it is likely that fluoxetine does not commonly produce akathisia at smaller dosages, which were the ones used by Maany and Dhopesh. The literature also suggests that fluoxetine-induced akathisia may be misdiagnosed or missed altogether. Ioannou (1992) reported a patient who developed a 'horrible feeling inside', which was not recognized as akathisia; rather, the suicidal ideas this patient subsequently developed were highlighted. That suicidal ideation sometimes seen in patients treated with SRIs (Teicher et al, 1990) may, at least in part, be due to akathisia has been suggested by Opler (1991), Wirshing et al (1992) and Hamilton and Opler (1992). This will be discussed further in Chapter 6.

Two cases (Klee and Kronig, 1993; Settle, 1993) of probable akathisia have recently been reported secondary to sertraline, a newer SRI. The author could not trace any reports of akathisia secondary to other SRIs, eg, paroxetine, fluvoxamine, indalpine. There is evidence, however, that these drugs worsen neuroleptic-induced parkinsonism or PD, thus suggesting a propensity to produce EPSE and possibly akathisia (Lipinski et al, 1990).

Serotonin antagonists

Cyproheptadine, a drug with histamine, 5HT and ACh antagonist properties, has been reported to cause akathisia in one case (Calmels et al, 1982). A case of akathisia has also been reported with methysergide, which, in addition to being a 5HT antagonist, is also a DA antagonist, while its metabolite, methergine, is a DA agonist (Bernick, 1988).

Akathisia has also been reported with buspirone, an azaspirodecanedione anxiolytic agent that reduces 5HT activity, enhances DA and norepinephrine (NE) cell firing, and may have additional effects on GABA systems. Ritchie et al (1988) reported a patient who developed generalized myoclonus, unilateral shoulder dystonia, and akathisia after 5 days of buspirone treatment. The symptoms resolved on drug withdrawal and short-term clonazepam treatment. Patterson (1988) reported another patient who developed akathisia in association with buspirone.

Heterocyclic antidepressants

Akathisia is not generally considered to be a complication of heterocyclic antidepressants. The literature with regard to the jitteriness syndrome has been reviewed in Chapter 2. At this stage, too little is known about the syndrome to lump it with drug-induced akathisia, and they will therefore be treated as separate syndromes in this book. However, a few reports of antidepressant-induced akathisia have appeared. Zubenko et al (1987) described the occurrence of antidepressant-induced akathisia that was indistinguishable from the neuroleptic-induced syndrome. Krishnan et al (1984) reported akathisia in three patients treated with clomipramine, amitriptyline and doxepin in conjunction with conjugated oestrogens. One patient developed akathisia when clomipramine was given simultaneously with the oestrogen; it disappeared when the latter was discontinued. In another case, akathisia occurred shortly after the patient took one dose of amitriptyline in the course of long-term treatment with conjugated oestrogens. These cases underscore the importance of the interaction of tricyclic antidepressants with oestrogens on DA-sensitive adenylate cyclase and on the modulation of DA receptors. Paik et al (1989) reported three patients who developed RLS in response to mianserin, a tetracyclic piperazino-azepine compound that is an established antidepressant drug. The authors argued that the nature of the syndrome produced was different from NIA in that the symptoms were confined to the lower limbs, were worse at night and disrupted sleep, thus resembling RLS. Mianserin is a moderate antagonist of presynaptic α_2 receptors, and a poor blocker of 5HT reuptake, but with no D_2 antagonist activity.

Akathisia has been reported with the tricyclic dibenzoxazepine antidepressant amoxapine. Barton (1982) reported four cases of amoxapine-induced 'agitation', although the descriptions of the symptoms resembled that of akathisia. Ross et al (1983) reported a case of akathisia which began on the third day of starting on amoxapine and responded to benztropine. Shen (1983) reported three further cases that responded to ACh antagonists. Hullett and Levy (1983) reported nine further cases and described two in detail. Amoxapine is an atypical antidepressant in this sense, and its intrinsic neuroleptic activity is recognized. It is the demethylated metabolite of the neuroleptic loxapine, and its 7-hydroxy metabolite is a DA antagonist (Donlon, 1981).

Anticonvulsants

Schwarcz et al (1986) reported a patient with left temporal lobe injury and intermittent bursts of polymorphic slowing on electroencephalogram (EEG) who developed 'jittery legs' and restless pacing due to a therapeutic dose of carbamazepine. Milne (1992) reported akathisia in two patients being treated with carbamazepine. The first was an 8-year-old girl with generalized epilepsy who developed restlessness in her limbs 2 months after initiation of the drug, the dosage of which was in the therapeutic range. This responded to dosage reduction, but the disorder recurred 8 months later when a further dosage reduction was warranted. The other case concerned a 38-year-old woman with partial complex epilepsy. There were no other organic factors. While other EPSE, including asterixis, dystonia, tremor and dyskinesia, have been reported with carbamazepine, these are the only reported cases of akathisia we could trace. This drug, on the other hand, has been used for the treatment of RLS (see Chapter 13).

Ehyai et al (1978) reported two children who developed generalized chorea and possibly akathisia when treated with ethosuximide. The report does not, however, permit a definitive diagnosis of akathisia.

Calcium channel antagonists

The calcium channel blocking agents are extensively used in cardiovascular medicine, and their tendency to produce EPSE is now well recognized. The commonly used drugs are cinnarizine, flunarizine, nifedipine, verapamil and diltiazem. Movement disorders have been most commonly reported with flunarizine and cinnarizine. The former is a difluorinated derivative of the latter and has a greater potency and a longer half-life. In addition to being calcium antagonists, these drugs have varying degrees of histamine, 5HT and D_2 antagonist properties.

Jacobs (1983) reported a patient who developed AA on the day following the introduction of diltiazem and improved promptly upon its cessation. Kuzuhara et al (1989) reported 31 patients with flunarizine-induced parkinsonism, 5 of whom also had akathisia. Chouza et al (1986) reported 12 patients who developed extrapyramidal motor signs and depression induced by flunarizine. Two of these patients had akathisia, and for one the problem persisted for 20 months after withdrawal of the drug. Further reports of flunarizine-induced akathisia have subsequently appeared (Meyboom et al, 1986; Micheli et al, 1987). AA seems to develop within hours or days, and there does not seem to be a relationship with dosage. Gimenez-Roldan and Mateo (1991) reported two predisposing factors to cinnarizine-induced parkinsonism: older age, and a history of essential tremor in the patient or an immediate family member. Whether this is also true for akathisia is unknown. To date, the incidence of akathisia in response to these drugs has not been published.

Lithium carbonate

While lithium is known to produce mild EPSE (Engel and Berggren, 1980) and exacerbate NIP, only a few case reports of akathisia have been published and no data on any large series are available. Channabasavanna and Goswami (1984) reported a patient who developed akathisia during lithium prophylaxis, and Price and Zimmer (1987) reported another patient who, after only 10 days of lithium treatment, developed akathisia, which responded to trihexyphenidyl. A case of lithium-induced RLS has also been reported (Terao et al, 1991).

The following conclusions can be reached with regard to akathisia secondary to non-neuroleptic drugs: (i) The evidence is preliminary, and larger epidemiological studies are necessary. (ii) The clinical characteristics should be systematically examined to determine if the akathisia secondary to neuroleptic or nonneuroleptic drugs is similar. (iii) Care should be taken when drugs are used in combination, eg, lithium and haloperidol in a bipolar disorder patient, calcium antagonist and neuroleptic drug in a hypertensive patient with psychosis.

Incidence and prevalence of tardive akathisia

A caveat

Even more than that of AA, the epidemiology of TA suffers from the limitations outlined at the beginning of this chapter. Many authors, while examining akathisia in long-term-medicated patients, did not examine the relationship of akathisia with the history of neuroleptic use in any great detail. The sample therefore tends to be a heterogeneous mix of AA, WA and TA. Diagnostic criteria for TA have been recently proposed by Burke et al (1989) and our group (Sachdev, 1994a), but their application to published studies has as yet been limited. In much of the literature, the chronicity of akathisia, variously defined, or its occurrence in a long-term-medicated population, is conceptualized to suggest a tardive syndrome, without regard to the more restricted 'delayed onset' meaning of the term *tardive*. The following published studies should be considered in the light of these limitations.

Some relevant studies

Case reports of 'late-onset and persistent' akathisia have appeared since 1960, when Kruse published three case histories of 'muscular restlessness' that persisted for 3–18 months after the cessation of the phenothiazines. All patients had associated dyskinesias.

An early study was performed by Hunter et al (1964), who surveyed 450 chronically ill patients in a mental hospital. The authors reported that no male patient ($n = 200$) and 13 (5%) female patients ($n = 250$) had dyskinesia, and all of the dyskinetic patients also had akathisia. The study is, of course, deficient for not using a precise definition of akathisia or a systematic examination procedure, but it is an early recognition that long-term-medicated patients can have akathisic symptoms.

In one study in their hospital, Kennedy et al (1971) examined all chronic schizophrenic inpatients ($n = 63$; 32 men, 31 women; age range 32–88 years) for akathisia, again not specifying the subtype. Twelve (38%) male and 12 (39%) female patients had akathisia. The study included a number of items that represented 'involuntary coordinated semipurposeful motor restlessness', and a factor analysis performed on the data essentially yielded three factors, with the first factor having high loadings on the motor restlessness items and accounting for 32.5% of the variance. The authors also attempted to identify risk factors, which will be discussed in Chapter 7.

In the 1970s, little was published with regard to late-onset akathisia, although it was becoming accepted as a distinct syndrome. Simpson (1977) referred to late-onset akathisia in his review, discussed its association with TD and drew attention to the possibility that its subjective aspects may be less prominent than in AA. The latter observation has been subsequently repeated but has not been empirically evaluated.

One of the more influential studies on TA was published by Barnes and Braude (1985). They examined 89 schizophrenic patients (age range 21–73 years) attending two outpatient depot neuroleptic clinics with a semistructured questionnaire (Braude et al, 1983) and compared them with 54 patients attending a surgical outpatient clinic. Twenty-nine (35%) of the schizophrenic patients and none of the controls met both subjective and objective criteria for the diagnosis of akathisia. In 6 cases, the akathisia had occurred in the preceding 6 months, coincident with an increase in drug dosage, and was diagnosed to be AA. The remaining 23 cases were diagnosed as CA, which was considered to be a mixture of tardive and acute persistent akathisia. There was an additional group of 10 patients who had motor restlessness without the subjective report of restlessless or distress, which was referred to as 'pseudoakathisia'. If the latter are included, the total number of patients with chronic akathisia was 33 out of 89, a prevalence of 37%. This was the first major study to examine akathisia systematically, using both subjective and objective phenomena, and to be sensitive to the possible subtypes.

Another significant report in this regard was published by Gibb and Lees (1986a). The authors performed two separate studies. In the first, they examined the subjective phenomena of akathisia, elicited by a semistructured interview, in schizophrenic outpatients, and in the second the motor phenomena of akathisia were examined in an inpatient population in order to distinguish it from TD. The first study involved 95 patients (54 men, 41 women) attending community clinics or psychiatric day hospitals for depot neuroleptics; all had attended the clinic for at least 1 year, and 50 (52.6%) for over 10 years. All were on stable medication, with none having been admitted to hospital in the preceding year. Fourteen items on the questionnaire were analysed, and the details will be discussed in Chapter 7. Thirty nine patients (41%) experienced a compulsion to move, and 52 (55%) complained of restlessness in the body and 44 (47%) in the mind. In the second study, 171 inpatients in a psychiatric hospital who had been there for at least 1 year were selected (out of a total of 842 potential subjects) for the presence of prominent hyperkinetic movements (patients with orofacial dyskinesia alone, or mild hyperkinesis, were excluded). Of the 171 patients, 12 were further excluded because they could not be definitely categorized. The majority of the remaining 159 suffered from schizophrenia (73.6%), with the rest diagnosed with dementia (22.6%) or affective disorder (3.8%). The subjects were divided into three groups on the basis of the presence or absence of oral TD, subjective akathisia and walk-ing in one spot (objective akathisia). The definite akathisia group comprised 27 (17%) patients who had both subjective and objective features of akathisia without orofacial dyskinesia. The TD group ($n = 79$) had orofacial dyskinesia and motor restlessness but without the characteristic subjective or objective features of akathisia. The indefinite group ($n = 53$) exhibited motor restless-ness but without either orofacial dyskinesia or the subjective or objective fea-tures of akathisia. If only the definitive group is considered, the prevalence of akathisia in this study is 27 (3.2%) out of 842.

Sandyk and Kay (1990b) conducted a study of elderly schizophrenic patients in a psychiatric hospital in Rome and reported that 40 (32.5%) of 123 patients on long-term treatment with neuroleptics had akathisia. No attempt was made to distinguish TA from AA, although the neuroleptic history (mean duration of use 25.5 years, SD 6.8) makes TA or CA the more likely diagno-sis in the majority.

A study of drug-induced movement disorders from a psychiatric hospital in Japan (Inada et al, 1991) reported 4 (0.6%) of 716 patients with akathisia, 1 (0.1%) of whom was diagnosed as TA since his akathisia was initially noted upon withdrawal of the neuroleptics and continued for several years.

Other studies have examined the side-effects of neuroleptic medication in long-term-medicated patients, without necessarily focussing on akathisia or trying to distinguish AA from TA. Curson et al (1985) followed up patients who had been treated with antipsychotics over 7 years. Of the original 81 patients, 64 were fully assessed at follow-up, and 73% of these had been maintained on depot neuroleptics. Of the 51 patients currently receiving antipsychotics, 10 were clinically diagnosed to have akathisia, based on the presence of both subjective and objective features, but no rating scales were used.

McCreadie et al (1992) interviewed 88% ($n = 146$) of all patients with a case record diagnosis of schizophrenia living in Nithsdale, south-west Scotland, and diagnosed them using the Barnes Akathisia Rating Scale (Barnes, 1989). It is one of the few studies in which a measure of interrater reliability was incorporated in the design. At the time of assessment, 18 sub-jects were not on any antipsychotic medication. Twenty seven (18%) were diagnosed to have at least mild akathisia, 5% pseudoakathisia (objective but not subjective features) and 10% had 'questionable akathisia'. Akathisic patients were more likely to be inpatients or day patients and had a trend towards more EPSE.

Two reports have presented clinical data. Davis and Cummings (1988) reported that 18% of the patients evaluated in their Los Angeles TD clinic suffered from TA. Burke et al (1989) presented their clinical data from the Movement Disorder Group of the Columbia-Presbyterian Medical Center in New York and the Baylor College of Medicine in Houston between 1974 and 1986. Tardive syndromes had been diagnosed in 114 patients, and 31 of these had TA with or without oral–lingual–buccal dyskinesia or tardive dystonia (TDt). Since these were large tertiary referral centres with a presumably unlimited catchment area, it is not possible to draw any conclusions regarding prevalence from these figures. The study does highlight, however, the frequency, relative to TD and TDt, with which TA may become a serious clinical problem requiring expert opinion.

TA has not been reported in relation to drugs other than the antipsychotics. The exception is perhaps metoclopramide, a substituted benzamide referred to earlier. Shearer et al (1984) reported two patients whom they diagnosed with TA in response to treatment with metoclopramide. A review of the case histories, however, leaves some doubt with regard to the appropriateness of the TA diagnosis. One patient had episodic symptoms of anxiety, motor restlessness, panic attacks and insomnia that started quite suddenly 4 months after the initiation of treatment and were not typical of akathisia. In the second patient, the symptoms were more suggestive of akathisia and developed 4 months after starting the drug, but again developed suddenly and subsided completely on the cessation of medication. Miller and Jankovic (1989) reported a patient with metoclopramide-induced akathisia in conjunction with TD and EPSE, but it is again not clear whether this was TA. While the occurrence of AA with metoclopramide is well established, TA nevertheless remains to be adequately documented although there is no theoretical argument why it should not occur.

TA has similarly not been documented with the newer antipsychotic drugs, and further exploration of this area is awaited. A summary of these studies is presented in Table 5.5. Our investigation (Sachdev, unpublished data) of TA in a sample of long-term-medicated schizophrenic patients on stable medication is briefly discussed in the following section.

Tardive or chronic akathisia study

Sample

One hundred patients from community health centres of the Eastern Sydney Area Health Service volunteered to participate. All patients had a DSM-III-R diagnosis of schizophrenic disorder, chronic, were between 18 and 60 years

Table 5.5. *Epidemiology of tardive or chronic akathisia*

Population	N	Prevalence (%)	Comment	Reference
—	3	Case reports	Persistence of 'muscular restlessness'	Kruse (1960a)
Chronic mental hospital patients	450	Male, 0 Female, 5	All dyskinetic patients also had akathisia	Hunter et al (1964)
Chronic schizophrenic inpatients	63	Men, 38 Women, 39	Clinical assessment; no rating scales	Kennedy et al (1971)
Outpatient schizophrenics	89	37	Semistructured questionnaire; includes 'pseudoakathisia'	Barnes and Braude (1985)
Outpatients on depot neuroleptics	95	41	Compulsion to move	Gibb and Lees (1986a)
Chronic psychiatric inpatients	171	3.2	Definite akathisia (both subjective and objective)	Gibb and Lees (1986a)
TD clinic	?	18	Proportion of tardive syndromes	Davis and Cummings (1988)
Elderly schizophrenic patients	123	32.5	Italian hospital	Sandyk and Kay (1990b)
Psychiatric hospital inpatients	716	0.1	5 (0.6%) in all had akathisia; Japanese study	Inada et al (1991)
Outpatients on depot neuroleptics	51	19.7	13 patients not currently on neuroleptics were not akathisic	Curson et al (1985)
Schizophrenic outpatients	146	23	Another 10% questionable	McCreadie et al (1992)
Specialist movement disorders clinic	114	27.2	Proportion of tardive syndromes	Burke et al (1989)
Chronic schizophrenic outpatients	100	31	TA/CA study	Sachdev (unpublished)

of age, were currently on neuroleptic medication that had not been changed in type or dosage in the preceding 6 weeks (or 3 months if on depot neuroleptic) and did not suffer from another neurological disorder.

Assessment

Subjects were assessed in the early afternoon, and those on a depot drug were seen before its administration. The charts were reviewed and the community nurse interviewed. Information was collected on a range of sociodemographic as well as illness- and treatment-related variables. Additionally, the following rating scales were administered: (i) an akathisia rating scale similar to the PHH Scale (Appendix B), except that each item was rated on a scale of 0–4 (nil, minimal, mild, moderate, severe) rather than 0–3 (this study was initiated before we decided to abandon the fence rating of 'minimal'; Sachdev, 1994c); (ii) Barnes Akathisia Rating Scale (Appendix C; Barnes, 1989), global rating only; (iii) AIMS; (iv) the Simpson and Angus scale for EPSE; (v) a 10-item negative symptom rating scale (Iager et al, 1985); (vi) six items of the Brief Psychiatric Rating Scale.

Subjects were videotaped during the akathisia and dyskinesia ratings. One in three video recordings was subsequently rated independently by three investigators in order to establish interrater reliability for the global ratings for TA and TD, with demonstrated high kappa coefficients (0.80 and 0.85, respectively). The subitems of the Barnes Akathisia Rating Scale were rated independently by the author and a research assistant trained in the ratings of akathisia, and again a high interrater reliability was established.

Results

The sums of the scores on the subjective items (Sum-Sub), the objective items (Sum-Obj) and all items (total) were used to categorize subjects as akathisia or nonakathisia. A score of 2 or more on the Barnes scale was used to define a 'global akathisia' group. Different diagnostic criteria were applied to the sample, and the resulting prevalence figures are presented in Table 5.6. Since there was a considerable overlap of akathisia with OBLF dyskinesia, a 'pure akathisia' group was also identified that had akathisia with no dyskinesia. It was considered impossible to establish accurately the point of onset of the akathisia in the patients, and therefore no attempt was made to try to separate patients with an acute or tardive onset. However, since there had not been a recent change in medication, the sample was conservatively assessed as chronic.

Table 5.6. *The TA/CA study: prevalence of akathisia in chronic, stably medicated schizophrenic outpatients* (N = 100)

Criterion	Description of criterion	Prevalence (%)	Comment
A	Akathisia Sum score >4	31	Total TA
B	Barnes akathisia score ≥2	33	Global TA
C	Sum-Obj score ≥4	24	Objective TA
D	Akathisia Sum score ≥4 and AIMS severity score ≤1	13	Pure TA

Source: Sachdev (unpublished).

Our study provides prevalence estimates of akathisia in a long-term medicated stable schizophrenic population using strict diagnostic criteria. It suffers from some of the limitations of the other TA studies. The akathisia we saw is possibly a mixture of CA and TA, which cannot be clearly separated since only one examination was performed. Strictly speaking, the prevalence refers to 'akathisia in chronic schizophrenia', rather than TA. A selection bias cannot be ruled out because chronic schizophrenic patients with negative symptoms, who may in fact be more susceptible to the disorder, do not often agree to participate in such studies. Further, only a longitudinal study can address the issue with regard to subtypes of CA and provide incidence figures. We are currently conducting such a study.

In conclusion, the literature on the epidemiology of CA and TA is deficient, and a longitudinal study of patients initiated and subsequently maintained on neuroleptics in the long term is necessary to provide an accurate estimate. Most reported studies have based their estimates on cross-sectional examinations. The studies do suggest that a significant proportion of patients on neuroleptics for the long-term suffer from akathisia, perhaps as high as 40%, although more conservative estimates would be closer to 20–30%. TA therefore occurs on a similar magnitude as does TD, and its lack of recognition and consequent neglect is difficult to understand.

Withdrawal akathisia

While the syndrome of WA is becoming increasingly accepted as a distinct subtype of akathisia, at least in the acute stage of its manifestations, the literature on its epidemiology is extremely limited. A careful examination reveals, however, that the observation that motor restlessness related to neuroleptics may sometimes worsen or appear for the first time on cessation of the drug has been reported since the mid-1960s. Many early papers (eg, Judah et al, 1961; Rothstein et al, 1962; Whittacker and Hoy, 1963) reported symptoms such as restlessness, pacing, agitation and hyperactivity after phenothiazine withdrawal. In most of these cases, the symptoms were construed as an exacerbation of the primary psychiatric disorder or as an autonomic and behavioural withdrawal syndrome (Gardos et al, 1978), not as neurological side-effects. Gardos et al (1978) did refer to motor restlessness as a withdrawal phenomenon, which they considered to be part of withdrawal dyskinesia.

Demars (1966) was one of the earlier authors to examine the effect on EPSE of the discontinuation of neuroleptic medication. The motor restlessness of 3 of his patients became worse, while for 1 it improved, for 3 it disappeared and for 13 it remained unchanged. Pryce and Edwards (1966) reported that 4 of their 21 patients became very restless over a period ranging from 3 weeks to 2 years after stopping the medication. Several other studies examined EPSE, including dyskinesia as well as akathisia, and reported both the exacerbation of symptoms upon cessation and their persistence subsequently (Hunter et al, 1964; Evans, 1965; Kennedy, 1969).

Hershon et al (1972) examined 63 chronic schizophrenic patients at baseline and a few months after withdrawal from trifluoperazine. In the double-blind study of withdrawal, half the patients were given placebo and the other half continued on trifluoperazine. The syndrome of motor restlessness was significantly worse at the end of the drug-free period in the placebo group ($n = 32$). The group mean rating increased, 6 preexisting cases became worse, and 5 new cases developed.

A few case reports of WA have been published which do not provide insight into the overall prevalence of this syndrome. Braude and Barnes (1983) reported two patients in whom akathisia developed many years after antipsychotic drug treatment had been started. The signs and symptoms of akathisia appeared only at the end of the depot injection period or after drug withdrawal, and were ameliorated by further antipsychotic drug administration. Other cases have been subsequently described (Lang, 1994).

The study by Dufresne and Wagner (1988) is of note for its more systematic examination of patients recently withdrawn from neuroleptics. The authors examined 33 schizophrenic patients who had been withdrawn off all antipsychotics for a minimum of 2 weeks before the assessment. The DiMascio Reversible Extrapyramidal Symptom Scale (Chien et al, 1974) rating akathisia on a scale of 0–3 was used (see Chapter 9 for details). Thirteen (39.3%) patients were diagnosed to have akathisia, and these patients also had more dyskinetic movements, but not dystonia or parkinsonism. Unfortunately, the patients were not assessed prior to the withdrawal, and it is uncertain how many had WA and not a persistence of AA or TA. As well, the authors do not state whether antiparkinsonian medication was also withdrawn at the time as were the antipsychotic drugs. Since the half-life of most antiparkinsonian drugs is shorter than that of the neuroleptics, the cessation of both types of drugs simultaneously may lead to an emergence of akathisia simply because of the wearing off of the antiakathisia medication while high levels of neuroleptics persist (Klawans et al, 1973).

Akathisia in special populations

Children and adolescents

Neuroleptic drugs are used in children not only for psychotic disorders but also for a number of nonpsychotic conditions, eg, Tourette's syndrome, autism, conduct disorder, ADHD and some paediatric neurological disorders. Despite this broad use, drug-induced movement disorders have been poorly documented, and akathisia has been relatively neglected. Polizos and Engelhardt (1978) reported that akathisia did occur in children treated with neuroleptics, but it was infrequent. In their large series ($n = 284$) of children (mean age 8.8 years) treated with a range of high- and low-potency neuroleptics for 'childhood schizophrenia with autistic features', while 23% of patients developed EPSE, only 2 cases of akathisia were reported. Chiles (1978) used high-potency antipsychotics to treat 11 adolescents and reported that all of them developed EPSE within 48 hours of drug treatment, with only 1 (7%) patient experiencing akathisia. Bruun (1988) described subtle akathisia that may occur in children with Tourette's syndrome treated with the neuroleptics haloperidol or pimozide. In her study, 9 of 208 patients developed akathisia, usually when the neuroleptic dosage was increased above the 'threshold' (1–20 mg/day for haloperidol and 4–15 mg/day for pimozide). That akathisia may worsen the Tourette's syndrome was also recognized by the same author (Weiden and Bruun, 1987). The latter was a retrospective case record study of 100 patients who had been treated by the authors. Six patients, after an initial improvement with the neuroleptic, reported a worsening of their Tourette's syndrome, and in all cases the worsening could be attributed to akathisia.

In one of the few prevalence studies of EPSE in children, Richardson et al (1991) examined 104 children and adolescents admitted over a 6-month period to a state-operated child psychiatric centre. At the time of evaluation, 61 patients were receiving neuroleptics and 11 antiparkinsonian agents. Akathisia symptoms were seen in 2 adolescent patients and were mild in both.

The literature, therefore, is too scant to draw any definitive conclusions with regard to the vulnerability of children to akathisia relative to that of adults, and prevalence and incidence studies are needed. Our own experience with the use of haloperidol and pimozide in Tourette's syndrome suggests that even though side-effects are common, typical akathisia is not so. While this may be a consequence of the low dosages used, the possibility that the very young are less vulnerable to akathisia cannot be ruled out.

Individuals with mental retardation

Neuroleptic medication is commonly used in mentally retarded individuals, especially in institutions (Sachdev, 1991), and a number of studies have examined drug-induced movement disorders in this group. Most studies have focused on TD, in particular withdrawal dyskinesias, or parkinsonian side-effects (eg, Gualtieri et al, 1980, 1986; Rao et al, 1987, 1989; Stone, Alvarez and Ellman, 1989; Stone, May and Alvarez, 1989; Sachdev, 1992). The examination of akathisia has not been adequate. This may partly be explained by the fact that hyperactivity and pacing can be present in this population for a variety of reasons, and a definitive diagnosis of akathisia is therefore difficult, with the patient often being unwilling or unable to provide a subjective account. Nevertheless, a few reports have been published.

Stone, May and Alvarez (1989) examined the entire population ($n = 1,227$) of a state facility for the developmentally disabled in California for dyskinesia, dystonia, akathisia, parkinsonism and paroxysms, using a special examination to facilitate the evaluation of noncompliant subjects. Akathisia was defined as an abnormal urge to move expressed as motor restlessness, and psychic agitation was not considered. Akathisia was diagnosed in 155 patients (13%). In 85 (7%), it coexisted with dyskinesia, and in 25 (2%) with dystonia. There were no sex differences, but akathisia showed a curvilinear relationship with age, increasing up to 40 years and then decreasing with age ($p < .0003$). Akathisia had a significant relationship with previous antipsychotic drug exposure.

The study by Ganesh and associates (1989) is of interest because of its special focus on akathisia in a population of mentally handicapped individuals. The authors examined 69 subjects in a long-stay hospital for motor restlessness, using a modified version of the checklist described by Barnes and Braude (1985). Five subjects were judged to have objective akathisia, 2 with coexistent TD. In those who had akathisia without TD, the clinical picture was typical of akathisia. All subjects had been on neuroleptics for over 3 years, and 25 were considered to have overt brain damage. The authors could not identify any significant predictors of akathisia, except for a possible effect of younger age.

Sachdev (1992) examined all residents (n = 53) in a facility for the developmentally disabled located within a large psychiatric hospital in New South Wales, Australia. Akathisia was diagnosed only if the subject complained of restlessness, particularly referable to the legs, and showed evidence of increased lower limb movements while sitting. Two (3.7%) subjects had definite but mild akathisia, and another 3 had a questionable presence of akathisia. The two with akathisia also had mild orolingual dyskinesia and had not had a change in neuroleptic dosage in the preceding 3 months, suggesting that the akathisia was chronic.

Gualtieri (1993) reported the results of the examination of residents in a large facility for mentally retarded adults in Louisiana. Of the 180 residents on long-term treatment with neuroleptics, 25 (14%) were diagnosed with TA. During the three-year study, only 10 (40%) could be completely withdrawn from the neuroleptics. The authors argue that a major reason for the lack of successful withdrawal was an exacerbation of akathisia.

In conclusion, akathisia appears to be common in retarded adults on long-term medication, but the overall data are too few to make comparisons with nonretarded populations. This is of interest since the issue of whether mental retardation is a risk factor for TD is still unresolved (Waddington, 1989; Sachdev, 1992), and the study of TA may offer some insights into this debate. The literature on AA in this population is minimal. Nevertheless, it is certainly true that akathisia does occur in mentally retarded individuals, and since their abilities to communicate their distress are usually poor, it may manifest as behavioural disturbance, with important implications for correct diagnosis and management.

Geriatric populations

Sandyk and Kay (1990b) published a study of akathisia in the geriatric population from a psychiatric hospital in Rome. They examined 123 patients suffering from chronic schizophrenia, with a mean age of 63.9 (SD 8.9) years, and diagnosed akathisia in 40 (32.5%). The akathisia was not subtyped, but since all the patients had been on long-term medication, it is likely to have been largely TA or CA. Akathisic patients were more likely to be women, who did not necessarily have more parkinsonism.

In a small study from Oregon, Ganzini et al (1991) examined 17 elderly individuals (mean age 77 years) who were treated with neuroleptics (range 25–250 mg chlorpromazine equivalents per day) for various reasons. Three

(18%) developed AA as judged on the St. Hans Hospital scale (Gerlach et al, 1993).

In general, reports of akathisia in the elderly have been few. The reasons for this are uncertain. It may reflect a failure of reporting or neuroleptic drug practices in this population (low-potency drugs in small dosages for short periods) or indeed a lower vulnerability. In Ayd's (1961) series, the oldest person with akathisia was 64 years old, even though a number of subjects were in their seventies and eighties. More systematic studies are necessary to establish the relationship between old age and vulnerability to akathisia.

6

Clinical characteristics and diagnosis of acute akathisia

It is well recognized that even experienced psychiatrists can make errors in the diagnosis of akathisia. This is because the diagnosis is primarily clinical and no laboratory indices are available. While some clinical features are distinctive, none is pathognomonic, and considerable overlap occurs with restlessness due to other causes. Many case descriptions of akathisia have been published, but few studies have systematically examined the clinical features, and even these suffer from the lack of specific diagnostic criteria and subtyping, as discussed previously.

In this book the clinical features of AA and TA are discussed separately. This separation reflects the view that the two syndromes can be distinguished by pathophysiology, longitudinal course and pharmacological profile. WA is described in association with TA for two reasons: Its clinical descriptions are few and do not produce a distinctive picture, and a parallel exists in the TD literature in which withdrawal dyskinesia is described as a subsyndrome of TD (Schooler and Kane, 1982).

Demographic factors

Age

The relationship between age and AA has not been adequately examined. Ayd (1961) suggested that akathisia was most prevalent between ages 12 and 65 years in his sample, in distinction with dystonia (more likely in the young) and parkinsonism (more likely in the elderly). The oldest person with akathisia in this series was 64, even though a significant number of subjects (not stated) were in their seventies and eighties.

In the Braude et al (1983) study, the age range of the sample was 19–72 (mean 40.6, SD 15.0) years, and there was no significant difference in age between the akathisic ($n = 24$) and nonakathisic ($n = 23$) groups. In our own

118

AA study (see Chapter 5 for a description), the subjects had a mean (SD) age of 34.4 (10.8) years (range 16–59). The akathisics did not differ significantly from the nonakathisics. On logistic regression analysis to assess for predictors of akathisia, age was not significant in most cases, with the exception of akathisia at day 7 using the global criterion for diagnosis, for which age was significant at the .15 level with an odds ratio of 1.034. Our study, however, was deficient in not including the very young or the elderly.

As discussed in Chapter 5, there are only a few studies of akathisia in children, and these suggest a lower incidence and prevalence than those in the adult populations. The literature on the elderly is even more scanty.

In conclusion, while the investigations that have examined this aspect seem to indicate that age is not a significant risk factor for akathisia, the few reports in the children and the elderly deserve to be followed up with more systematic epidemiological studies. If the incidence is indeed low at the extremes of the life span, it would be unique for any drug-induced movement disorder.

Sex

The relationship between akathisia and sex, like that between akathisia and age, has not been adequately investigated. Ayd (1961), in his sample of 48.5% men and 51.5% women, found the male–female ratio for akathisia to be 35:65. Sarwer-Foner (1960b), on the other hand, stated that 'akathisia . . . tend(s) to prevail in men' (p. 316) but did not provide any figures to support this. Most epidemiological studies have not reported any sex differences in the vulnerability to akathisia (Braude et al, 1983; Van Putten et al, 1984c). Our own AA study did not reveal any sex differences between akathisics and nonakathisics, and sex did not emerge as a significant predictor on logistic regression analysis. An exception is the study by Sandyk and Kay (1990b) in which a larger proportion of women (40.6%) than men (20%) resident in a long-term unit of a psychiatric hospital was found to have akathisia. The patients were elderly (mean age 63.9, SD 8.9 years), and no attempt was made to separate AA from TA.

From the limited data available, one must conclude that sex does not seem to significantly determine the occurrence of AA. As a caveat, however, it is possible that sex interacts with age as a vulnerability factor, such that its importance may become apparent in the very young or the old. This must be empirically examined using well-diagnosed AA populations.

Race

Akathisia has been reported in many racial groups (Sandyk and Kay, 1990b; Inada et al, 1991), although comparative studies examining incidence have not been published. There is no suggestion that any particular racial group is more vulnerable to AA.

Psychiatric diagnosis

Most of the epidemiological studies of AA have been performed in patients suffering from schizophrenia (see Chapter 5). Some studies, however, included mixed psychiatric populations. The Braude et al (1983) study included patients with affective disorder and personality disorder, as well as a few with 'other neurotic conditions' and alcoholism. There was no suggestion that any diagnostic group was particularly vulnerable. Our AA study included 25 patients with nonschizophrenic psychotic disorders; psychiatric diagnosis was again not a significant predictor. The data would, therefore, suggest that the nature of the psychiatric disorder is probably not important. It must be pointed out that neuroleptic drugs tend to be used at different dosages in different disorders, and since akathisia is dose-related, this aspect needs to be taken into consideration in the analysis. The report by Galdi and Bonato (1988) is of interest, although the implications of their finding are difficult to assess. While examining the relationship of adverse drug reactions and the length of stay in hospital, they found that akathisia was associated with an increased hospital stay in only the schizophrenics who had a family history of affective disorder. Gardos et al (1992), in their study that attempted to quantify psychomotor activity in akathisia by monitoring ambulatory activity, reported that the clinical ratings of akathisia tended to be higher in depressed patients, even though they were on smaller dosages of neuroleptics than the manic and schizophrenic patients. This therefore raises the possibility that depressed patients may be more vulnerable to akathisia, as has been suggested for TD (Khot et al, 1992) and possibly drug-induced parkinsonism (Friedman, 1992). This suggestion should be examined more systematically in a larger sample. The Gardos et al study also suggested that the manifestations of akathisia interact with those of the primary psychiatric disorder. The latter should therefore be taken into consideration, particularly if quantification of the movements is intended.

As already pointed out, akathisia frequently occurs in healthy individuals challenged with neuroleptics or other drugs known to cause akathisia, or in patients suffering from medical or surgical illnesses. Akathisia in response to metoclopramide or calcium antagonists bears testimony to this (see Chapter 4). There is, additionally, no suggestion that the akathisia seen in normal individuals is phenomenologically different from that seen in psychiatric patients.

Onset

There is general agreement that akathisia develops within hours or days of the initiation of a neuroleptic drug or an increase in its dosage or a switch to a high- from a low-potency drug. Ayd (1961) reported that akathisia developed within days, and 90% of the cases developed in the first 73 days of initiation of treatment. Akathisia developed slightly before EPSE in this study. In the Braude et al (1983) study, 85% of patients with akathisia developed EPSE within a week of the maximum dose being prescribed, with 3 developing it within 12 hours. Van Putten et al (1984c) reported that with a single oral haloperidol (5 mg) challenge, 40% developed akathisia in the first 6 hours, and then on maintenance treatment (10 mg/day) 76% developed akathisia in the first 7 days. With thiothixene (0.22 and 0.44 mg/day, respectively), the figure was 20% in the first 6 hours and 63% in the first 4 weeks. In our AA study, patients were started on a neuroleptic on day 1, and the first cases of akathisia were usually diagnosed by the day 3, and an initial peak was reached by day 6 (see Fig. 5.1). A second, but smaller, peak was seen by days 10 and 11 and was probably related to an increase in neuroleptic dose from days 4 to 6. This suggested a 5- to 6-day delay between an increase in the neuroleptic dosage and the maximum likelihood of akathisia occurring. Levinson et al (1990) reported that the akathisia typically developed 2–3 weeks after treatment with neuroleptics.

The speed of development of akathisia does, to some degree, depend on the type of drug, the rate of increase of dosage and, more importantly, the route of administration. That high- rather than low-potency drugs may be likely to cause akathisia earlier is suggested by clinical experience and the Van Putten et al (1934) study. Ayd (1974) reported that with depot fluphenazine enanthate or decanoate, 90% of akathisia developed in the first 1–4 days. Challenges with iv neuroleptics can produce akathisia in minutes. Jungmann and Schoffling (1982) reported that their subjects, following an iv bolus of 10 mg metoclopramide, developed akathisia after 15–30 minutes which lasted for 3–4 hours. Kendler (1976) reported his experience of akathisia following an im haloperidol 1 mg injection, which began about 30 minutes after the injection, reached a peak by 90 minutes and lasted about 5 hours.

Subjective features: symptoms

The description provided here draws largely from the two major studies of AA, the Braude et al (1983) study and our AA study, and the reports of behavioural toxicity provided by Van Putten and colleagues. As already discussed in Chapter 4, the clinical features of akathisia may be subjective or objective, and these will be discussed separately.

Perhaps the most outstanding feature of AA is the subjective distress. In its milder form, it is experienced as a vague feeling of apprehension, irritability, dysphoria, impatience or general unease (Van Putten, 1975). Almost all patients describe a feeling of 'inner restlessness', especially if this description is suggested to them. In the AA study, 35 of 40 akathisic patients described themselves as being restless on direct questioning. On further enquiry, 15% said that this restlessness stemmed from the mind, 30% said that it was in the body and mind and 55% said that it was in the body, primarily the legs.

Patients describe their experiences of akathisia in a variety of ways:

I feel . . . restless; nervous; fidgety; unable to keep still; compelled to move; like my legs are jumping; on the go; uncomfortable; like there are ants in my trousers; on edge. My nerves are jumping. I feel like I'm wired to the ceiling. My legs want to keep moving. I feel impatient and nasty. I can't concentrate. I can't describe the feeling, it's so terrible. I'm quivering from the waist up. I want to climb the walls. I feel all revved up. If this continues, I'd rather be dead.

The more colourful descriptions reflect the level of distress akathisia can cause. An experience of akathisia lucidly described by Kendler (1976), a medical student, that was induced by 1 mg haloperidol im is worthy of note:

. . a diffuse, slowly increasing anxiety. My uneasiness soon began to focus on the idea that I could not possibly sit for the rest of the experiment. I imagined walking outside; the idea of walking was particularly attractive. I could not concentrate on what I had been reading. . . . As soon as I could move, I found myself pacing up and down the lab, shaking and wringing my hands. Whenever I stopped moving, the anxiety increased. . . . I imagined bicycling home rapidly – the thought of rapid motion was again appealing. . . . Two features of this akathisia reaction impressed me. First, the intensity of the dysphoria was striking. . . . Second, the sense of a foreign influence forcing me to move was dramatic. Long before I thought of akathisia, or even discovered that moving made me less anxious, I was pacing and wringing my hands. (pp. 454–455)

While the restlessness of akathisia may be felt in the mind or body or both, the characteristic that distinguishes it from restlessness of other aetiology is its reference to the lower limbs (Braude et al, 1983; Van Putten and Marder, 1986). Patients complain that the greatest difficulty is in keeping their legs still. While sitting, they are compelled to move the legs constantly, either flexing–extending at the knees, or inverting–everting at the ankles, or abducting–adducting at the hips, or crossing–uncrossing. Pacing is one common consequence of this urge, and if asked to stand in one spot, these patients fidget, shift their weight repeatedly and complain of increasing distress. The movements are described as a response to an irresistible urge to move, but the movement alleviates the urge and the distress only temporarily. The urge can therefore becoming unrelenting and may preoccupy the person's thinking. As will be discussed later, this could lead to adverse behavioural consequences. Kalinowsky (1958) stated that akathisia can be 'more difficult to endure than any of the symptoms for which ... (the patient) was originally treated' (p. 295).

Patients often say that they cannot maintain one posture for long periods. If they are sitting, they have to get up periodically, move around and then sit again. Mild cases can often be detected by asking patients if they have any difficulty in queueing at supermarkets, cooking a meal while standing or watching television. The amount of time a patient is able to stay in a particular posture without being compelled to move may be an indication of the severity of akathisia. While some authors have reported that patients find standing in one spot to be the most distressing (Braude et al, 1983; Barnes and Braude, 1985), our patients (AA study) reported standing to be the worst position in 40% of cases, and sitting in 60%. There is agreement in the literature that lying provides some relief to the majority of the patients, although those with severe akathisia may even find this position distressing and may periodically get up to move around. This feature distinguishes akathisia from RLS, the latter being at its worst when the patient is in a recumbent position.

In addition to restlessness, 'tension' was described by 52.5% of our patients – 25% experiencing it in the mind or body, and the rest in both mind and body. A number of our patients (42.5%) described discomfort in the arms or legs, and a few (12.5%) experienced paraesthesiae. The latter is not, however, as prominent a feature of akathisia as of RLS. Patients may rub their legs and arms to relieve themselves of the distress, and face rubbing may also occur. Some of our patients (4%) describe an uncomfortable feeling in the abdomen. Table 6.1 gives a list of the signs and symptoms described in AA. Table 6.2 gives the percentages of patients with akathisia who manifested the various signs and symptoms in two studies (Braude et al, 1983; AA study, Sachdev and Kruk, 1994).

Patients, especially those suffering from psychosis, may not always articulate their distress as restlessness. Some may experience their internal distress in the form of apprehension, irritability, impatience or general unease. Others may exhibit fear, anxiety, terror, anger or rage, or experience vague somatic symptoms. One of Van Putten's (1975) patients described her akathisia as follows:

I just get these attacks of tension. I don't feel right. My stomach feels strange. It's like I'm churning inside. I feel hostile and I hate (with intense affect) everybody. I'm in a homosexual panic. As soon as I sit down, the voices start ... they call me names like

Table 6.1. *Signs and symptoms of neuroleptic-induced akathisia*

Symptoms (subjective features)

Inner restlessness
Inability to remain still (fidgetiness)
Inability to keep legs still
Inability to maintain one posture (eg, sitting, standing, lying)
Feeling of tension in body or mind
Apprehension, irritability, general unease, dysphoria
Anxiety, tremor, rage, fear
Uncomfortable limb sensations
Vague somatic sensations
Worsening of psychotic symptoms
Aggressive thoughts and actions
Suicidal thoughts and acts
Sexual craving
Poor concentration and memory
Unwillingness to take medication
Sleep difficulty

Signs (objective features)

While sitting
Lower limbs
  Abduction–adduction; lateral movement of knees
  Crossing–uncrossing at knee or ankles
  Pumping legs up and down
  Swinging or kicking crossed leg
  Lifting foot or part of foot with tapping or bouncing movements
  Plantar flexion/dorsiflexion of feet
  Sliding foot forwards, backwards or laterally
  Inversion–eversion and writhing of ankles
  Toe movements
  Sudden jerks of legs or toes
  Spontaneously rising from chair
Arms and legs
  Crossing–uncrossing of arms
  Rubbing, caressing or shaking of arms or hands
  Rubbing or massaging of legs
  Fidgeting movements of hands, wrists, fingers
  Tapping, picking on clothes
  Gesticulation
  Distressing sensations in arms or hands
Head and trunk
  Nodding, shaking of head
  Neck writhing
  Trunk rocking
  Sitting up, straightening motions
  Shifting body or trunk
Vocal/respiratory
  Grunting, shouting, moaning
  Irregular respirations

Table 6.1. (*cont.*)

While standing
  Marching or walking in one spot
  Changing stance, shifting weight, slow treading
  Swaying
  Flexing–extending knees
  Wriggling toes
  Sudden jerks, especially of legs
  Arm, hand, trunk and head movements as earlier

While walking
  Pacing, repetitive walking, wandering
  Stomping
  Fidgetiness of hands, clapping
  Sighing, irregular respiration
  Walking sideways
  Exaggerated hand swing

When lying
  Crossing–uncrossing of legs
  Shifting position of buttocks or torso
  Lateral movements of legs
  Toe movements
  Sudden jerks of legs or feet
  Coarse tremor of legs or feet
  Inability to remain lying
  Arm and hand movements as earlier

---

queer. I feel afraid. I want to fight. I just get these hurry up feelings. I'm frantic. I just can't get my emotions under control. All of a sudden I feel terrified and I want to run. (p. 44)

It is partly the patient's inability to distinguish clearly the distress caused by akathisia from that due to other causes, as well as appropriately attribute it, that can lead to atypical and bizarre manifestations of akathisia. Some examples are the exacerbation of psychosis, violence, suicide, sexual torment and other 'paradoxical behavioural reactions'. Some of these will be discussed in detail.

Akathisia manifesting as an exacerbation of psychosis

That neuroleptics may on occasion exacerbate psychosis has been recognized for some time. Sarwer-Foner and Ogle (1956) reported, without referring to akathisia, that chlorpromazine and reserpine may lead to increased anxiety and psychotic exacerbation. Sarwer-Foner (1960b) described 'paradoxical

Table 6.2. *Percentage of akathisic (global rating ≥ 1) and nonakathisic subjects (global rating = 0) with positive rating (≥ 1) on the items of the PHH Akathisia Scale on day 7 in the AA study*

| Symptom/sign | AA study (Sachdev and Kruk, 1994) | | Braude et al (1983)[a] |
	Akathisic (n = 32)	Nonakathisic (n = 68)	Akathisic (n = 27)
Subjective			
Distressing sensations in the limbs	43.7	10.3	55.5
Feeling of inner restlessness	86.2	35.3	81.5
Inability to remain still, standing			
or sitting	59.4	19.1	92.6
Inability to keep legs still	56.2	10.3	96.3
Objective			
Sitting			
Inability to remain seated	37.2	2.9	18.5
Semipurposeful or purposeless			
normal leg or feet movements	65.6	20.6	37.0
Inability to keep toes still	43.7	10.3	—
Shifting body position in chair	58.1	14.7	40.7
Semipurposeful hand or arm			
movements	31.2	8.8	22.2
Standing			
Shifting weight from foot to foot			
and/or walking on the spot	65.6	7.4	55.5
Other purposeless (normal) foot			
movements	53.1	11.8	37.0
Inability to remain standing in			
one spot (walking or pacing)	31.2	4.4	29.6
Lying			
Coarse tremor of legs or feet	18.1	0	51.9
Myoclonic jerks of the feet	19.4	2.9	59.3
Semipurposeful or purposeless			
leg or feet movements	45.2	7.4	33.3
Inability to remain lying down	25.8	4.4	7.4

[a]Data of Braude et al are shown for comparison.
Source: Sachdev and Kruk (1994).

behavioural reactions' to neuroleptic drugs leading to a 'turbulent' phase in schizophrenic patients. He offered psychodynamic explanations for most of these reactions but added that the neurological side-effects may secondarily produce psychodynamically determined reactions. Other authors discussed the subtle interactions between premorbid personality and drug effect in producing phenothiazine-induced exacerbations (Klerman et al, 1959; Henniger et al, 1965). It has long been recognized that neuroleptics, like most other psychotropic drugs, could produce a toxic psychosis, in particular because of the anticholinergic properties (Lang and Moore, 1961; Chaffin, 1964; Bucci, 1969). Certain other cognitive side-effects like depersonalization, unreality feelings, and depression may also be construed as psychotic exacerbations (Hollister, 1957; Sher, 1962).

Van Putten et al (1974) were the first to suggest that neuroleptic-induced exacerbations of psychosis may result from akathisia. They described 9 (11%) patients in their study of 80 who suffered exacerbations, and all were being treated with piperazine phenothiazines. These authors argued that the exacerbations were indeed caused by akathisia, because (i) they occurred with high-potency drugs, also likely to cause more akathisia; (ii) they were always associated with akathisia, even though mild and subtle, rather than any other side-effect; (iii) the exacerbations, like EPSE, were dose-related; (iv) they were promptly reversed by an antiparkinsonian drug, biperiden, which is also effective against akathisia; and (v) similar syndromes have been described in association with PD, postencephalitic parkinsonism and other basal ganglia disorders. Van Putten (1975) and Van Putten and Marder (1987) provided further reports of patients who, while previously stable in their psychosis, demonstrated exacerbations of their psychotic symptoms in clear consciousness that were temporally related to recent neuroleptic introduction or dosage increase and that responded to biperiden. The clinical importance of this observation is that such an exacerbation of psychosis may be construed as a lack of responsiveness to the neuroleptic, prompting an increase in dosage, which may only worsen the problem. If the clinician is sensitive to the subtle manifestations of akathisia, they can usually be identified so that appropriate action, which often is a reduction in neuroleptic dosage, can occur. As previously stated, the error is more likely to occur in acutely psychotic individuals who do not usually provide an accurate account of their subjective experiences and may otherwise be agitated. Kumar (1979) provided an example of a man with severe mental retardation whose behaviour worsened episodically in response to thioridazine, which was being used to treat aggressive behaviour.

Over the years that he took this drug, he had periodic episodes during which he disrobed, ran or paced from door to door, tried to climb up walls and doors, tried to reach the nearest exit and get out through windows, stared into space, breathed heavily, and sweated profusely. . . . These episodes occurred every few weeks and lasted for a few hours.

The episodes subsided after treatment with benztropine.

Akathisia manifesting as violence

Van Putten (1975) described aggressive and self-destructive behaviour as a result of akathisia. Keckich (1978) published the case history of a patient with a characterological and social predisposition to violence who was initially treated with imipramine with an exacerbation of his anger and hostility. He was subsequently treated with haloperidol and became agitated, with an inability to sit and a jumpy feeling inside. He also developed urges to assault anyone near him, culminating in an assault on his dog with an intent to kill. The author argued that this violence was a manifestation of akathisia. Schulte (1985) reported five patients who developed homicidal or suicidal ideation and action as a result of akathisia produced by haloperidol. One patient made the following statements: "The only reason I knifed the guy was Haldol [haloperidol] messed me up. . . . Plolixin [fluphenazine decanoate] makes me want to kill too. . . . Mellaril [thioridazine] makes good for me and makes me smooth" (p. 7). Shaw et al (1986) reported that in their double-blind cross-over study comparing haloperidol with BW-234U, an experimental neuroleptic with little affinity for DA receptors, a patient showed rapid clinical decline during haloperidol treatment including moderately severe akathisia, suicidal and homicidal ideation, increased paranoia, and an intensification of anxiety, tension and agitation.

These few case reports in the literature have been used as an argument to suggest that violence may be one manifestation of akathisia. The association between akathisia and violent thoughts or actions has been interpreted in the following manner: (i) Akathisia leads to marked internal distress, and in a predisposed individual this may manifest in the form of aggression and violence. Keckich's case perhaps exemplifies this. The inability to distinguish the restlessness of akathisia from general distress contributes to this problem. (ii) The association is a chance one. Given that akathisia and aggressive behaviour are both common phenomena in neuroleptic-treated patients, it is not inconceivable that an association may be observed in a few patients. However, the attribution by patients of their aggression and violence to the ill effects of medication cannot be easily dismissed. (iii) Akathisia, violence and suicide are common but independent consequences of neuroleptics owing to their pharmacological effects. (iv) Akathisia reduces impulse control in individuals, leading to violent acts. These four possibilities will be discussed later in relation to suicide, where the same arguments apply. At this stage, it is perhaps reasonable to say that the most likely possibility is that akathisia can produce marked distress, and in some patients this may be expressed in the form of aggression and violence. This is not a common occurrence but is worthy of recognition so that appropriate action may result.

Akathisia and suicide

The literature on suicidal ideation and attempts in relation to akathisia is similar to that for violence. In the Van Putten et al (1974) report on 'behavioural toxicity' of neuroleptics, three of the nine patients developed suicidal ideation de novo. Shear et al (1983) drew attention to this association in their report of two patients who jumped to their deaths when suffering from akathisia and who had previously not been recognized as having suicidal thoughts. Drake and Ehrlich (1985) reported two further cases. One patient, a 25-year-old schizophrenic man, was described as follows:

The patient received 2 intramuscular injections of 5 mg haloperidol and . . . was left in a room to relax. Within an hour he became acutely agitated and felt that he would 'jump out of (his) skin'. He tried pacing around the room, then escaped from the emergency ward and ran home in the hope that talking with his roommates would calm the unbearable inner restlessness. When this did not yield any relief, he went up to his third floor apartment and leaped out of the window, breaking his arm and leg. (p. 500)

The patients reported by Schulte (1985) and Shaw et al (1986) had suicidal ideation, as already mentioned. Weddington and Banner (1986) treated a patient suffering from hiccups with chlorpromazine and metoclopramide; on day 3 of treatment, the patient developed restlessness, a feeling that he was 'going crazy' and had an intense suicidal preoccupation.

The possible interpretations of this association are the same as that for violence. Ayd (1988) criticized the tendency to attribute suicidal ideation to the akathisia, citing his own experience of an initial survey of 3,775 patients (21.2% had akathisia) and a later survey of 5,000 patients (36.8% had akathisia), with no report of suicide or suicidal or homicidal ideation attributable to akathisia. We do not consider it reasonable to dismiss the association, especially because in the cases reported, akathisia was usually not recognized. We consider suicidal and homicidal ideation as the particular individual's response to subjective distress. The distress may also lead to greater impulsivity so that any propensity to suicide or homicide may become manifest because of disinhibition. That suicide has been reported with akathisia, and not with the other side-effects of neuroleptics, probably reflects the intensity of the unrelenting distress of akathisia. We have, nevertheless, treated a patient who tried to hang herself because she 'could no longer put up with the shakes'. This patient had developed moderately severe resting tremor of the upper and lower limbs and the jaw because of depot neuroleptics which had failed to respond to benztropine. We therefore recommend that any patient who develops suicidal or aggressive thoughts in the context of neuroleptic treatment should be examined for akathisia or other significant drug effect, and the appropriate remedial action must be taken if they are present.

The recent debate on the relationship between SRIs and suicide has added another dimension to this issue. Akathisia has been reported to occur during treatment with fluoxetine (Lipinski et al, 1989; Hamilton and Opler, 1992; Wirshing et al, 1992) and other serotonergic antidepressants (Zubenko et al, 1987). Fluoxetine has also been linked with suicidal ideation since the paper by Teicher et al (1990). It has been argued by some authors that suicidal ideation and akathisia related to fluoxetine or other SRIs may be linked and that it is the akathisia that causes the suicidal ideation. Wirshing et al (1992) described 5 patients, all women, who had no suicidal behaviour in the past and developed akathisia with the characteristic restlessness and the urge to pace when treated with fluoxetine. All experienced suicidal ideation at the peak of their agitation, and both the restlessness and suicidal ideation improved after the cessation of fluoxetine. Hamilton and Opler (1992) reported a similar patient. Many of these patients clearly recognized that the suicidal ideation was related to the distress caused by the restlessness. The association of fluoxetine with suicidal ideation and akathisia has also provoked speculation on the role of 5HT in both akathisia and suicide, and this will be discussed in Chapter 10 on pathophysiology.

Other atypical subjective manifestations

Akathisia may first become apparent when the patient refuses drugs. It has been recognized as an important cause of noncompliance in schizophrenic patients (Van Putten, 1975; Van Putten et al, 1976).

Van Putten (1975) reported the case of a 52-year-old women who experienced extreme sexual cravings on day 9 of treatment with haloperidol. These feelings were ego-alien, were associated with a vague inner restlessness and responded selectively to im biperiden but not to placebo. The background history of guilt over homosexual urges is noteworthy.

Raskin (1985) argued that akathisia may arise as cognitive impairment (a form of pseudodementia) in the elderly, especially in those who are nonverbal or already suffer from dementia.

Objective features: signs

The objective manifestations of akathisia are the motor and behavioural features that are observable by an examiner. Traditionally, the objective features of akathisia were not accorded the same importance as the subjective ones, and there was a belief that the motor features were a response to the inner distress and were therefore of secondary importance. There has been a recent move to consider the motor features to be equally important and to regard akathisia as both a mental and a motor disorder (Stahl, 1985; Burke and Kang, 1988). This issue is discussed later.

The observable features are various motor phenomena that are listed in Table 6.1. Fidgetiness is perhaps the most common sign, and the fidgetiness of akathisia is most commonly manifest as semipurposive or purposeless movements of legs, feet and toes. These are usually complex and repetitive, but lack the stereotyped quality of a dyskinesia or dystonia. When patients are sitting, they are likely to move their legs, wriggle their toes, pump their legs up and down or cross and uncross them, tap the toes, or invert and evert the feet. In the standing position, the leg movements are typically in the form of shifting one's weight from foot to foot, marching on the spot or moving the feet and toes. Restless movements are also seen in the lying position. In addition to the fidgetiness, the characteristic feature is the difficulty in maintaining a posture. While sitting, the patient may shift body position repeatedly and may have the classical 'inability to sit' (from which the disorder gets its name), although the latter symptom was present in only 18.5% (Braude et al, 1983) and 37.2% (AA study) of patients in two series. The patient usually prefers to walk, and inability to remain standing was present in 18.5% and 31.2% patients in the two series, respectively. In severe cases, the patient may be completely unable to sit or lie down.

While the emphasis is on leg and postural movements, semipurposeful or purposeless arm and hand movements may occur (18.5% and 31.2% in the two series, respectively). These may take the form of fidgeting, finger tapping or rubbing of the hands or other parts of the body (usually the legs and sometimes the face). Upper limb movements are less prominent and virtually never occur in isolation. Walters et al (1989) described a patient with TA who had restlessness of the arms as the principal manifestation, but such a presentation has not been reported for AA. Truncal movements in the form of rocking or twisting have been described in some patients, again more commonly in TA.

There is no consensus regarding which movements, if any, are characteristic of akathisia or, indeed, specific to it. Barnes and Braude (1985) considered shifting weight from foot to foot or walking on the spot while standing as fairly characteristic. In our own study, when a discriminant function analysis was performed on the various scale items to determine the items that best distinguished akathisia from nonakathisia, those items most consistently differentiating akathisia were (i) shifting weight from foot to foot or walking in one spot, (ii) inability to keep legs still (subjectively), (iii) feelings of inner restlessness and (iv) shifting of body position in a chair. Since these features are not present in all patients, their clinical utility is limited. Table 6.3 gives the

Table 6.3. *Percentage of subjects with a positive (1 or more) rating on the different items of the PHH Akathisia Scale on days 1 (baseline), 7 and 14*

Symptom/sign	Day 1 ($n = 100$)	Day 7 ($n = 100$)	Day 14 ($n = 91$)	Days 7 and 14 (rank order of frequency)
Subjective				
Distressing sensations in the limbs	3	21	31.9	5
Feeling of inner restlessness	18	52	53.8	1
Inability to remain still, standing or sitting	9	32	36.6	3
Inability to keep legs still	6	25	25.3	6
Objective				
Sitting				
Inability to remain seated	6	14	9.9	13
Semipurposeful or purposeless normal leg or foot movements	12	35	45.1	2
Inability to keep toes still	1	21	25.3	9
Shifting body position in chair	13	27	29.7	4
Semipurposeful hand or arm movements	4	16	17.6	10
Standing				
Shifting weight from foot to foot and/or walking in one spot	6	26	20.9	8
Other purposeless (normal) foot movements	4	25	25.3	6
Inability to remain standing in one spot (walking or pacing)	8	13	12.1	12
Lying				
Coarse tremor of legs/feet	0	5	3.4	16
Myoclonic jerks of the feet	1	8	8.0	15
Semipurposeful or purposeless leg or foot movements	2	19	12.5	11
Inability to remain lying down	4	11	12.5	14

Note: No subjects received a clinical diagnosis of akathisia on day 1.
Source: Data from AA study (Sachdev and Kruk, 1994).

relative frequency of the different signs and symptoms for the subjects on days 1, 7 and 14 in the AA study, as well as their ranking jointly on days 7 and 14.

There is a suggestion from the literature, supported by clinical experience, that the nature of the movement disorder may to some degree depend on the severity of the disorder. In the Braude et al (1983) series, features such as an inability to remain seated or standing, as well as rocking from foot to foot, were more common in the severe group. Movements in the lying position were absent in mild akathisia in this study. In the AA study, the ratings in the lying position were positive in fewer subjects (see Table 6.2) and tended to be less intense. The global ratings in the different positions again supported the finding that akathisia was least prominent in the lying position, with the mean global ratings on day 7 being 0.41, 0.32 and 0.23, and on day 14 being 0.47, 0.34 and 0.21 in the sitting, standing or lying positions, respectively. Furthermore, the motor features of akathisia may be totally absent, at least on brief examination, in the mild cases. In these cases, prolonged observation on the ward may reveal the fidgetiness and inability to maintain posture that is readily apparent in the more severe cases.

The effect of 'activating' manoeuvres

It has long been recognized that the performance of voluntary movements, especially those involving concentrated effort, affects the manifestations of involuntary movements. An examination of dyskinetic movements in TD is instructive. Movements like tongue protrusion, finger tapping or walking may bring out movements not otherwise apparent. We have, in our studies, used two manoeuvres in the assessment of akathisia: finger tapping with either hand for 30 seconds, and listening to a reading or watching a video clip for 2 minutes. It is our observation that the movements of AA are usually diminished, and may disappear completely, during such activities. The exception is with severe akathisia, in which case, interestingly, the performance of these simple manoeuvres may be impaired because of poor concentration. While patients may complain of difficulty in performing the manoeuvres, it is rare for the motor disorder to worsen. This may, to some extent, be also true of TA, which will be discussed later. While the adjective *activating* has been retained to describe these manoeuvres, in the case of akathisia they tend to produce the opposite effect, ie, diminishing or suppressing the movements.

A recent study by Fleischhacker et al (1993) partly supports this observation. They found a reduction of akathisic movements during a motor task (finger tapping), but mental activation (serial 7s task) led to an increase of symptoms in one sample and produced no change in another. Further work is necessary to determine whether the results of such procedures can be used diagnostically.

Is the motor disorder of akathisia voluntary or involuntary, or 'intentional and involuntary'?

The majority of the patients report that akathistic movements are voluntary and in response to subjective distress. They report a strong urge to move prior to the movements which can become irresistible. With sustained voluntary effort, the movements can be suppressed for varying periods of time, but at the expense of increasing discomfort. Even in the few patients who do not have a prominent subjective component to their disorder, the movements can usually be suppressed temporarily. The duration for which movements can be completely suppressed by voluntary effort may be an indicator of the severity of the disorder. There are, however, some patients, mostly at the very severe end of the spectrum, who report a complete lack of control over the movements and perceive them as involuntary. The question of voluntariness may, therefore, be one of degree. One must certainly recognize that the movements are ego-dystonic, ie, the patient does not wish to have these movements.

A parallel can be drawn with motor and vocal tics, which are also experienced by many patients as being in response to an irresistible urge to move and can be voluntarily suppressed temporarily (Kurlan et al, 1989). Many patients are distressed at not being able to control their tics in view of the fact that they can suppress or modify them briefly. Much recent attention has focussed on the sensory phenomena that precede some tics. Shapiro et al (1988) coined the term *sensory tics* to describe 'recurrent involuntary somatic sensations in joints, bones, muscles or other parts of the body' that lead to dysphoria and a voluntary movement or vocalization to relieve the abnormal sensation. Bliss (1980) gave an introspective account of his experience as a Tourette's syndrome sufferer: 'Each movement is the result of a voluntary capitulation to a demanding and restless urge accompanied by an extraordinarily subtle sensation that provokes and fuels the urge. . . . The intention is to relieve the sensation, as surely as the movement to scratch an itch is to relieve the itch'. He asked, 'If the itch was so subtle and fast that it escaped detection, would that make the act less voluntary?' One patient's experiences cannot, however, be generalized to all others. Kurlan et al (1989) found that while most patients with sensory tics reported that their movements occurred in response to an abnormal sensation, they had difficulty in stating that the movements were truly voluntary. The findings of Lang (1991) were slightly different. He carefully questioned 170 patients with various hyperkinetic disorders. Of the 60 patients with tics, 41 felt that their tics were 'voluntary' or intentionally produced, and 15 described them as having both voluntary and involuntary components, the former predominating. Of the 110 patients with other hyperkinetic movement disorders, 102 described their movements as involuntary; the remaining 8 were patients with akathisia who felt that their movements were completely voluntary.

This information is clinically useful in trying to distinguish akathisia from other movement disorders but does not necessarily settle the voluntary vs involuntary debate. The older literature considered tics to be voluntary, representing a weakness of the will (Wilson, 1955). The DSM-III-R describes them as involuntary movements (American Psychiatric Association, 1987). The truth is somewhere in between. Akathisic movements may be even closer to the voluntary end of the spectrum. A difference is that tics are more stereotyped and are obviously abnormal, whereas akathisia movements are semi-purposive and readily mistaken for anxiety and agitation. Some recent authors have emphasized the distinction between the terms *voluntary* and *intentional* (Freyhan, 1961). It is useful to consider the philosophical approach to voluntariness (Culver and Gert, 1982). For an act to be truly voluntary, as this argument goes, the individual must possess both the will to perform the act and the will not to perform it. By this argument, akathisic movements are not truly voluntary but would be categorized as 'intentional and involuntary', as the affected person lacks the ability to will to not perform the movements. Two movement disorders have been described in relation to akathisia that are more appropriately described as involuntary—myoclonus and tremor—and these will now be discussed.

Myoclonus in akathisia

The term *myoclonus* is used to describe sudden, brief, shocklike involuntary movements caused by active muscle contraction or inhibition of ongoing muscle activity. The frequency may vary from rare, single jerks to frequent, repetitive contractions, and the amplitude may range from a small contraction that is too weak to move a single joint to massive jerks that move the whole body. The many causes of myoclonus have been described by Fahn et al (1986). Periodic myoclonic movements are an important feature in many patients with RLS, as will be discussed in Chapter 12. Myoclonic movements are known to be caused by many drugs (see review by Klawans et al, 1986).

Myoclonic jerks have been described in patients with akathisia, although they are generally not a prominent feature. Braude et al (1983) described myoclonic jerks in the feet in 16 of 27 patients with akathisia. All the patients experienced myoclonic jerks that were moderate to severe in their intensity and were best seen when the patients were in the lying position. In the AA study, myoclonic jerks of the legs and feet were observed in 5 patients, all of them with severe akathisia. A number of patients were also observed to have jerky toe movements, but since the ratings of these movements demonstrated a poor interrater reliability and could not be readily distinguished from normal toe movements, they were excluded from analysis. Braude et al (1984) used an accelerometer to record finger and toe movements in akathisic patients and control subjects. They recorded the presence of large-amplitude, low-frequency (<4 Hz) rhythmic foot movements in akathisia, the amplitude and frequency of which varied with changes in akathisia severity. They suggested that these movements had features common with segmental myoclonus, a phenomenon characterized by jerky, rhythmic, low frequency (<3 Hz) motor activity (Marsden et al, 1982). Ritchie et al (1988) reported a patient who developed prominent myoclonus along with akathisia and dystonia in response to the anxiolytic drug buspirone.

A few polysomnographic studies of akathisia have been reported. Nishimatsu et al (1992) performed all-night polysomnography in a patient with AA on two occasions, before and after treatment with clonazepam. The pretreatment study revealed frequent nocturnal myoclonus, associated with arousal reactions in the mental electromyogram (EMG) and the EEG. After clonazepam therapy, the akathisia improved, the sleep efficacy increased and the total number of episodes of nocturnal myoclonus decreased considerably. Walters et al (1991) performed polysomnography on 9 akathisic patients and compared them with 11 RLS patients. The akathisia patients had both subjective and objective features, did not have a sleep abnormality clinically, did not suffer from other drug-induced movement disorders and were not currently psychotic, but the authors do not state whether the features were acute or tardive in onset. Periodic movements in sleep or nocturnal myoclonus was present in 5 of 9 akathisia patients (cf the fact that 1.4 of 9 normals of comparable age would be expected to have such movement) and in all 11 RLS patients. Presence or absence of current neuroleptic treatment did not seem to make a difference. In 3 akathisic patients, a few repetitive, rhythmical bursts of 0.5–2 cps activity were present in the legs during wakefulness as documented by EMG. These were characterized by co-contractions of agonist and antagonist muscles, much like what has previously been described in TD (Bathien et al, 1984). However, the multiple, large-amplitude, violent myoclonic jerks seen in the prone RLS patients were not present in any patient with akathisia. The study by Lipinski et al (1991) produced somewhat different findings. In their 9 patients with akathisia (how many were acute is not known), leg movement activity during sleep was generally within normal limits and differed little from that seen in healthy individuals or patients with depression. It must be pointed out that the difference between the two studies could be related to age differences. The Walters et al (1991) subjects were older (mean age 49 years, range 36–63) than the latter subjects (mean age 31 years, range 19–47), and it is notable that the only subject in the Lipinski et al study with an abnormal myoclonus index was also the oldest (age 45 years). Moreover, the full medication status of the Walters et al subjects is not known. Further studies using clearly defined populations and larger samples are necessary to resolve these discrepancies.

In conclusion, the issue of myoclonic jerks as a feature of akathisia is unresolved. Jerks of the legs and feet may be present in akathisia, as well as occur during both waking and sleep hours, but they are not a prominent feature. They are more likely to occur in moderately severe to severe akathisia. High-amplitude myoclonic jerks frequently seen in RLS are not a feature of akathisia. Further studies are necessary to determine whether the jerks seen in some akathisic patients are abnormal relative to a healthy population.

Tremor

Tremors are characterized by rhythmic, regular, oscillatory movements varying in frequency from 3 to 20 Hz. The aetiology of tremor is varied, and a classification has been proposed by the ad hoc Tremor Investigation Group (Bain et al, 1993) of the International Tremor Foundation. Neuroleptics are well known to produce a tremor which typically involves the fingers or the hands, but may involve the jaw, feet or tongue. This tremor, which is evident at rest, is classically a part of drug-induced parkinsonism (DIP), and not a feature of akathisia. It is seen in akathisia insofar as there is an overlap between akathisia and DIP. A number of akathisic patients also show rigidity, bradykinesia and tremor of DIP, and the extent and nature of this relationship will be discussed later. We found a correlation of .3 between akathisia and EPSE scores in the AA study, the latter largely made up of rigidity and tremor. The correlation between tremor and elbow rigidity was higher ($r = .53$).

Braude et al (1983) described a 'coarse' tremor of the feet in patients with akathisia, which was a low-frequency (<4 Hz), large-amplitude, relatively irregular but rhythmic motor activity localized to the feet. They demonstrated this by accelerometry in six patients with akathisia (Braude et al, 1984), the coarse tremor not being evident in the finger recordings. The frequency spectra of the toe recordings showed characteristic wave forms, with peaks at 3–4 Hz, which were different from those in the nonakathisia patients, the latter showing relatively flat tracings of toe movements. The authors also demon-

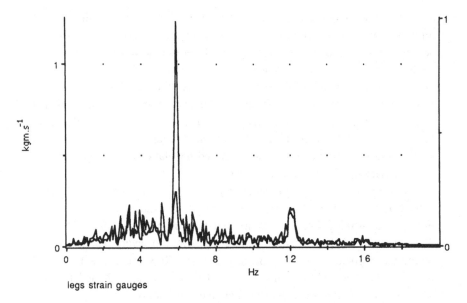

Fig. 6.1. Power spectrum of movements recorded from the legs (left and right tracings superimposed) using strain-gauge measures in a patient with akathisia. The tracing is a fast Fourier transform of the mean record obtained in 6 epochs of 30 seconds each.

strated that the tremor was sensitive to change in the severity of akathisia and argued that this coarse, jerky tremor was an objective sign of akathisia, which was distinct from the restless fidgety movements, as well as the resting tremor of parkinsonism. They likened this tremor to segmental myoclonus (Marsden et al, 1982), suggesting spinal drug effect as the aetiology.

Our own tremographic investigation of akathisia did not support the finding of a low-frequency tremor. The power spectrum showed increased activity in the low-frequency range (<3 Hz) but without any definitive peak (Fig. 6.1). This was consistent with the restless leg movements of akathisia and did not suggest a distinct, involuntary tremor. The finger demonstrated a medium-frequency tremor consistent with DIP. The issue of tremor therefore remains unresolved, but on balance it appears that a rhythmic tremor does not occur in *akathisia,* which has movements that are irregular and nonrhythmic.

Variability of the movements

Any clinician familiar with akathisia will testify to the marked variability in its expression, especially in the mild cases. This variability is apparent over

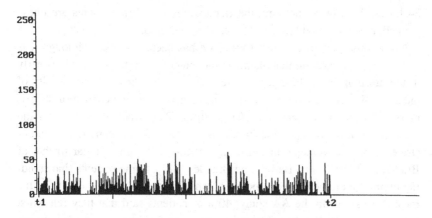

Fig. 6.2. Record of movements of left leg in a patient with akathisia over 4 hours by actigraphy. The units in the abscissa are arbitrary, indicating relative extent of movement.

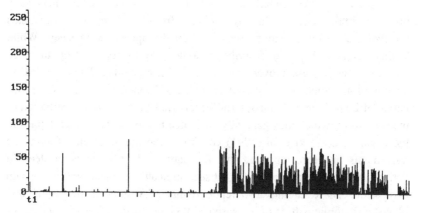

Fig. 6.3. Record of movements of left leg in a patient with akathisia over 24 hours by actigraphy (same patient as in Fig 6.2).

time, but even within one brief observation akathisic movements are manifest only intermittently unless the disorder is severe in intensity. This can lead to significant difficulties in the diagnosis of akathisia, if it is to be based on a single, brief examination. Longitudinal studies, in particular those involving treatment, are also complicated by this variability. The variation is best demonstrated by ambulatory activity monitoring using a piezoelectric device strapped to the ankle (see Chapter 9 for details). Figure 6.2 shows a tracing over 4 hours from one patient with AA, and Fig. 6.3 of the same patient over

24 hours. To a large measure, the fluctuations in the movements are unexplained, but some modifying factors can be identified.

No definite pattern of diurnal variation has been described, although it is our clinical observation that akathisic movements may be less obvious early in the morning for a short period after the patient wakes up. The activity of the akathisic patient should, of course, be considered in the context of the primary disorder the patient is suffering from. The effect of posture on the movements has been previously discussed. Our akathisic patients demonstrated fewer movements in the lying position, a finding similar to that of Braude et al (1983) and Barnes and Braude (1985). Some patients find standing in one spot to be the worst position, while others consider sitting to be the most distressing. In the AA study, 40% of patients said that they felt worst when standing, 60% when they were sitting. As Tables 6.2 and 6.3 indicate, the ratings on items were positive in fewer subjects when lying down, and less intense. All subjects who had positive ratings on these items were also rated at similar or greater severity on the other items.

Sleep has a marked ameliorating effect on akathisia, and this may have important implications for its differentiation from RLS. Figure 6.3 illustrates the fact that akathisic movements virtually disappear during sleep. While Walters et al (1991) did describe periodic movements in sleep in some patients, overall these movements were not prominent and represented an amelioration compared to daytime movements. In their questionnaire examination of 20 patients with NIA, 6 (30%) reported a night-time exacerbation of the symptoms, which they generally attributed to the intake of neuroleptics in the evening. Lipinski et al (1991) confirmed the improvement of akathisic movements in sleep, reporting that the pattern of movements in sleep in patients with NIA was similar to that seen in healthy subjects and those with depression. These authors also reported that NIA subjects frequently displayed a rhythmic pattern of increased EMG tone lasting 10–40 seconds, during which the EMG amplitude would wax and wane in bursts of markedly increased tone followed by periods of moderately increased tone. This pattern occurred before sleep onset and disappeared during sleep, occasionally reappearing after brief awakenings. The authors described this in 8 of 9 NIA patients on at least one night, compared with 1 normal control subject and 1 depressed patient. This finding was described earlier from the same laboratory by Cunningham et al (1991) in 2 other akathisia patients.

Other factors that modify the expression of akathisia have not been systematically studied. The effect of activating manoeuvres has been discussed previously, and the suggestion is that, unlike TD, the movements of akathisia decrease when the individual performs a task that requires concentration or

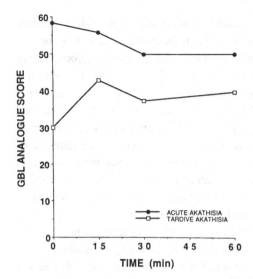

Fig. 6.4. Mean global analogue akathisia ratings (0–100) after challenge with 1 ml saline iv in six patients with acute akathisia (solid circles) and seven patients with tardive akathisia (open squares). Data from Sachdev and Loneragan (1993a,b).

the activation of specific muscle groups. Anxiety interacts with akathisia such that the presence of akathisia leads to an increase in anxiety, which in turn worsens the distress and movements of akathisia. Our AA study demonstrated, however, that it is possible for patients to distinguish the subjective experience of akathisia from that of anxiety.

The variability of akathisia complicates the treatment studies. Our studies (Sachdev and Loneragan, 1993a,b,c) have demonstrated a significant placebo effect even over short periods, as well as random variation in both baseline and repeat recordings (Fig. 6.4). The determinants of this variability need to be systematically investigated.

Relationship of AA to EPSE

Acute akathisia and EPSE share some clinical and pathophysiological features, and there is overlap between the two syndromes. Both are acute side-effects of neuroleptics, with a roughly similar time of onset after drug initiation and relationship with drug dosage and type (more with high potency). Like akathisia, the majority of patients develop EPSE in the first 2–3 weeks after drug initiation (Freyhan, 1959; Ayd, 1961; Medinar et al, 1962). Ayd (1961) reported that EPSE developed slightly later than akathisia, but 90% of his patients had developed it, like akathisia, in the first 72 days. It is therefore not surprising that the two often co-occur in the patient. There is some evidence that there may be a shared vulnerability to the two syndromes, since they have a better than chance correlation. In the AA study, the objective akathisia score had a significant correlation with the EPSE score on days 7 ($r = .25$, $p < .05$) and 14 ($r = .40$, $p < .001$). The same was true for the total akathisia scores (.30 on both days, $p < .01$). The correlations were significant ($p < .01$, .05) for elbow rigidity and tremor, respectively. In the same study, the EPSE score emerged as the most significant risk factor for akathisia. In other words, patients who developed marked EPSE were also more likely to develop akathisia. In the Braude et al (1983) study, while there was no association between the severity of akathisia and the peak parkinsonism scores, one-third of patients had a peak parkinsonian score of 1.6 or more on the Simpson and Angus scale. The authors reported that the subgroup of akathisics who also had EPSE tended to respond to anticholinergic drugs (6 out of 9) whereas the others did not (0 out of 12). This study, therefore, suggested that there may be two subgroups of akathisia – those with and without EPSE – with different pharmacological profiles. The latter observation remains to be systematically examined. In a double-blind, iv challenge study (Sachdev and Loneragan, 1993b), 3 of the 4 patients who responded to benztropine had tremor and 2 had rigidity, and both conditions improved. The results were, therefore, consistent with the preceding suggestion, although our sample was too small to address the question specifically. Sandyk and Kay (1990b) examined the relationship between akathisia and parkinsonism in 123 long-term-medicated elderly schizophrenic patients and found no significant differences in akathisia in patients with and without parkinsonism. The parkinsonian patients were older, however. It must be stated that the authors were possibly dealing with CA or TA rather than AA.

In conclusion, the research evidence suggests that there may be an overlap between the two syndromes, with possibly some shared vulnerability. It is also possible that the akathisics with EPSE may show a different pharmacological profile. In spite of this, the two should be considered pathophysiologically different syndromes, and akathisia should not be considered another symptom of parkinsonism. The classical literature considers bradykinesia, tremor, rigidity and postural instability as the characteristic features of parkinsonism. In the AA study, tremor and elbow rigidity showed a higher correlation with each other (day 7, $r = .53$, $p < .001$) than with akathisia (correlation of tremor and rigidity with global akathisia scores on day 7, .44 and .25, respectively). Akathisia is not a prominent feature of idiopathic parkinsonism (PD), although it is known to occur (see Chapter 8). The majority of patients with akathisia do not have EPSE, and the pharmacological responsiveness of the two are different, with EPSE usually showing an excellent response to ACh antagonists, from which only a proportion of akathisics derive benefit. This distinction has implications for the understanding of the pathophysiology of akathisia as will be discussed in Chapter 10.

Acute akathisia and tardive dyskinesia

Both the AA and the Braude et al studies suggested a lack of association of AA with orofacial dyskinesia. This is not surprising since AA is an acute syndrome, whereas the latter is a late-onset side-effect, often occurring months or years after the initiation of medication. It is possible, however, for a patient with orofacial TD to develop AA due to recent drug exposure or change in type or dosage of neuroleptic. This is analogous to the co-occurrence of TD and DIP. In the AA study, while no subjects met the diagnostic criteria for TD, a number of them received positive scores on some items, in particular those pertaining to limb and truncal movements. The limb–truncal dyskinesia scores had a positive correlation with the sum of objective akathisia item scores (day 7, $r = .29$, $p < .01$; day 14, $r = .23$, $p < .05$). This was interpreted to reflect the difficulty in distinguishing some akathisic movements from dyskinetic ones when they involved the limbs, in particular the lower limbs.

It has been suggested that the development of severe akathisia as an acute side-effect may be a risk factor for the later development of TD. This hypothesis was originally put forward by Crane (1972), who regarded vulnerability to severe early-onset EPSE as a risk factor for subsequent TD. Chouinard et al (1979) added their clinical observations to suggest that patients with 'hyperkinetic' symptoms (tremor or akathisia) were more likely to develop TD than those with 'hypokinetic' symptoms such as bradykinesia and rigidity. DeVeaugh-Geiss (1982) suggested that akathisia may be a stage in the progression from parkinsonism to TD. Goswami, Channabasavanna and Gaswami (1984) reported a patient with bipolar affective disorder who, on therapeutic doses of lithium, developed severe akathisia which worsened with a chlorpromazine challenge, and 2 weeks later developed orofacial and lower-limb dyskinesia following the addition of an anticholinergic drug. Barnes and Braude (1984) reported two patients who developed AA that persisted, despite the reduction of drug dosages to maintenance levels, and seemed to herald the onset of TD. In chronic schizophrenics, TA and TD often coexist (Barnes and Braude, 1985; Gibb and Lees, 1986a; Burke et al, 1989; TA study). A proportion of this so-called TA is chronic persistent akathisia, ie, akathisia that develops as AA but tends to become chronic. This may be argued to suggest that some AA may lead to CA and TD. Longitudinal studies specifically examining early AA as a risk factor for TD are lacking. A few investigators have examined EPSE in general. Jus, Pineau and colleagues (Jus et al, 1976; Pineau et al, 1976), in a retrospective study of 300 subjects, found that past history of EPSE was the same in those with or without TD. In two separate studies from the Hillside Hospital in New York (Kane et al, 1986; Kane, 1990; Saltz et al, 1991), the early occurrence of EPSE was found to be associated with at least a threefold increase in the risk of TD in both young adult and elderly subjects. Nasrallah et al (1980) and Munetz (1980) made similar observations with regard to acute drug-induced dystonia.

In conclusion, while there seems to be little association between AA and TD cross-sectionally, there is a suggestion that longitudinally such an association may exist, with AA being a forerunner of TD in some cases. The frequent overlap between CA and TD is well recognized, and the persistence of some AA into chronicity may explain the association of AA with later TD. That akathisia is a transitional state between EPSE and TD has very limited support in the literature, and the course of development of EPSE and akathisia, as discussed earlier, argues against this hypothesis.

Differential diagnosis

The subjective and motor behaviours associated with akathisia must be distinguished from those of a number of other disorders. In addition, some disorders manifest both features. The diagnosis can therefore be difficult, and the following features should be recognized so that an early diagnosis of AA can be made.

Distinctive features

While no one feature of AA is diagnostic, the combination of an experience of restlessness especially referable to the legs and an inability to keep the legs still, with some characteristic movements – such as shifting weight from foot to foot, crossing/uncrossing of legs, shifting of body position in a chair and pacing – is very suggestive of akathisia. The patient is, except in the very severe cases, able to suppress the movements voluntarily for at least a short period. There is, nevertheless, a driven or unnatural quality to the restlessness in akathisia (Kendler, 1976) which may help to distinguish it from other kinds of restlessness. The movements are semipurposive and give the impression of voluntariness to an observer, while also being usually accepted by the patient as voluntary. Some involuntary movements in the form of myoclonic jerks may, however, occur in akathisia. The movements show considerable variation with posture, time of day, mental state and extraneous activities the patient is engaged in. Repeat examinations, and observation of the patient in an informal setting, may therefore be of assistance. The diagnosis is especially difficult in very mild cases and for acutely psychotic individuals who do not provide a very detailed account of their subjective experience or are unable to distinguish the distress of the psychiatric disorder from that produced by akathisia.

Proximity to the drug

The knowledge that the patient was recently treated with a neuroleptic or other drug known to cause akathisia should result in a high index of suspicion for the disorder. A recent introduction or dosage increase or change in type of drug may be responsible. By definition, this is an essential, though not sufficient, cause of AA. By the definition proposed in this book (Chapter 4), the drug event (introduction or change) should have happened in the preceding 6 weeks, and certainly in the preceding 3 months, with the patient currently on the drug.

Pharmacological response

In case of doubt about the diagnosis, a reduction in the drug dosage is helpful and will improve AA but worsen psychiatric agitation or anxiety. An increase in dose will usually lead to a worsening of AA, which is unacceptable as a diagnostic strategy. The response to ACh antagonists has previously been proposed as a diagnostic test, but this is likely to result in a number of false negatives, as not all patients with AA respond to these drugs. Further, an iv challenge may be inferior to a trial of oral medication, but the latter will be a much slower diagnostic process and may function more appropriately as a 'therapeutic trial of medication' which will in turn reinforce the diagnosis. A response to βA drugs has similar limitations and is also complicated by the anti-anxiety effect of these drugs. Adler et al (1986) reported that propranolol was more likely to benefit akathisia than anxiety. The reverse holds for an anxiolytic drug like lorazepam.

Disorders that produce similar subjective distress, with or without the motor features

These disorders, which should be considered in the differential diagnosis, were discussed in Chapter 2 under restlessness. They will be mentioned only briefly here.

Psychotic agitation

Since patients in whom akathisia is suspected are usually also psychotic, the differentiation between the two is paramount. The patient may be unable to distinguish akathisia from psychotic agitation but may complain of worsening because of the medication. The presence of the agitation prior to neuroleptic treatment and its improvement with the drugs helps the differentiation. The patient with psychotic agitation will not localize the symptoms especially to the legs and will not complain of an inability to keep the legs still. The motor disturbance of agitation is more generalized and is often chaotic, disorganized and even frenzied. It does not have the typical features of akathisia described earlier.

Anxiety

The subjective experience of anxiety is qualitatively different from that of akathisia, with the former leading to worry and inner turmoil. The anxious individual may pace restlessly, moving arms and legs aimlessly, but the characteristic movements of akathisia are usually lacking, as is the reference to the lower limbs. The autonomic arousal of anxiety is not a prominent feature of akathisia, although akathisia may secondarily produce anxiety. The setting, the usual absence of drugs that produce akathisia, history and exacerbating and relieving factors will usually help distinguish anxiety from AA, but the two may co-occur. Further, the cognitive symptoms of vigilance and scanning associated with anxiety are not present in akathisia. A trial of a benzodiazepine drug may be helpful.

Nonakathisia neuroleptic dysphoria

Patients may have a dysphoric response to neuroleptic drugs from a variety of causes, as has been discussed in Chapter 3. They may be distressed by the bradykinesia, rigidity or tremor produced by the drugs or may complain of cognitive slowing, lack of concentration, derealization, etc as side-effects with consequent dysphoria. They may also misattribute their illness-related restlessness or dysphoria to the neuroleptics. A detailed analysis of the symptoms should, however, distinguish these reactions from akathisia without much difficulty except for the very mild cases. The relationship of both akathisia and other drug-induced dysphoria with drug dosage makes pharmacological strategies less easy to apply.

Agitation associated with organic disorders

As discussed earlier, agitation may be an important feature of delirium, dementia, head injury, hypoglycemia, etc, as discussed in Chapter 2. This agitation is qualitatively different from akathisia and often manifests in the form of general restlessness, pacing, complaining, repetitive sentences or questions, negativism, constant requests for attention and cursing or verbal aggression. The typical motor symptoms of akathisia, with their reference to the lower limbs, are usually lacking. There is an associated disorientation and confusion in most cases that will help one arrive at a diagnosis. Neuroleptics control the agitation, but ACh antagonists will often make it worse. A difficulty arises in situations in which the possibility of superimposed akathisia exists, when a reduction of neuroleptic dose may be necessary for the diagnosis to be clarified.

Agitation of affective disorder

Agitation is a feature of both endogenous and nonendogenous depressions and has been described in Chapter 2. The typical picture of agitation is seen in endogenous depression. Patients usually fidget a great deal, shift position continually in a chair, play with their fingers or whatever they are holding and rock, and in more severe cases may have an inability to sit, with a tendency to pace up and down and tear at their hands and face, manifesting a picture of extreme anguish. The particular reference to the legs, as in akathisia, is usually lacking, but if the agitated person tries to control his or her agitation by gripping something or holding on firmly to the arms of a chair, the motor activity in the arms and body may cease but may become apparent in the form of restless legs and feet. The agitation usually responds to neuroleptic drugs.

The restlessness of hypomania may at first appear to be goal-directed and purposive, but as the disorder becomes severe, increasing disorganization sets in. The patient characteristically does not experience distress because of it and generally lacks insight.

Drug withdrawal syndromes

Withdrawal from alcohol, sedative-hypnotics, antidepressants, nicotine, opioids, etc can produce restlessness, but the differentiation from akathisia does not usually pose a problem when the appropriate history is available.

The 'jitteriness' syndrome

This syndrome (see Chapter 2 for details) was reported in some panic disorder patients who were treated with TCAs (Zitrin et al, 1978, 1980; Pohl et al, 1988), and comprises restlessness, trouble sitting still, 'shakiness inside', insomnia, increased energy and anxiety. While this closely resembles the subjective experience of akathisia, the reference to the lower limbs often seen in akathisia is usually lacking. The motor features of jitteriness have not been described in detail, but the suggestion from the reports is that the characteristic lower-limb movements and inability to maintain posture of akathisia are mostly lacking. Jitteriness seems to respond to benzodiazepines and phenothiazines, arguing for a different pharmacological profile from AA.

Restless legs syndrome

The major differences between AA and RLS are presented in Table 12.5. A detailed history and examination of the features should enable a fairly definitive differentiation between the two syndromes.

Hysteria and malingering

It is interesting that Haskovec's diagnosis in one of his first two patients was hysteria. This probably reflected the diagnostic practices at the time, but it is not inconceivable that hysteria may mimic akathisia. Psychiatric patients have ready models for the disorder, either in a past experience of akathisia or by witnessing another patient suffer from it. Akathisia can be dramatic and attract considerable attention and intervention. In our experience, the occurrence of akathisia symptoms as a conversion reaction is rare. A careful history, an examination of the premorbid personality, exploration for any stressors and the establishment of secondary gain all help in the diagnosis.

Malingering is difficult to distinguish from a conversion reaction, and an obvious material gain will usually have to be demonstrated. One possibility to consider is that the patient abuses ACh antagonists, such as benzhexol, or benzodiazepines and uses the complaint of akathisia to obtain a prescription. This again is difficult to distinguish from a genuine response of akathisia to benzhexol, lorazepam, etc. The clinician should beware of an escalating dosage of benzhexol or benztropine. In case of doubt, it may be reasonable to treat the akathisia with a nonaddicting drug like propranolol.

Disorders with similar motor features but without the subjective distress

As discussed earlier, in AA, motor features are unusual in the absence of subjective distress. The subjective report may not always be available, however, especially in the psychotic patient, and the clinician may have to depend solely on observations to make a diagnosis. It is in such cases that differentiation from other disorders with similar movements becomes necessary.

Stereotypies and mannerisms

Psychotic patients untreated with medication may demonstrate a range of hyperkinesias. Stereotypies and mannerisms are of interest because of their superficial similarity with some akathisic movements. Stereotypies are spontaneous, goal-directed behaviours that are repeated in a uniform manner and often retain remnants of purposive behaviour or symbolic significance (Manschreck, 1986). Some common stereotypies seen in schizophrenic patients are continuous movement in and out of a chair, crossing oneself, waving repeatedly in the air, touching objects over and over and grasping one's hands or clothes continuously. Mannerisms are unusual, frequently stilted variations in the performance of normal, goal-directed movements such as greeting, shaking hands or writing. Stereotypies and mannerisms are ego-syntonic, and the individual derives satisfaction from their performance or at least does not exhibit any distress because of them. They are more likely to occur when the patient is otherwise unoccupied and may not be prominent during a formal examination by the doctor. A history from an informant will suggest their presence prior to the initiation of neuroleptics, and these drugs are likely to reduce their frequency and intensity. Stereotypies and mannerisms are more difficult to differentiate from TA rather than AA.

Tremors

A tremor is a regular, rhythmic movement of a part of the body, resulting from alternate contractions of agonist and antagonist muscles. Generally, tremors are not likely to be confused with akathisic movements, with the latter being irregular and arrhythmic. The tremor of NIP most commonly involves the hands, tongue, jaw and toes, but the lower limbs and the whole body may be involved. It is best seen during voluntary movement but may be present at rest. The patient may be distressed, but this is usually secondary to the presence of tremor. It has a high correlation with other parkinsonian features such as rigidity and bradykinesia. There are a number of other causes of tremor (Young, 1992) and many manifestations of it, but these are unlikely to be confused with akathisia. Essentially, it is severe neuroleptic-induced tremor that affects the limbs or the whole body that may occasionally be misdiagnosed as akathisia. Additionally, it may coexist with akathisia, when both should be diagnosed.

Drug-induced dyskinesia

Dyskinetic movements are choreic (rapid, jerky, nonrepetitive), athetoid (slow, sinuous, continuous) or choreoathetoid and may affect any part of the body. They are reduced by voluntary movement of the body part, and increased when unaffected parts are moved. When dyskinesias affect the limbs, they may be confused with akathisia. A close examination of the phenomenology, as well as the drug history, will usually reveal the true diagnosis.

The most important syndrome in this category is TD, which is a delayed side-effect of chronic neuroleptic use and is important in the diagnosis of TA rather than AA. Acute akathisia may, however, develop in patients who suffer from TD, and it may become important to differentiate the features of the two. Dyskinesias may occur less commonly early in the course of neuroleptic treatment, with a prevalence of 2.3% reported in one study (Ayd, 1961). These dyskinesias are dosage related and respond well to ACh and histamine antagonists. They may be associated with acute dystonias that commonly affect the eye, neck and throat.

Dyskinesias may develop secondary to drugs other than neuroleptics. Acute dyskinesias have been described with L-dopa, amphetamines, caffeine, phenytoin, oestrogens, lithium and chloroquine. L-Dopa and amphetamines can also lead to a delayed development of dyskinesias, which still improve upon dosage reduction.

Myoclonus

Myoclonus refers to a sudden, irregular contraction of a muscle or a group of muscles, triggered by an event in the CNS (Marsden, 1980). The presence of myoclonic jerks in akathisia has already been discussed earlier in this chapter. Myoclonus may be associated with generalized epilepsy or with a number of other neurological disorders. In itself, myoclonic jerks are unlikely to be mistaken for akathisia, but their occurrence in delirium or dementia may sometimes create diagnostic difficulties.

Other movement disorders

Some patients with chronic motor tic or Tourette's syndrome may appear restless and have movements associated with a subjective feeling of distress, a compulsion to move and an ability to suppress the movements for short periods. The presence of facial and vocal tics as well as other symptoms such as coprolalia, echophenomena, an onset in early childhood, a remitting and relapsing but chronic course, the familial loading and the response of the tics to neuroleptics all help to distinguish this from akathisia.

Other movement disorders such as Huntington's disease, Wilson's disease, Sydenham's chorea and Fahr's syndrome rarely pose any diagnostic problems with akathisia except in the rare case when psychosis coexists with these disorders. Features resembling akathisia may occasionally occur in encephalitis, and in fact some of the early descriptions of akathisia were in relation to epidemic encephalitis.

Endocrine/metabolic disorders

Patients with hyperthyroidism may exhibit restlessness and choreiform movements of the limbs that may be confused with akathisia (Klawans, 1973). The presence of other features of thyrotoxicosis, and laboratory tests, will quickly establish the diagnosis.

Some features of hypoparathyroidism, such as numbness and cramps of the limbs, paraesthesiae and, uncommonly, choreiform movements may rarely signify a differential diagnosis. Laboratory evidence of hypocalcaemia, hyperphosphataemia, decreased urinary calcium and increased calcifications in the brain will establish the diagnosis.

7

Clinical characteristics of tardive and chronic akathisia

Introduction

The evidence for a tardive akathisia syndrome

There are a number of reasons why TA has not been universally accepted as a distinct syndrome. First, there is a relative dearth of investigations into this disorder. While TD has been extensively studied and a number of monographs on it have been published, only a few studies on TA have appeared in print. Second, no one feature of TA (discussed later) is pathognomonic of the disorder. While certain subjective reports and some motor signs can be considered to be highly characteristic, similar features can be seen in a number of other disorders. Akathisia is often mistakenly diagnosed (and dismissed) as restlessness or agitation, without a close analysis of the clinical features. A diagnostic laboratory investigation is not available, leaving the diagnosis to the vagaries of clinical judgement. Third, the strong overlap between TA and TD has suggested to some authors that TA should not be categorized as a separate disorder, but rather as a variation of the manifestations of TD. This has resulted in a reduced emphasis on the investigation of TA. Fourth, a temporal cause-and-effect relationship between neuroleptics and TA is difficult to establish. Not all patients treated with neuroleptics develop TA. It is a side-effect that develops after months or years of neuroleptic use. This is in contrast to AA, which develops within hours or days of drug initiation, thus establishing a more definitive causal relationship. Further, it may persist for months or years after the withdrawal of the neuroleptic drug and may possibly become irreversible, further confounding the temporal relationship. Fifth, the pharmacological profile of TA is not clearly understood, and no one drug is uniformly successful in its treatment. Dopaminergic, noradrenergic, cholinergic, opioid and other neurotransmitter systems have been implicated. Akathisia may first become apparent upon the reduction or cessation of medication, and neuroleptic drugs may in fact mask the symptoms of the disorder.

This phenomenological heterogeneity is similar to that of TD and has further hampered the recognition of TA as a distinct syndrome.

In spite of these difficulties, there is increasing acceptance that a syndrome of TA does exist. Some of the evidence presented in its favour follows.

There is convincing anecdotal evidence that akathisia can develop as a delayed side-effect of neuroleptic medication, may first become evident upon reduction of neuroleptic dosage and may persist for months or years after the drug is no longer administered. This is similar to the clinical profile of TD.

Kruse (1960a) first reported three patients who developed 'muscular restlessness' (he did not use the term *akathisia*) that persisted for 3–18 months after the cessation of phenothiazines. Braude and Barnes (1983) reported two patients who developed late-onset akathisia characterized by emergence towards the end of each depot neuroleptic injection interval. Gardos et al (1987) reported two cases of TA, although it is uncertain if these patients did not have an acute-onset akathisia that became chronic. Yassa and Bloom (1990) reported a patient who developed an acute-onset akathisia 3 months after the initiation of 75 mg/month pipotiazide but which persisted for 6 months after the cessation of the drug. Sachdev and Chee (1990) reported a patient with a delayed-onset and persistent akathisia, and Sachdev and Loneragan (1993c) investigated seven patients who met the modified Burke et al (1989) criteria for TA. Some other anecdotal reports suggesting late onset and persistence are described in Chapter 5 on epidemiology (see also Hunter et al, 1964; Kennedy et al, 1971; Shearer et al, 1984; Barnes and Braude, 1985; Gibb and Lees, 1986a; Yassa et al, 1988; Burke et al, 1989; Yassa and Groulx, 1989; Miller and Jankovic, 1990; Sachdev and Loneragan, 1993a,c).

Onset of akathisic symptoms upon drug withdrawal has also been described by a number of authors (Hunter et al, 1964; Evans, 1965; Demars, 1966; Kennedy, 1969; Braude and Barnes, 1983; Lang, 1994). Dufresne and Wagner (1988) systematically examined for akathisia patients recently withdrawn from a neuroleptic, but unfortunately they did not report patients' status at baseline.

The most detailed evidence of the persistence of TA comes from the study by Burke et al (1989). In the 26 patients with TA in whom the neuroleptic drug was discontinued, akathisia persisted for 2.7 ± 0.4 years (range 0.3–7 years).

The phenomenological examination of patients on long-term neuroleptic medication suggests that TA is distinct from TD, with overlap between the two. TA has a characteristic profile of signs and symptoms, which will be detailed in this chapter. Later, the relationship between TA and TD and TDt is examined. TA can occur in the absence of TD, and vice versa, but the two often co-occur.

The pharmacological profile of TA is probably distinct from that of both AA and TD, although this awaits further research. While some aspects, such as a therapeutic response to DA-depleting drugs (eg, tetrabenazine, reserpine) (Burke et al, 1989; Sachdev and Loneragan, 1993c) and an improvement with a low-dosage apomorphine challenge (Sachdev and Loneragan, 1993c), are similar to TD, the improvement of some patients with ACh antagonists (Sachdev and Chee, 1990; Sachdev and Loneragan, 1993a) is contrary to the expectation for TD. The response to βA antagonists, benzodiazepines, opiates, etc is variable, but the suggestion is that TA behaves differently from AA (Sachdev and Chee, 1990; Sachdev and Loneragan, 1993a).

The prevalence studies of TA have been discussed in Chapter 5 and highlight the fact that given the limitations of the definition, the syndrome that meets the description of TA is common, perhaps as common as TD in some patient populations. Regarding it as a distinct syndrome has the added advantage of promoting further research.

Direct evidence for the existence of the TA syndrome can come from prospective long-term studies of patients assessed at baseline and followed up while being maintained on neuroleptics. Strictly speaking, the studies should have a control group of patients treated with a placebo, and be double-blind. However, such a study would be impossible because of the ethical and practical objections. There are currently some longitudinal studies of schizophrenia in progress, and the issue of tardive emergence of akathisia could be addressed in these studies (eg, Kane et al, 1988; Morgenstern and Glazer, 1993).

Tardive and chronic: is there a difference?

In this book, we have proposed a differential usage of the two terms; *tardive* denotes a delayed onset, whereas *chronic* refers to the duration of akathisia irrespective of the nature of onset. It is possible that much of TA reported in the literature is also chronic (ie, present for more than 3 months). The reverse, however, is not true, and descriptions of CA do not necessarily imply a tardive onset. Akathisia differs from drug-induced dyskinesia in this respect. Whereas dyskinesia (excluding dystonia) due to neuroleptics is almost invariably (with the rare exception of 'paradoxical dyskinesia') a delayed-onset side-effect, akathisia may start early and persist, or may develop later. Akathisia in long-term-medicated patients can therefore be of either acute or delayed (tardive) onset. The research literature is deficient in that it does not attempt to distinguish clearly between a late onset and a chronic course. For purposes of clinical description, therefore, the two terms are used interchangeably in this section of the book. Further, some investigators (eg, Gibb and Lees, 1986a) describe akathisia in chronic schizophrenic patients without attempting to exclude AA consequent upon recent drug administration. These deficiencies limit the description of TA, a clearer description of which will emerge as more studies using strict criteria become available.

Important studies

The following description is derived largely from four studies – Barnes and Braude (1985), Gibb and Lees (1986a), Burke et al (1989), and the TA/CA study – which are first briefly outlined.

Barnes and Braude (1985) examined 82 depot clinic patients over 3 months and diagnosed 23 to suffer from CA and 10 from pseudoakathisia. The CA subjects had both subjective and objective symptoms of akathisia, while the pseudoakathisia subjects had only the objective features.

Gibb and Lees (1986a) studied the subjective and objective features of akathisia in two separate populations. The subjective symptoms were studied by questionnaire completed at an informal interview with 95 young schizophrenic patients attending a depot neuroleptic clinic. The motor symptoms were investigated in 171 long-term (>1 year) inpatients of a psychiatric hospital who were noted to be hyperkinetic, a proportion of whom were akathisic. The majority (73.6%) of the latter were also schizophrenic, with the rest suffering from dementia (22.6%) or affective disorder (3.6%). While this study offers an excellent description of the phenomena, its main limitation for our purposes is the lack of any attempt to subtype akathisia. The authors purportedly described 'akathisia', not any particular subtype, but since the patients were long-term-hospitalized patients on neuroleptics and often suffered from orofacial dyskinesia, it can be argued that the akathisia in them was probably of the chronic or tardive subtype.

Burke et al (1989) described the clinical features of 52 patients – seen in two specialized movement disorder clinics (31 at Columbia-Presbyterian Medical Center in New York and 21 at Baylor College of Medicine in Houston) – who met diagnostic criteria for TA on retrospective chart review. The diagnostic criteria used are listed in Chapter 4, and TA referred to all DA-antagonist-induced, persistent (>1 month) akathisias, regardless of their time of onset in relation to drug treatment. The major limitations of the study were that it was retrospective and conducted in tertiary neurological centres, making it possibly unrepresentative of the true TA population.

The TA/CA study was briefly described in Chapter 5. Signs and symptoms were examined in TA/CA patients using research criteria for the diagnosis in a sample of 100 stable, long-term-medicated schizophrenic patients.

Much of the description of AA also applies to TA, at least as far as current empirical observation is concerned. The following description will emphasize the features that distinguish the tardive syndrome from the acute one.

Demographic factors

Age

Since increasing age has consistently emerged as a risk factor for TD (Jeste and Caligiuri, 1993), the relationship between age and TA is of interest. The research data are, however, insufficient to make any definitive statement on this. In the Barnes and Braude study, the CA subjects (mean age 44.4 ± 12.9 years) were somewhat older than the AA subjects (33.5 ± 9.1 years), but no different from the nonakathisics (44.2 ± 12.1 years). The younger age of the AA group probably reflects the recent onset of illness in them. Interestingly, the pseudoakathisia group was older (51.0 ± 13.0 years). In our TA/CA study, the TA group ($n = 31$, mean 40.1 years) was not different from the non-akathisic, nondyskinetic group ($n = 35$, mean 38.9 years), whereas the TD subjects were older ($n = 23$, mean 43.3 years, $p < .1$), in particular those with the OBLF syndrome ($n = 15$, mean 47.2 years, $p < .01$). The age of onset in the Burke et al subjects ranged from 21 to 82 years, with a mean of 58.4 ± 2.0 (SEM) years, with the men (54.1 ± 4.2 years) having a slightly earlier onset than women (60.9 ± 1.9 years). The age of first treatment in 44 patients was 53.2 ± 2.5 years.

In conclusion, two prevalence studies do not suggest that TA subjects are different in age from nonakathisic patients similarly exposed to neuroleptics. A retrospective clinic-based study found TA subjects to be mostly over 50 years of age, and they had been exposed to an average 5.2 years of neuroleptic treatment. It is possible that this reflects a selection bias, and further studies examining a wide age range are necessary. As will be discussed later, there is a strong overlap between TA and TD. If TD shows a strong association with age and TA does not, it would suggest two possible subsyndromes of TD, with or without akathisia. Previous investigators have argued for this subtyping, reporting differences between the OBLF and the limb–truncal (LT) dyskinesias (Kidger et al, 1980; Brown and White, 1992). Nine of the 11 TD dyskinesia patients in the TA/CA study had a global rating of mild to moderate akathisia. While the overlap between the OBLF syndrome and TA was also common, the greater overlap of TA with LT dyskinesia supports the notion that OBLF dyskinesia may indeed be a distinct syndrome. A note of caution is in order here: the movements of LT dyskinesia may be mistaken for akathisia and vice versa, thus making for diagnostic uncertainty that may erroneously present a picture of overlap.

Sex

The sex ratio of patients with TA in the Barnes and Braude and the TA/CA studies was similar to that in the control populations. It must be pointed out that the two samples comprised relatively young subjects, and it can be argued that sex may interact with age as a risk factor for TA. In the TD litera-ture, female sex as a vulnerability factor is robust only for the geriatric age group (American Psychiatric Association, 1992). There are a few studies on older, but not necessarily geriatric, populations in which the sex ratio was reported. In the Kennedy et al (1971) study which examined chronic schizo-phrenic inpatients, men (mean age 53.6 years) and women (mean age 60.4 years) were equally represented. In the Hunter et al (1964) study, patients in the 56–84 age group were examined, and all 13 patients with akathisia (possi-bly TA) were women. In the Burke et al series, the female to male ratio was 1.9:1, and this was, again, an older group of patients. The question of whether older women are more prone to TA, just as they are to TD, therefore remains open and further research is warranted.

Race and ethnicity

No published information on race and ethnicity is available.

Psychiatric diagnosis

Both the Barnes and Braude and the TA/CA studies were conducted on schiz-ophrenic patients, thus disallowing any examination of the role of the primary psychiatric disorder. The Gibb and Lees study did not examine the role of this variable. Burke et al reported that while all disorders treated with neuroleptics were represented, there was a notably high proportion of patients with depres-sion (47%). Further study to examine this latter observation is warranted.

Onset

In retrospective studies, it is extremely difficult to establish the time of onset of TA with certainty. Barnes and Braude reported that 12 of 23 CA patients reported onset soon after a marked increase of neuroleptic drug, with the akathisia persisting for 7 months to many years. They called this 'acute persistent' akathisia. The remaining 11 patients reported the onset of symptoms in relation to dosage reduction, or in the week before the regular depot injection, thus suggesting a withdrawal onset. In the TA/CA study, we could not establish the onset with certainty. The TA subjects had been exposed to neuroleptics for a mean 14.0 (SD 9.0) years, which was not different from that of the nonakathisic nondyskinetic controls. Burke et al reported that the duration of exposure prior to onset ranged from 2 weeks to 22 years, with a mean of 4.5 (SD 0.75) years. The patient with onset after 2 weeks of exposure could be described as 'acute persistent'; she went on to have akathisia for 5 months even though neuroleptics were curtailed a month after onset. Tardive akathisia occurred in the first year of exposure in 15 patients, but they were not different in age from those who developed TA after more than 1 year's exposure.

The relationship between the duration of treatment with DA antagonists and the cumulative onset of TA in the Burke et al subjects is given in Fig. 7.1. About one-third of patients developed it in the first year, over one-half in the first 2 years. This may reflect a vulnerability to TA in these subjects, but no other features suggesting such a vulnerability were reported. TA continued to appear for the first time after 5 or 10 years of exposure, with one-fourth of patients developing it after 5 years, suggesting that the risk does not disappear after many years of treatment. The retrospective nature of this study limits its usefulness, and a prospective study is necessary to examine the development and natural history of TA.

Clinical features

As with AA, subjective and motor or behavioural manifestations of TA have been described in the different studies. The range of symptoms in the two syndromes is the same, but there is some difference in the relative prevalence of different symptoms. There may also be qualitative differences in the manifestation of some symptoms and signs. We will examine this later.

Subjective features

The patient reports are very similar to those in AA, with spontaneous complaints of 'feelings of restlessness', 'legs go all the time', 'feel compelled to move my legs', 'cannot stop pumping my legs', 'feelings of fidgetiness or

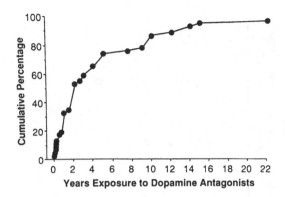

Fig. 7.1. The cumulative percentage of patients ($N = 45$) with tardive akathisia in relation to the years of exposure to a dopamine antagonist as reported by Burke et al (1989). (Reproduced with permission.)

nervousness', 'cannot sit in one place', compelled to get up and walk', 'a tortured sort of feeling', etc. Patients are frequently distressed by inner restlessness and complain of an inability to remain still or to keep their legs still. Burke et al reported that all their patients experienced inner restlessness. In our series, an inability to keep legs still was the most common subjective report, with the complaint of inner restlessness being present in about 55% of cases, by one diagnostic system. Table 7.1 gives the percentage of patients with different subjective features in two studies. It has been suggested that the subjective distress of TA is not as great as that of AA (Barnes and Braude, 1985), and our clinical experience and findings from the TA/CA and AA studies point in the same direction. Table 7.2 presents a comparison of the symptoms of TA/CA and AA in our two studies. The proportion of patients with the different symptoms in the two studies was not significantly different, with the exception that inner restlessness was more common in AA. The figures do not refer to the severity of the particular symptoms, but this was greater in the AA group. In the Barnes and Braude report, 4 of 6 AA subjects and only 6 of 23 CA subjects had moderate to severe associated distress. These authors also reported less limb paraesthesiae in TA. The theme of reduced distress in CA or TA will be taken up later in regard to the longitudinal history of akathisia and the concept of pseudoakathisia. The reasons for this reduced distress could be varied: the development of 'tolerance' over a period of time, reduced emotional responsiveness because of flattening of affect in chronic schizophrenia or a lack of reporting because of apathy and

Table 7.1. *Percentage of akathisic and nonakathisic patients with different subjective and objective features*

Feature	TA/CA study		Barnes and Braude		
	Akathisia (TA/CA) (n = 31)	Nonakathisia (n = 68)	Chronic akathisia (n = 23)	Pseudo-akathisia (n = 10)	Nonakathisia (n = 43)
Subjective					
Distressing sensations in the limbs	35.8	14.7	30	0	9
Feeling of inner restlessness	54.9	13.2	87	20	30
Inability to remain still, standing/sitting	61.3	22.1	87	0	19
Inability to keep legs still	74.2	19.1	96	0	14
Objective					
Sitting					
Inability to remain seated	6.5	0	9	0	0
Semipurposeful/purposeless normal leg/foot movements	93.5	44.1	91	80	33
Inability to keep toes still	38.7	10.3	—	—	—
Shifting body position in chair	54.8	10.3	39	20	0
Semipurposeful hand/arm movements	—	—	65	60	33

Standing					
Shifting weight from foot to foot and/or walking in one spot	29.0	3.0	83	100	0
Other purposeless (normal) foot movements	54.8	4.4	9	20	0
Inability to remain standing in one spot (walking or pacing)	3.2	0	22	0	0
Lying[a]					
Coarse tremor of legs/feet	0	0	—	—	—
Myoclonic jerks of the feet	4.2	0	—	—	—
Semipurposeful or purposeless leg/foot movements	2.5	0	34	10	0
Inability to remain lying down	0	0	4	0	0

[a]Some data are missing ($n = 7$–12) on these items in the TA/CA study.
Source: Data from the TA/CA and Barnes and Braude (1985) studies.

Table 7.2. *A comparison of the clinical features of acute akathisia (AA study) and tardive/chronic akathisia (TA/CA study) (percent)*

Feature	Acute (n = 32)	Tardive/chronic (n = 31)
Subjective		
Distressing sensations in the limbs	43.7	35.8
Feeling of inner restlessness	88.2	54.9
Inability to remain still, standing/sitting	59.4	61.3
Inability to keep legs still	56.2	74.2
Objective		
Sitting		
Inability to remain seated	37.2	6.5
Semipurposeful/purposeless normal leg/foot movements	65.6	93.5
Inability to keep toes still	43.7	38.7
Shifting body position in chair	58.1	54.8
Semipurposeful hand/arm movements	31.2	—
Standing		
Shifting weight from foot to foot and/or walking in one spot	65.6	29.0
Other purposeless (normal) foot movements	53.1	54.8
Inability to remain standing in one spot (walking or pacing)	31.2	3.2
Lying[a]		
Coarse tremor of legs/feet	18.1	0
Myoclonic jerks of the feet	19.4	4.2
Semipurposeful or purposeless leg/foot movements	45.2	2.5
Inability to remain lying down	25.8	0

[a]Some of these items are missing in the TA/CA study.

poverty of speech. In the TA/CA study, the ratings of TA showed a robust association with negative symptoms and a consistent association with poor performance on some neuropsychological tests.

Behavioural analogues of tardive akathisia

Unlike AA, TA has not been generally associated with behavioural symptoms. This is difficult to understand if one accepts that subjective distress is a significant aspect of TA. It may be because of a lack of appreciation by psychiatrists of the frequency with which TA occurs. More probably, it is because AA is more distressing, occurs acutely and is more likely to be misconstrued by the patient because of its overlap with an acute psychiatric disturbance. Furthermore, some of the behavioural analogues of AA, as discussed previously, were accurately diagnosed when the response to an anticholinergic drug or a reduction in the neuroleptic dosage was used as diagnostic information. Such a strategy is unlikely to work in the case of TA (since the pharmacological responsiveness in TA is much less predictable), making any behavioural analogue of TA more difficult to recognize. There is no theoretical reason why TA cannot or should not lead to an exacerbation of psychotic symptoms, although in our TA/CA study, akathisic and non-akathisic subjects did not differ in their scores on the 'psychosis' items of the Brief Psychiatric Rating Scale (Overall and Gorham, 1962). Similarly, it is possible that TA leads to impulsivity, thus causing aggressiveness or violence. Whether TA, like AA, leads to increased noncompliance remains to be investigated.

A syndrome of tardive dysbehaviour has been described which may be argued to have some overlap with TA or, more correctly, with WA. Gualtieri et al (1984), in their study of the effects of the cessation of neuroleptics in children and adolescents, reported acute behavioural deterioration in 4 of 41 subjects. This manifested as insomnia, hyperactivity, aggression, screaming, running and agitation, symptoms that were clearly different from the ones that had led to the original treatment. The deterioration lasted less than 8 weeks. A similar case was reported by Caine et al (1978) in a 15-year-old Tourette's syndrome patient, but no such cases have been reported in adults. Other tardive behavioural syndromes have been described as analogous to TD and TA, after the initial suggestion for the existence of such syndromes was made by Davis and Rosenberg (1979). Two syndromes have particularly been debated: supersensitivity psychosis (SP) and tardive dysmentia (TDys).

The existence of SP has been argued mainly by Guy Chouinard and his colleagues (Chouinard et al, 1978, 1982, 1986; Chouinard and Jores, 1980; Chouinard, 1982), who emphasized the following features: (i) a rapid return of psychotic symptoms during or following withdrawal or dosage reduction of the neuroleptic (within 6 weeks for oral and 3 months for depot neuroleptic); (ii) exacerbations of psychosis characterized by positive symptoms; (iii) tolerance to the antipsychotic effect of neuroleptics, necessitating an increase of neuroleptic dosage; and (iv) dramatic improvement usually shown when antipsychotic drugs are readministered. Chouinard et al (1986) surveyed 234 schizophrenic patients attending day care and reported that 22% had definite and 21% borderline SP. The borderline cases had either relapsed slowly or shown only tolerance without evidence of relapse upon dosage reduction. In spite of the first Chouinard paper on this topic appearing in 1978, only a few case reports supporting the concept have been published by other investigators (Csernansky and Hollister, 1982; Cole et al, 1984). Some other case reports of a rapid relapse of psychosis (manic or schizophreniform), or its emergence for the first time, have been published (Sale and Kristall, 1978; Kent and Wilber, 1982; Ekblom et al, 1984; Witschy et al, 1984; Perenyi et al, 1985). In none of these reports was there any suggestion that the patients suffered from WA that could have led to the exacerbation of psychosis. The argument generally presented by the proponents of the concept is that SP is a consequence of the supersensitivity of limbic DA receptors. By this argument, if the disorder does exist, it is likely to co-occur with WA rather than be a consequence of the distress seen in the latter.

Following Chouinard's reports, three groups of investigators examined their data for the evidence of SP. Weinberger et al (1981) noted that of the 20 chronic schizophrenic patients withdrawn off neuroleptics, 10 worsened, 5 of them markedly, and 3 improved in the subsequent 4 weeks. Four had an initial worsening followed by an improvement. Schooler et al (1982) assigned 67 patients, who had been on maintenance oral fluphenazine or fluphenazine decanoate for 1 year, to oral fluphenazine or placebo. Over the succeeding 15 weeks, the oral fluphenazine patients who were given the active drug had a relapse rate of 33% and the placebo group 59%, with most relapses occurring in the first 3 weeks. The relapse rate had a modest correlation with the emergence of dyskinetic symptoms, although akathisic symptoms were not described. This study supported the presence of some form of DA supersensitivity. However, the placebo patients also had their antiparkinsonian medication suspended, which complicates the interpretation of the results. Borison et al (1988) reported a rapid worsening of psychosis following the cessation of clozapine, but this may be related to the pharmacokinetics of the drug.

In summary, the evidence for the existence of SP is tentative, and since the natural history of untreated schizophrenia, or that treated only with small doses of low-potency neuroleptics, is far from clear, the concept is extremely difficult to establish with certainty. The suggestion to date is that WA does not make any significant contributions to its occurrence.

The concept of TDys was proposed by Wilson et al (1983), who noted that some patients with TD had hypomanic symptoms in addition to their schizophrenia and did not have a history of schizoaffective disorder. The features described were euphoria, labile mood, loud speech, circumstantiality and aimlessness in conversation, use of excessive words and intrusiveness with invasion of others' privacy. In a chronic ward, they studied 29 patients with a minimum of 2 years of exposure to neuroleptics and found that the symptoms correlated significantly with each other, and three symptoms (loud speech, labile mood and intrusiveness towards examiner) had significant but smaller correlations with AIMS scores. Mukherjee (1984) criticized the concept of dysmentia, stating instead that the features suggested dyscontrol and were part of the schizophrenic illness. He reported the absence of behaviour resembling dysmentia in his TD patients suffering from bipolar disorder. Goldberg (1985) presented a similar argument against the TDys concept. Chard et al (unpublished data, 1986) compared nine TD patients with six non-TD matched patients on the Multiple Affect Adjective Checklist (MAACL) (Zuckerman and Lubin, 1965). The two groups did not differ on the Mini-Mental State Examination (Marsden et al, 1969) scores, but the TD group scored higher on many items of MAACL, in particular tension, aggression and euphoria. The authors argued that this supported Wilson et al's suggestion of euphoria as a tardive effect. Much literature has been published on the 'anosognosia' of the TD patient, especially in relation to his or her motor abnormality (Myslobodsky, 1986, 1993). Some literature has also been published on the 'stimulus-boundedness' or 'environmental dependency' of TD patients (Myslobodsky, 1993), but empirical data are scant. In conclusion, the concept of TDys is interesting but needs much more study and documentation before it can be either established or discredited.

Objective features

The description of the movement disorder of TA is very similar to that of AA, with some qualitative differences. The movements as described in the different studies are listed in Table 6.1. Tardive akathisia movements, like those in AA, are complex and repetitive, but not as stereotyped as those in dyskinesia or dystonia. They involve all parts of the body, particularly the legs. Patients complain of an inner distress or tension that is partially relieved by the movements. The movements can be suppressed for at least a short period by concentrated effort and are affected by 'activating' or 'distracting' tasks and by certain body postures.

Gibb and Lees analysed the motor phenomenon in three categories of patients, divided on the basis of (a) subjective desire to move, (b) observable walking in one spot and (c) orofacial TD, into three groups: (1) 'definite' akathisia ($n = 27$) with (a) and (b); (2) TD group ($n = 79$) with (c) but without (a) or (b); and (3) 'indefinite' group ($n = 53$) with restlessness but without (a), (b) or (c). The prevalences of the different movements in this study are presented in Table 7.3. As is obvious from the table, the restless movements of

Table 7.3. *Percentage of patients with hyperkinetic movements*

Movements	Group 1 (n = 27)	Group 2 (n = 79)	Group 3 (n = 53)
Sitting			
Head and trunk			
Nodding head	3.7	6.3	3.5
Writhing neck	0	3.8	0
Rocking trunk	11.1	17.7	11.3
Sitting up	7.4	5.0	1.9
Shifting body	7.4	12.7	7.5
Arms and hands			
Crossing arms	3.7	0	1.9
Rubbing arms	11.1	30.4	15.1
Rubbing face	14.8	12.7	7.5
Fidgeting hands	18.5	38.0	24.5
Legs and feet			
Shifting knee laterally	18.5	7.6	11.3
Crossing knees	25.9	16.4	17.0
Swinging leg	25.9	7.6	28.3
Plantar flexion of crossed foot	25.9	19	18.9
Lifting forefoot	29.6	16.4	13.2
Sliding foot	18.5	8.9	1.9
Writhing foot	14.8	35.4	9.4
Standing/walking			
Walking in one spot	25.9	0	0
Changing stance	25.9	12.7	15.1
Flexing knee	3.7	2.5	3.8
Swaying	7.4	3.8	3.1
Pacing spontaneously	3.7	0	11.3
Walking fast	48.0	6.3	62.3
Walking slower	18.5	25.3	0
Wandering	0	8.9	3.8
Holding hands together	31.6 (of walkers)	21.9	9.8
Fidgeting hands	15.8	21.9	17.1
Lifting leg excessively	0	15.6	2.4

Source: Adapted from Gibb and Lees (1986a), with permission.

the legs and feet, with the exception of writhing foot movements, were more common in group 1. However, head and trunk movements (head nodding, neck writhing, rocking of the trunk, sitting up or shifting body movements), as well as fidgeting and rubbing movements of the hands, were more frequent in group 2. Group 3 had a greater similarity with group 1 than with group 2. The authors argued that while orofacial dyskinesia seemed to characterize patients with TD, walking in one spot and subjective restlessness were less

Table 7.4. *Frequency of motor phenomena among patients with tardive akathisia: chart and video analysis*

Motor phenomenon	Chart (n = 52)	Video (n = 17)
Marching in place	30 (58)	6 (35)
Crossing/uncrossing legs	25 (48)	6 (35)
Rocking trunk	23 (44)	6 (35)
Shifting trunk	18 (35)	5 (29)
Respiratory grunting	15 (29)	6 (35)
Pumping legs up/down	13 (25)	2 (12)
Pacing	13 (25)	3 (18)
Shifting weight from foot to foot (standing)	13 (25)	5 (29)
Rising from chair	11 (21)	1 (6)
Moaning	10 (19)	2 (12)
Abducting/adducting legs	10 (19)	4 (24)
Rubbing face	5 (10)	5 (29)
Rubbing hair	4 (8)	5 (29)
Picking at clothes	4 (8)	5 (29)
Shouting	3 (6)	2 (12)
Scratching	3 (6)	4 (12)
Folding/unfolding arms	3 (6)	1 (6)

Note: Data represent number of patients; numerals in parentheses are percentages.
Source: From Burke et al (1989), with permission.

selective of akathisia. They interpreted the data to suggest that akathisia and TD are distinct syndromes with considerable overlap, such that in the absence of orofacial dyskinesia, it was difficult to distinguish between the two. They also reported that the absence of the subjective component did not exclude the possibility of akathisia. The important question here is, can akathisic movements be distinguished from dyskinetic movements in the same patient?

Burke et al analysed the abnormal movements in their TA patients in detail, from charts on 52 patients and videotape records on 17 others (Table 7.4). Leg movements were the most common, in particular marching in place and crossing/uncrossing the legs while sitting. A number of patients also tended to pump their legs up and down, or abduct/adduct them, while sitting. In our experience, these movements are more common in TA than in AA but can be difficult to distinguish from stereotypic movements associated with an anxiety state or psychosis. The Burke et al patients commonly exhibited truncal movements (rocking back and forth, or shifting while sitting) and respiratory irregularities (including panting, grunting, moaning or even shouting). It is, however, uncertain whether the respiratory irregularities should be considered features of TA or TD or both. Respiratory dyskinesias have been described as features of TD in the absence of TA in a number of patients (Casey and Rabins, 1978; Weiner et al, 1978). In a prevalence study (Yassa and Lal, 1986), respiratory dyskinesias were diagnosed in 2.3% of a chronic schizophrenic population. The movements of the arms and hands (face rubbing, hair rubbing, scratching, picking at clothes, folding/unfolding of arms, etc) were less common.

The proportions of different movements in the TA subjects in the Barnes and Braude and the TA/CA studies are presented in Table 7.1. The semipurposeful or purposeless leg and foot movements were again the most common. Inability to maintain posture (sitting, standing or lying) was not a very common feature. Table 7.2 contrasts the movements of TA with those of AA, and a number of differences are obvious. The TA patients are more likely to have stereotyped movements in one position, whereas the AA movements are less stereotyped, and an inability to maintain posture is a more prominent feature.

We performed a discriminant function analysis to determine the items that best distinguished akathisia from nonakathisia as diagnosed by various criteria. While all 12 items were significant discriminating variables, the top 5 items were (in order of the size of Wilks' lambda): semipurposeful/purposeless normal leg/foot movements while sitting; inability to remain still, subjectively; purposeless foot movements while standing; semipurposeful/purposeless hand/arm movements; and shifting body position in a chair while sitting. An interesting observation in this study was that if the patients with TD, as diagnosed by a severity rating of 2 or more on the AIMS, were excluded from the discriminant analysis, the first 5 items were as follows: subjective feeling of an inability to keep legs still; shifting weight from foot to foot while standing; myoclonic jerks of the feet while lying; distressing sensations in the limbs; and inability to remain standing in one spot. These items are more suggestive of AA, thereby suggesting that pure TA, in the absence of concomitant TD, may closely resemble AA.

Effect of position on signs and symptoms

All three studies that addressed the significance of position came to the conclusion that TA symptoms were least prominent in the lying position. In the Burke et al study, of the nine patients asked about their most comfortable position, eight said it was lying down and one standing. Five found sitting, and two standing, as the most difficult position. In the TA/CA study, patients exhibited few if any movements in the lying position, and the motor features were most prominent when the patients were sitting. This postural difference was more marked for AA rather than TA. The mean (SD) global akathisia ratings in the sitting, standing and lying positions for TA in our study were 1.75 (0.72), 0.64 (0.82) and 0.17 (0.49), respectively. No patient had a higher rating for TA in the lying position compared with the other two. However, severely affected patients do manifest akathisia movements in the lying position in the form of flexion/extension at the knees, abduction/adduction at the hips and foot and toe movements. While toe movements are not uncommon in the lying position, to distinguish them from 'normal' fidgetiness is difficult.

Effect of 'activating' manoeuvres

Systematic data on this aspect is unavailable, but our studies suggest that the response of the movements of TA is similar to those of AA, with the diminution or disappearance of movements during the manoeuvres. If this is true, these manoeuvres may help distinguish these movements from dyskinetic ones, which are often unmasked or exacerbated by them (Jeste and Wyatt, 1982).

Other characteristics of the motor disorder of tardive akathisia

The issue of the voluntary vs involuntary nature of the movements has been previously discussed with regard to AA, and the same arguments apply to TA. Barnes and Braude (1985) reported a coarse, jerky tremor in 9 (39%) of 23 CA patients, compared with 6 of 6 AA subjects. In our series, more TA subjects had a tremor, compared with nonakathisics, but the tremor was always mild in intensity.

There are no studies that have examined for myoclonic jerks in these patients. However, myoclonus has been described as a tardive complication of neuroleptics (Little and Jankovic, 1987; Tominaga et al, 1987; Burke, 1992), and it is therefore unclear whether myoclonic jerks, if seen in a patient with TA, should be considered evidence of coexisting tardive myoclonus or a feature of TA. The myoclonic jerks described by Tominaga et al were in the arms and shoulders and were elicited by holding the hands up and forward. Little and Jankovic described myoclonic jerks in the neck and lower face upon neuroleptic withdrawal in 1 patient. Burke (1992) observed myoclonus in 158 patients with tardive syndromes referred to a neurological clinic. An association of the jerks with TDt, but not TA, was described.

The movements of TA show variability over time, even in one brief observation period. Using a stopwatch to clock the pattern of movements in four patients with chronic schizophrenia and CA while they watched a videoclip, Nemes et al (1990) observed that these movements occurred in bursts which

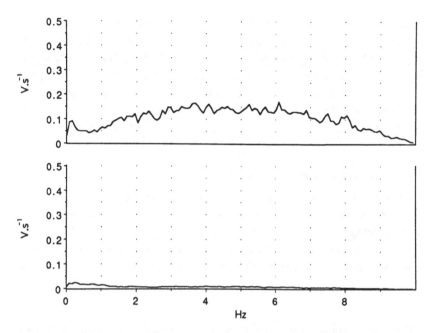

Fig. 7.2. The power–frequency spectrum of akathisic movements. The patient sat in a chair with both feet resting on plates bearing strain-gauge measures. Data were recorded for 6 epochs of 30 seconds each, averaged and fast Fourier transformed. The akathisic movements are not represented by any definite peak. Top, right leg; bottom, left leg.

ranged from 6 to 100 seconds (median 24), with 5 to 221 (median 25) movements per burst. During the bursts, the movements were noted to occur with great regularity. This observation has not been replicated. Our own studies of patients with TA using a piezoelectric device strapped to the ankle, or a strain-gauge platform on which the patient sits or stands, do not support this burst pattern. We have observed the movements to be much more irregular, as demonstrated in Fig. 7.2. Table 7.5 highlights the diversity of the tardive syndromes.

The overlap of tardive akathisia with other tardive syndromes

TA patients often manifest dyskinetic (and less commonly dystonic) movements that in many cases are orofacial. Gibb and Lees divided their patients into akathisia and TD groups depending on whether they had the typical oro-facial (buccal–lingual–masticatory) dyskinesia and found that a number of TD patients also had the subjective and objective features of akathisia, such

Table 7.5. *Neuroleptic-induced tardive syndromes described in the literature*

Tardive dyskinesia (orofacial, LT or mixed) (TD)
Tardive akathisia (TA)
Tardive dystonia (TD)
Tardive tics and Tourette's syndrome
Tardive myoclonus
Tardive tremor
Tardive parkinsonism
Tardive dysmentia (TDys)
Supersensitivity psychosis (SP)

---

that TA could arguably be diagnosed in these cases. Barnes and Braude reported moderate to severe orofacial dyskinesia in 9 (39%) and choreo-athetoid limb dyskinesia in 13 (56%) of 23 CA patients. The limb dyskinesia involved lower limbs in 7 and both upper and lower limbs in the remaining 6. In patients with pseudoakathisia, dyskinesia was even more common: of 10 patients, 7 had orofacial and 5 limb dyskinesia. Overall, 16 (41%) patients with akathisia and 5 (12%) without it had orofacial dyskinesia; and 30 (77%) with akathisia and 4 (9%) without it had limb dyskinesia. The akathisic patients with orofacial dyskinesia tended to have more chronic symptoms.

The overlap was also noted by Burke et al (1989), who found that 51 of their 52 TA patients also had either TDt or TD: 14 (7%) had both dystonia and dyskinesia at some time during their illness, 4 (8%) had dystonia alone and 33 (63%) had OBLF dyskinesia. The patients with TA and TDt had an earlier age of onset (39 ± 7 years) than the TA with OBLF dyskinesia patients (62.2 ± 1.7, $p = .0002$), with the TA plus TDt plus OBLF dyskinesia patients being in between (55 ± 4.4 years).

In the TA/CA study, 18 of the 31 TA subjects also met the criteria for TD. The TA patients had mean (SD) ratings on the AIMS as follows: sum of seven items was 4.6 (3.8); sum of four items (OBLF dyskinesia) was 2.2 (2.1); sum of three items (LT dyskinesia) was 2.4 (2.1). The TA subjects with ($n = 18$) and without ($n = 13$) TD did not differ on sociodemographic or illness- and treatment-related variables. The association of akathisia was most robust with LT dyskinesia, with 9 of 11 LT dyskinesia patients having a global rating of mild to moderate akathisia.

This overlap between TA and TD can be interpreted in various ways: (i) TA and TD are separate syndromes that often co-occur; (ii) TA is a subsyn-drome of TD; (iii) some TD patients have LT movements that are misdiagnosed as being akathisic; or (iv) some TD patients respond to the presence of limb dyskinesia with restless feelings and movements that resemble akathisia. We will discuss the evidence for and against these possibilities. Our conclusion from the evidence is that TA and TD are likely to be separate syndromes with considerable overlap.

The first issue is whether it is possible to distinguish choreoathetoid limb dyskinesia from akathisia. The description of akathisic motor disorder that has preceded this section would suggest an answer in the affirmative. Dyskinetic movements are choreic (rapid, jerky, quasi-purposive and non-rhythmic) or athetoid (slow, sinuous or writhing) or choreoathetoid. They are recognized by the patient as being involuntary, cannot be readily suppressed by voluntary effort and increase when the patient is engaged in 'activating' manoeuvres. Akathisic movements are more complex and less stereotyped, tend more commonly to involve the lower limbs, are usually preceded by a feeling of subjective distress (the patient often recognizes the movements as being voluntary in response to the distress) and can be suppressed for at least short periods. Some akathisic movements, such as moving from foot to foot, marching on the spot, inability to sit or stand in one place or crossing/uncrossing of legs, cannot be mistaken for dyskinesia and are recognized to be typical of akathisia. It is therefore possible to distinguish limb dyskinesia from akathisia in most cases. Arguably, if the subjective aspect of the akathisia is mild and the movements are relatively simple, a difficulty may arise. There will therefore be borderline cases, but in our experience these are in the minority. The overlap between LT dyskinesia and TA in our study may partly be because of a lack of concerted effort to distinguish limb movements as definitely akathisic or dyskinetic. Also, there are sufficient data to support the similarity between the outstanding features of AA and TA, to characterize them as different from anxiety and agitation and to suggest that the akathisia seen in TD patients cannot be merely construed as a response to the dyskinesia.

Whether TA is considered to be a subsyndrome of TD or a separate syndrome depends, to some degree, on the definitions used and the attribution of primacy. The various arguments to be considered in this debate are as follows.

The primacy argument

Tardive dyskinesia has been well recognized as a drug-induced syndrome since its first report in the 1950s (Schonecker, 1957), whereas TA has been recognized with certainty only recently. There is therefore a tendency to classify the syndromes discovered subsequently, including TDt and tardive tics, as subsyndromes of TD, especially because the other syndromes often coexist with dyskinetic movements. In our view, this primacy argument is weak, because it merely reflects a historical fact rather than a clinical or pathophysiological argument on which such decisions should rest.

The prevalence argument

It was earlier supposed that TA was an uncommon disorder that sometimes occurred in patients with TD, the latter being much more common. Recent prevalence studies, as discussed in Chapter 5, reveal the error in this argument, as TA is relatively common and can occur quite independently of TD.

The clinical argument

Some authors conceptualize TD as a broad disorder which subsumes various kinds of disordered movements. The term *dyskinesia* can be strictly applied to any kind of movement disorder (Caine, 1992), and by corollary so can TD be applied to any movement disorder that is a delayed side-effect of neuroleptic medication. It is, according to this argument, not necessary to restrict the use of the term *TD* to disorders that manifest as choreoathetoid movements. Dystonia, tics, myoclonus or tremor could therefore be subsumed under TD by this definition. We argue that akathisia is different: not only are the movements 'intentional and involuntary' (as distinguished in Chapter 6) rather than involuntary, but akathisia is more than a movement disorder; it is also a mental disorder (see Chapter 4 for discussion).

An early study that employed factor analysis to subdivide neuroleptic-induced movement disorders in chronic schizophrenia into subsyndromes was published by Kennedy et al (1971). They obtained a three-factor solution: a restlessness factor which included all LT movements, an orofacial movements factor and a parkinsonian factor. Their first factor could be labelled akathisia, although they did not seek confirmatory reports from the patients. Following drug withdrawal (Hershon et al, 1972), the parkinsonian and orofacial movement factor scores were unchanged, but the motor restlessness scores increased significantly. In light of current knowledge, one can argue that this could represent a withdrawal exacerbation of TA or perhaps an increase in anxiety or psychotic agitation that interacted with akathisia. There is evidence from a number of studies (Barnes and Braude, 1985; Burke et al, 1989; TA/CA study) that TA may occur in the absence of any dyskinetic movements, arguing for a distinct syndromal status.

There is some evidence that choreoathetoid TD may also be validly divided into subsyndromes. Three studies have been published to this effect (Crane et al, 1971; Kidger et al, 1980; Glazer et al, 1988). The first two studies yielded three factors: an orofacial movement factor, an LT movement factor and a parkinsonian factor. The third study (Glazer et al, 1988), which factor-analysed the seven anatomical variables of the AIMS, and did not include EPSE, yielded two orofacial factors and an LT factor. Some other studies have suggested that these two TD subsyndromes may have different risk factors, clinical concomitants, treatment response and prognostic implications. For example, orofacial, but not LT, TD is associated with increasing age (Barnes et al, 1983; Glazer et al, 1988) and cognitive dysfunction (Waddington et al, 1987) as risk factors. Several studies using pharmacological probes have reported discrepant findings for the OBLF and LT syndromes (Fann et al, 1974; Gardos et al, 1976; Casey and Denney, 1977; Simpson et al, 1977). A more detailed discussion of this subtyping is beyond the scope of this book, but it highlights the point that even the well-accepted features of TD may not constitute a unitary syndrome, and the symptoms need to be studied separately. Furthermore, the movements rated as LT dyskinesia may, in many studies, include akathisic movements, thus explaining part of the inconsistency in the associations.

The pathophysiology argument

Both TA and TD are side-effects of neuroleptic drugs. They do not occur in all individuals at risk, suggesting that there is a vulnerability which at present is poorly understood. With OBLF dyskinesia, an additional factor is the occurrence of spontaneous orofacial dyskinesia, especially in the elderly. It can be argued that neuroleptics bring out this predisposition, thereby explaining the high prevalence of OBLF dyskinesia in the elderly. A spontaneous or idiopathic counterpart of TA does not exist, as was emphasized by Burke et al (1989). This would suggest that TA is a purer drug-induced syndrome.

Increasing age, female sex, affective disorder diagnosis, diabetes, alcoholism, etc have not emerged to be risk factors for TA as they have for TD (Jeste and Caligiuri, 1993), although this may merely reflect a lack of adequate research into TA.

The pharmacological response argument

The pharmacological and biochemical characteristics of TD have been extensively studied (Khot et al, 1992), but relatively little is known about TA. A few studies have examined the pharmacological responsiveness of TA patients (Burke et al, 1989; Sachdev and Chee, 1990; Yassa and Bloom, 1990; Kuniyoshi et al, 1991; Sachdev and Loneragan, 1993a,c). There is no clear evidence from these studies that TA is different from TD, but there are some pointers: ACh antagonists may be effective in treating some TA patients, whereas TD is usually worsened by these drugs (Jeste and Wyatt, 1982); noradrenergic mechanisms seem to be more important for TA than for TD. Further research is necessary to investigate the biochemical profile of TA.

Considering all of these arguments, it would be reasonable to treat TD and TA as two syndromes with some common clinical and pathophysiological features.

TA and EPSE

The significant overlap of AA and EPSE is generally accepted, as discussed in Chapter 6. That CA or TA patients may also have increased parkinsonian side-effects was pointed out by Barnes and Braude (1985). Their CA patients had a mean (SD) rating on the Simpson and Angus scale of 0.61 (0.63) vs the nonakathisia group with a rating of 0.32 (0.4) ($p < .05$). The TA subjects in our TA/CA study, with or without TD, had a significantly higher Simpson and Angus scale score compared with schizophrenic control patients without TA or TD. The groups did not differ on the total neuroleptic dosage or type of drug (high vs low potency) or the proportions of patients on antiparkinsonian medication. A multiple regression analysis suggested that the EPSE score related significantly to the severity of TA and the LT dyskinesia, but not to the OBLF syndrome.

The significance of this finding is unknown. Various explanations for this overlap are possible. It may be that the TA group is heterogeneous and includes some patients with AA who were misdiagnosed. We consider this unlikely, as the patients in the TA/CA study were on stable medication, and akathisia was not of recent origin. It is possible that some had a chronic, acute-onset akathisia rather than TA, but they would still be categorized as CA. The natural course of EPSE in patients maintained on neuroleptics for the long term is unknown. One study (Azima and Ogle, 1954) suggested that EPSE resolve within 2 months, and others have suggested that chronic antiparkinsonian treatment is rarely needed (DiMascio and Demirgian, 1970). This has led to a common belief that EPSE are temporary phenomena that correct themselves over time. This may not be true or perhaps may apply only to the more severe form that needs treatment. Kennedy et al (1971) found that in their 63 patients treated with trifluoperazine over 3 years, 27 continued to have a tremor and 24 had rigidity. More research on the natural history of EPSE is clearly indicated, but the current data do suggest that mild forms of EPSE may persist in some patients. If this is the case, then the patients with CA or TA could also have chronic, mild EPSE. One can speculate that this reflects a common vulnerability to movement-related side-effects in some patients.

The coexistence of EPSE and TA may seem to be a contradiction if EPSE are seen as a DA-deficient state and TA (like TD) a DA-excess state. There is enough evidence that simplistic formulations of the pathophysiology of these syndromes are frequently violated. It is well recognized that TD may co-occur with EPSE (Crane, 1972; Fann and Lake, 1974; Richardson and Craig, 1982; Kucharski et al, 1987). In our TA/CA study, EPSE were more common in the patients with TD that could not be explained on the basis of current neuroleptic medication. Furthermore, the coexistence of dyskinesias and bradykinesia is often seen in PD patients being treated with L-dopa (Nutt, 1992). It is therefore possible that relative DA excess in one part of the brain may coexist with relative deficiency in another. Further, since the DA-excess hypothesis of TD, and even more so of TA, is on somewhat shaky ground, any theoretical objections to an empirical observation are not valid.

Tardive akathisia: subjective, objective or both; the concept of 'pseudoakathisia'

While subjective and objective features characterize TA, there is no consensus on whether both need to be present for a diagnosis. In Chapter 4, we put forward a conservative proposal that both are necessary for a definitive diagnosis. The diagnostic criteria adopted by Burke et al (1989) for TA and Barnes and Braude (1985) for CA also included both features. Since the clinical features of TA overlap with those of other syndromes, thus making the diagnosis difficult, and there are no external validators in the form of abnormal laboratory tests, a conservative approach is reasonable.

Cross-sectional studies of TA suggest that there are some patients who have either the subjective or the objective features of akathisia alone. In the TA/CA study, 20 subjects each had a score on subjective items of 2 or more (subjective akathisia) without the objective features. The major difficulty in diagnosing these patients as having TA is in the fact that the subjective report is often unreliable, especially in chronically ill schizophrenic patients. Patients find it difficult to distinguish akathisia from other causes of internal distress. If the akathisia has developed acutely and clearly in association with a change in neuroleptic dosage, as is usually the case with AA, the subjective report is much more reliable. Only prospective longitudinal studies can help decide the real status of subjective akathisia.

There are other patients who manifest the characteristic movements of akathisia but report no subjective distress and often are unaware of the movements. When their attention is drawn to the movements, they may suppress them temporarily or dismiss them as 'habits'. What is striking is the stereotyped, but voluntary and semipurposive nature of the movements (eg, crossing/uncrossing of legs, shifting weight from foot to foot, pacing), which set them apart from agitation and dyskinesia. In the Barnes and Braude study, 10 of 82 patients met this description, and in the TA/CA study, there were 9 such patients. Again, only a longitudinal study can help decide if this is true akathisia. Barnes and Braude used the term *pseudoakathisia* to describe these patients. They *did not,* however, imply that these patients were not suffering from akathisia but from some other disorder that resembled it. Their use of the term was, therefore, different from that of Munetz and Cornes (1982), as we have already discussed in Chapter 4. The latter authors were referring to lower-extremity TD, or a form fruste of TD, that was mistaken for akathisia and was therefore 'pseudoakathisia'. We consider the use of the term *pseudoakathisia* by Barnes and Braude as inappropriate because it begs the question, Is it, or is it not, akathisia? In Chapter 4, we suggested the term *probable akathisia (objective)*, which summarizes the concept underlying the description.

What is the basis of objective akathisia? In the absence of longitudinal data, one can only speculate. It is possible that some patients with schizophrenia have a predominance of negative symptoms and a flattening of affect such that they express little in the form of subjective experience. In such cases, objective akathisia represents a relative dearth of subjective manifestations rather than a true entity. There is some evidence to suggest that TA subjects have more negative symptoms (Brown and White, 1991a; TA/CA study), which would support this suggestion. It has also been suggested that objective akathisia may be a later stage in the natural history of akathisia, which begins with AA and proceeds to CA and later objective akathisia. Both the Barnes and Braude and the TA/CA studies supported the notion that subjective distress was less prominent in TA than in AA, but only a prospective longitudinal study can validly address the issue. Such a study is yet to be published.

We cannot dismiss the possibility that at least a part of what is considered objective akathisia is a misdiagnosis. The possibilities to consider include dyskinetic movements affecting the limbs, and stereotypies seen as part of schizophrenia. Even when attention is paid to the nature of the movements in systematic detail, confident differentiation of the various kinds of movements is extremely difficult in some cases.

Differential diagnosis

The major issues in the differential diagnosis of TA are similar to those of AA and have been discussed at length in Chapter 6. The following special points should be considered for TA:

1. The subjective distress in TA may not be as severe as in AA. The nature of the distress is not different, however. The motor features may be the ones that draw attention to the akathisia. Since these features may resemble fidgetiness or restlessness, TA is more likely to be overlooked than AA.
2. TA occurs most often in chronic schizophrenic patients who are more likely to manifest stereotypies and mannerisms, especially if they are institutionalized. The reduced distress and the associated negative symptoms of the schizophrenic illness can make it quite difficult to distinguish the movements of akathisia from stereotypies and mannerisms. As well, there is a suggestion that the movements of TA may be more stereotyped and less purposive than those of AA, although definitive data on this aspect are lacking.
3. The co-occurrence of a number of tardive syndromes may make it difficult to categorize the different movements present into separate syndromes. The dyskinetic and dystonic movements are more likely to attract an observer's attention than akathisic movements, thus leading to the latter being ignored.
4. Other basal ganglia disorders, such as Huntington's chorea, figure more prominently in the differential diagnosis of TA than AA. The characteristic features of Huntington's chorea are chorea and dementia, but the chorea may precede the dementia by months or years. Choreic movements, especially when they involve the limbs, may be mistaken for akathisia. They are, in most cases, suppressed by haloperidol and other neuroleptics. Huntington's chorea may, in some cases, manifest as a psychiatric disorder, including schizophreniform psychosis, which may in turn be treated with neuroleptics, making it difficult to attribute appropriately the movement disorder that develops later. The family history, evidence of cognitive decline, atrophy of the caudate nuclei on brain scan and the presence of an expanded and unstable CAG repeat sequence in a gene (IT15) on chromosome 4 (MacMillan et al, 1993) will help establish the diagnosis of

Huntington's chorea. Other disorders affecting the basal ganglia that should be considered are encephalitides, collagen vascular diseases (eg, systemic lupus erythematosus), metabolic encephalopathies and vascular, demyelinating or degenerative disorders. It is interesting that some of the early descriptions of akathisia were associated with epidemic encephalitis.

5. Hysteria and malingering must occasionally be considered in the differential diagnosis. A patient's previous experience of akathisia, or a fellow patient's suffering, may serve as a model. A careful history, an examination of the premorbid personality, the patient's response to his or her akathisia and the evidence of secondary gain may help establish the diagnosis.

The natural history of akathisia

The longitudinal course of akathisia is largely unknown, with no systematic prospective studies having been conducted. Some impressions are based on retrospective accounts and a few treatment studies that followed up patients for some months. Acute akathisia may persist in some patients for months, perhaps years, becoming chronic in the process. The chronicity of the akathisia may manifest itself if a drug being used to treat akathisia, eg, benztropine or propranolol (see, eg, Dupuis et al, 1987; Hermesh et al, 1988), is withdrawn. It is not known, however, what proportion of AA becomes chronic and what further proportion persists after repeatedly administered neuroleptics are stopped. It is also not known what happens to the risk of akathisia upon repeated exposure to neuroleptics. Most clinicians are familiar with a few patients who develop marked akathisia upon each episode of neuroleptic treatment. Our AA study suggested that the risk for AA was reduced if the patient had had past treatment with antipsychotic drugs, but the effect was slight.

TA may develop months or years after the initiation of medication. The range in the Burke et al (1989) study was from 2 weeks to 22 years (mean 4.5 years), with 50% of patients developing it in the first year of exposure. Forty-eight TA patients were followed up for a mean of 2.3 ± 0.3 years by these authors. Of these, 32 (67%) continued to have akathisia for a mean of 4.2 years. In 26 patients, the neuroleptic drug had been discontinued, but their akathisia persisted at follow-up (2.7 ± 0.4 years later). Sixteen (33%) patients were free of akathisia at follow-up. Four of these were considered to have true remissions, having been tapered off all medication. They had taken a mean 1.2 ± 0.4 years to remit after the discontinuation of the neuroleptic. The 13 patients who had responded to medication had done so 2.4 ± 0.8 years after first developing akathisia. Those who responded to drugs or remitted completely had developed akathisia (and dyskinesia) at an earlier age, but did not differ in the years of neuroleptic exposure, the nature of the associated dyskinesia or other variables. The suggestion, therefore, is that TA is more likely to become persistent in older patients. This needs to be examined in a longitudinal study.

8

Akathisia due to a general medical condition

Some neurological disorders may be associated with the development of a syndrome resembling DIA. We will refer to this syndrome as *akathisia due to a general medical condition,* in keeping with the nomenclature adopted in the fourth edition of the *Diagnostic and Statistical Manual of Mental Disorders* (DSM-IV) (American Psychiatric Association, 1994). The akathisia in this case is judged to be a direct physiological consequence of the neuroleptic disorder, in the absence of a drug that could be causative. Using earlier nomenclature (eg, DSM-II-R, American Psychiatric Association, 1987), this syndrome would most appropriately be termed *organic akathisia.*

A review of the published literature suggests the following neurological causes of akathisia: (i) encephalitis lethargica and postencephalitic parkinsonism, (ii) PD, (iii) traumatic brain injury or (iv) subthalamic abscess.

Encephalitis lethargica and postencephalatic parkinsonism

Most neurologists are aware of the epidemic of encephalitis lethargica (EL; also called 'sleeping sickness'), which started in 1916–1917 and raged for about 10 years, becoming worldwide. Innumerable cases and small epidemics of a similar disease had been described for many centuries. The infectious nature of EL was demonstrated by Constantin von Economo, who was able to transmit the disease to monkeys, but the presumed viral agent has never been isolated. The outcome varied from death in about 25% of cases to complete recovery, but a number of patients showed postencephalitic sequelae affecting both cognitive faculties and motor control, with parkinsonism being most common (von Economo, 1931).

Clinical features resembling those of akathisia have been described both during the acute phase of the encephalitis and as part of the sequelae. In fact, as Breggin (1993) argues, 'Nearly all the cognitive and motor disorders commonly associated with neuroleptic treatment were also commonly associated with lethargic encephalitis' (p. 9). Several patients with EL suffered from compulsive hyperactivity in what Haase (1959) called the 'irritative hyperkinetic' form of the disease. The purposelessly hyperactive patients typically exhibited subjective and often extreme tension and anxiety, features resembling those of AA, at least in its superficial aspects. Von Economo (1931) described it as 'general mental unrest and ceaseless motor activity' (p. 36). Some patients had episodes of violent movements and frenzies (Jelliffe, 1932). It must be stated, however, that detailed descriptions of hyperactivity and inner tension in EL suggest only a superficial similarity with DIA, and since the epidemic ended in about 1930, a direct comparison between the two syndromes is not possible.

Patients may also exhibit hyperactivity and distress during the postencephalitic phase. This may occur in episodes, interspersed with 'obstructive', akinetic periods. Patients can move from states of 'frozen' catatonia to profound restlessness, often associated with bizarre perceptions, thoughts and emotions (Jelliffe, 1932).

Some patients developed an akathisia-like syndrome after being treated with L-dopa for the postencephalitic parkinsonism. Sacks (1983) provided some excellent descriptions of this in his book *Awakenings*. His patient Mrs. Y was 'terribly excitable' and 'hysterical', constantly kicking and crossing her legs. The observable agitation was combined with an intense feeling of inner distress, much like that of akathisia. Some of these phenomena occurred in episodes, seeming like 'physiological storms of an incredible ferocity and unpredictability' (p. 97). In another patient, the akathisia subsided, 'leaving behind a restless "pawing" movement of the right leg (suggestive of a high-spiritied, impatient horse)' (p. 110).

Breggin (1993) suggested that the EL model of drug-induced movement disorders is apt, and the common feature is possibly the involvement of the basal ganglia.

Parkinson's disease (Bing–Sicard akathisia)

As discussed in Chapter 1, the association of akathisia and PD was convincingly described by Sicard and Bing even though earlier descriptions of restlessness in PD, both historical and medical, exist. The restlessness observed in PD has been attributed to various causes. Wilson (1952) considered it to be a consequence of muscular discomfort due to rigidity and bradykinesia: 'The accumulation or summation of afferent excitations, derived from a largely motionless (though not resting) musculature, is such that the patient must rise and "work it off", only, however, to sink once more into the same state of motionlessness' (p. 3). Other causes of restlessness in PD that have been suggested are: (i) tremor if it is generalized; (ii) dyskinesia if misdiagnosed as restlessness, or the patient uses movement to decrease the dyskinesias or make them more tolerable; (iii) secondary to L-dopa used in the treatment; (iv) associated anxiety, depression, nervousness or claustrophobia; and (v) sensory symptoms (cramping, burning, itching, aching, pulling, drawing, crawling, hot/cold feelings, numbness, pins-and-needles, pain, etc) with secondary restlessness (Lang and Johnson, 1987).

Does true akathisia occur in the setting of PD? The only systematic study to answer this question was published by Lang and Johnson (1987). The authors interviewed 100 patients (62 men, 38 women; mean age 54.1, SD 11.8 years) with idiopathic PD and questioned them using a standardized questionnaire on restlessness, fidgetiness and/or an inability to remain still. When a positive response was obtained, the patients were further questioned about the possibility of this being attributable to the causes discussed in the preceding paragraph. Akathisia was diagnosed if the restlessness could not be attributed to any other definable cause.

Of the 100 patients, 68 periodically experienced the need to move, with an inability to sit, stand or lie still. Of these, the restlessness and need to move in 26 patients could not be attributed to any definable cause, and the authors argued that these had true akathisia. Another 17 had only a feeling of restlessness without movement, and these were considered to possibly have akathisia. The remaining 57 patients were nonakathisic with either no restlessness or having a definable cause for it. The akathisia group was more likely to be akinetic-rigid than tremulous compared with the nonakathisic group, but they did not differ in other clinical characteristics. The akathisic patients reported more crawling sensations ($p < .02$), but these were not relieved by the movements and could not account for the restlessness. Cramps, aching and numbness relieved by movement were more frequent in the patients without akathisia.

The onset of akathisia could be dated by retrospective enquiry in only 14 subjects. It was present at the onset of PD in 3; in 1 it developed within a week of starting L-dopa and in 10 within a variable time after the initiation of treatment. After its development, it gradually worsened in many cases. The manifestation of akathisia did not relate well with the 'on' or 'off' phases of PD, and most subjects showed no relationship between akathisia and the state of their mobility or the timing of the drug. Two patients had 'beginning-of-dose' akathisia without accompanying dyskinesia or sensory symptoms, which lasted for a shorter period than the motor effects of the L-dopa. No patient demonstrated an 'end-of-dose' akathisia. Only 1 patient obtained relief from L-dopa. One patient had a complete resolution of akathisia during two separate drug holidays, only to suffer a recurrence several months after reinitiation of treatment. Dopaminergic drugs like bromocriptine or pergolide did not improve the symptoms of akathisia in any patient.

Comment

This study, which remains to be replicated, provides fairly convincing evidence of the existence of restlessness and fidgetiness in PD that cannot be attributed to any identifiable cause. The range of the phenomena that constitute this akathisia have not been described, thus making a comparison with DIA difficult. More research is clearly indicated, which should include a comparison of PD-related akathisia and DIA.

The akathisia in PD may be attributable to treatment with L-dopa in some subjects, but the overall relationship with drug therapy is inconsistent. That PD can result in akathisia may have some implications for our understanding of the pathophysiology of akathisia. PD involves disturbance in many neurotransmitters, but DA deficiency, especially in the nigrostriatal area, correlates best with the characteristic symptoms of PD (Hornykiewicz, 1966). Cell loss and DA deficiency in the ventral tegmental area (VTA) is less severe in PD (Javoy-Agid and Agid, 1980; Scatton et al, 1982). If akathisia is due to reduced DA transmission in the mesocortical pathway, as has been suggested by some authors (Marsden and Jenner, 1980), this may explain the uncommon occurrence of akathisia early in the course of the disease, its development as the disease progresses and its greater likelihood in patients with the rigid-bradykinetic form of PD. The lack of responsiveness of the akathisia to L-dopa or other DA agonists may be because these drugs do not augment DA transmission in the mesocortical pathways as much as the nigrostriatal pathways. Encephalitis lethargica and neuroleptics affect all DA pathways in the brain, and this may explain why they more commonly cause akathisia.

It is equally possible that the akathisia in PD is due to disturbances in nondopaminergic pathways: NE, 5HT, ACh, GABA, substance P, endogenous opioids, etc. This will be taken up further in the discussion on the aetiology of DIA.

Traumatic brain injury

In Chapter 2, we discussed the relationship of head injury to restlessness. This restlessness was not described as having the characteristic features of akathisia, occurred usually in the recovery phase of the head injury and was often part of a delirium; as well, most patients had no definable brain lesions that could clearly explain its development. The report by Stewart (1989) is possibly an exception. He described a 61-year-old patient who was examined 1 year after traumatic brain injury at which time he was markedly restless, spending his entire day pacing or rocking in a chair. The patient described himself as 'fidgety but not nervous' (p. 1200) and denied anxiety or depression. On computerized tomography (CT) brain examination, there was a small right parietooccipital area of encephalomalacia and large bilateral orbitomedial lesions. The patient did not respond to alprazolam, improved subjectively with diazepam but had a complete resolution of symptoms with bromocriptine up to 15 mg/day. The author argued that the presence of bilateral prefrontal disturbance and the response to a DA agonist supported the hypothesis that akathisia was possibly caused by a reduction in mesocortical DA activity.

Subthalamic abscess

Attention was drawn to the association between a lesion in the subthalamic area and the development of akathisia in a report by Carrazana et al (1989). They described a 54-year-old man with a history of iv drug use and HIV infection who exhibited jitteriness, restlessness and frontal headache. The authors described his abnormal movements as follows:

He was noted to be restless, changing body position at least 6 times per minute. Abnormal upper extremity movements included stroking the face and hair repeatedly with the right hand, and almost constant fidgety motions involving his right fingers, hand, and wrist. Abnormal movements were also present in the right lower extremity and included rapid tapping movements of the foot and sliding the foot back and forth on the floor. In addition, the patient would repeatedly cross and uncross his right leg over his left. (p. 449)

The patient recognized these movements as being involuntary and was embarrassed by them. The neurological examination was otherwise normal except for an exaggerated swinging of the right arm during walking, and there was no hemiballismus. The CT brain scan showed an area of hypodensity predominantly in the left lentiform nucleus, adjacent to the third ventricle. With contrast, there was a nodular area of enhancement in the region of the left subthalamic nucleus and an area of ring enhancement in the left posterior parietal lobe with some adjacent oedema. The movement disorder worsened when he was treated with haloperidol. Toxoplasmosis was diagnosed and treated, but he deteriorated rapidly and died 6 weeks later. Autopsy revealed a 1.2-cm area of necrosis in the left subthalamic area with surrounding oedema involving the left basal ganglia. There was also a 1.5-cm area of necrosis in the left parietooccipital area.

The authors argued that the nature of the movement in this patient, and its worsening with haloperidol, suggested akathisia, and not hemiballismus, which has previously been reported in patients with subthalamic lesions (Gilbert, 1975; Casey and Rabins, 1978; Nath et al, 1987). The clearly involuntary nature of the movements in this report makes them unusual for akathisia, and this is the only case of 'unilateral akathisia' we are aware of. The movements of hemiballismus are different from those seen in this patient. They are usually wild, rapidly flinging movements that occur at irregular intervals, originating proximally in a limb. Abnormal facial movements may also occur. Movements of hemiballismus are exacerbated by stress and reduced by relaxation, disappearing in sleep. The movements can be controlled for seconds with great effort on the part of the patient. Since the studies conducted by Whittier and Mettler (1949), hemiballismus has usually been associated with subthalamic lesions. The subthalamic nucleus receives GABAergic inhibitory input from the lateral globus pallidus and some excitatory input from the cortex. The efferent connections to the medial and lateral globus pallidus are also GABAergic inhibitory. It also sends a glutamatergic excitatory efferent to the substantia nigra pars reticulata, with a branch to the medial globus pallidus. Lesions of the subthalamus will therefore lead to an increased activity of the globus pallidus, which is the output organ of the basal ganglia, leading to the development of ballismus. Why the Carrazana et al patient developed akathisia-like movements rather than a ballism is difficult to explain, except to point out the fact that their patient had oedematous lesions of the basal ganglia as well, and the lesion was not localized to the subthalamic nucleus.

Hemiakathisia and monoakathisia

Rapoport (1989) briefly reported two patients with focal akathisia, one with rhythmic leg swinging on sitting down and the other with periodic knee flexion on standing up. Both were young men being treated with a neuroleptic, with no reported evidence of an organic lesion. Rapaport called it *monoakathisia* in contrast with the *hemiakathisia* of the Carrazana et al patient. Carrazana and Rossitch (1989), in response to this report, rightly commented that the presence of a unilateral or focal movement disorder should raise the suspicion of an organic lesion, be it cerebrovascular, infectious, malignant or other in aetiology.

CT scan brain abnormality and drug-induced akathisia

Unlike TD, akathisia has not been the subject of brain imaging studies, with the exception of a case report by Sandyk and Kay (1990a), who investigated the relationship of akathisia with CT measurements in 25 chronic schizophrenic patients. Akathisia had a significant correlation with a measure of sulcal prominence ($r = .422$, $p < .025$), but not with the ventricle–brain ratio ($r = .19$). The authors agreed that preexisting brain damage may increase the risk of development of akathisia. Of heuristic importance would be the investigation of abnormalities in the neuronal circuits purportedly involved in the motor disorder of akathisia (see Chapter 10 for discussion of a model).

Comment

The association of akathisia with organic brain lesions or well-recognized neurological disorders is of clinical relevance and heuristic importance. Clinically, the importance of recognizing akathisia and appropriately managing it has already been stressed in preceding chapters. For example, its lack of recognition in PD may have serious implications for the patients' welfare. Heuristically, it permits one to speculate on the brain mechanisms that may be involved in the pathogenesis of the syndrome. In this context, the concept of akathisia predates the introduction of neuroleptic drugs. What should be appreciated, however, is that the diagnosis of akathisia is often tentative, and sometimes clearly inappropriate, in many of these cases. We are still at the stage when the phenomenon of restlessness associated with many neurological disorders needs to be systematically examined and its characteristics compared with those of DIA, before any general understanding of the processes becomes acceptable. It is possible that there are many different 'akathisias', sharing some common themes, yet differing in their causes and clinical characteristics. We highlight this to some degree in our discussion of restlessness (Chapter 2) and acknowledge this further in Chapter 10, in which a model of akathisia is presented that accommodates the diverse aetiology and recognizes the varied manifestations.

9

Assessment and measurement of akathisia

Measurement began our might . . .
> W. B. Yeats, *Last Poems* (1939)

Clinical and experimental research into akathisia depends on the reliable and accurate measurement of the disorder. Unfortunately, akathisia has proved to be notoriously difficult to quantify for a number of reasons.

Problems in assessment

The nature of the syndrome

Akathisia comprises both subjective and objective features; any attempt at measurement must take this fact into consideration. Methods that quantify the movements alone are inadequate, yielding only partial information of the disorder. It is for this reason that most research on akathisia has relied on rating scale measures, which can incorporate measures of both subjective and objective features. The movements of akathisia are complex, semipurposive and nonstereotyped, and resemble normal movements. An element of judgement is involved in deciding whether a certain movement should be considered akathisic. Instrumental methods of quantification are therefore prone to serious error and must be rigorously tested and validated before being accepted.

Tremor and myoclonic jerks can be quantified with greater ease because of their involuntary nature and reproducibility. But tremor is arguably not a feature of akathisia, and myoclonic jerks are variable, unpredictable and infrequent, occurring only in the more severe cases.

The lack of a definition

Even if methods to quantitate the clinical features of akathisia are reliably developed, what constitutes akathisia is an important clinical and research decision which, with our current knowledge, is uncertain. In Chapter 4, we have highlighted the characteristic features and proposed research diagnostic criteria. However, as akathisia needs to be distinguished from a number of other disorders (see Chapters 6 and 7 for differential diagnosis), a clinical judgement is involved in the final diagnosis. An instrumental or a rating scale measure cannot, therefore, yield definitive diagnosis of the disorder. Factors like exposure to neuroleptic medication and the absence of nondrug causes must be taken into account. The current drug status of the patient may influence the manifestations of the akathisia, and this influence may differ for AA, TA or WA.

In Chapter 4, cut-off scores on an akathisia rating scale were presented in order to diagnose akathisia with acceptable sensitivity and specificity. This approach can be criticized for its dependence on accuracy of ratings of the different items and an implicit acceptance of the relative specificity of the items to akathisia, both of which conditions may not be met.

The setting in which it occurs

Akathisia usually occurs in patients with an active psychosis. This presents a number of difficulties. The patient is often reluctant to cooperate with any measurements that may not clearly be seen as being helpful; the fact that the disorder is the product of a treatment that is resented in the first place makes cooperation even less likely. The patient additionally may exhibit agitation, hyperactivity or catatonic symptoms which resemble akathisia and may not be differentiated by the patient from the akathisia. Other abnormal movements are often present. The acute akathisic may manifest a tremor, and the tardive akathisic a dyskinesia, that will complicate any automatic quantification procedure.

The variability

Akathisia demonstrates marked variability over time, especially in the mild cases. Even within one assessment session, it may manifest only intermittently. Some of this variability may be explained by posture, time of day, level of anxiety, arousal, stress, etc, but much variability is unexplained. Furthermore, day-to-day drug changes in the acutely ill patient will produce an inconsistent clinical picture. This variation affects estimates of reliability and makes longitudinal and treatment studies difficult to interpret if they involve small numbers of subjects.

The measurement stance

Most clinicians are aware of the effect of 'being watched' on the manifestations of some movement disorders. It is not uncommon to see patients with Tourette's syndrome demonstrate few tics in the doctor's office, even when not actively trying to suppress the movements. Akathisic patients, when being videotaped or asked to sit or stand on a strain-gauge platform, tend to show far fewer movements than when sitting in the lounge room relatively free of close scrutiny. This can frustrate many attempts at quantification.

Measurement methods

The various methods of measuring akathisia can be broadly classified as (i) instrumental methods, (ii) frequency counts of movements, (iii) videotape assessments and (iii) multi-item rating scales. The methods are applicable to all subtypes of akathisia, but the choice of particular items for the scales for different subtypes remains to be empirically examined.

Instrumental methods

The utility of automated techniques in the measurement of movement disorders has received increasing attention (Symposium, 1989). Traditionally, electrophysiological techniques used in movement disorders have involved EMG of the muscles involved and the correlation of the EEG with abnormal EMG. Analysis of reflexes as well as kinematic (including accelerometry) and kinetic analyses of the movements are increasingly being used with the growth in computer technology. Acceleration transducers have been the most popular tool, but many investigators have used ultrasound, pneumatic transducers, photographic tracings, load cells, capacitance circuits, electromagnetic moving coil circuits and photodetectors.

Instruments offer an objective assessment, without bias, carry-over or halo effects. They can be extremely useful for measuring drug effects, especially over short periods of time. They cannot, however, replace clinical diagnosis since judgement is usually involved in the latter. Patient-generated artefacts due to talking, smoking, humming, etc have to be accounted for, and the clinical validity of any measurement should be carefully established.

As May et al (1983) point out, only a few investigators have paid sufficient attention to the calibration of instruments against known standards of amplitude and frequency. For example, the response of many transducer–amplifier systems is not linear and flat, such that the high-frequency tremors tend to be exaggerated and the low-frequency ones underestimated. Magnetic and coil devices have a similar problem (Caliguiri et al, 1991). Further, attention must be given to the measurement conditions, eg, limb position in tremor measurement (Findley et al, 1981). Different methods of measurement must be compared for replication of the findings.

Accelerometry

Acceleration transducers are extensively used in the general measurement of motion. They all use Newton's law $F = Ma$, by measuring the force required to accelerate a known mass M. Accelerometers have been successfully used in the measurement of tremor (Marsden et al, 1969) and have been applied to TD with less success (Fann et al, 1977; Wirsching et al, 1991). They were first used in the assessment of akathisia by Braude et al (1984), who recorded finger and toe tremor in six akathisia patients and reported that akathisia was characterized by the presence of large-amplitude, low-frequency (<4-Hz), rhythmic foot movements, changes in the frequency and amplitude of which reflected the changes in severity. Our own studies of akathisia patients using hand and toe accelerometers suggest that while the associated tremor is well delineated, akathisic movements do not produce a characteristic pattern and are merely reflected by an increased force in the lower-frequency spectrum. This pattern cannot be differentiated from normal restless movements.

Accelerometry has many limitations in its application to akathisia. It is best designed to measure rhythmic movements such as tremors, not the arhythmic, semipurposive akathisic movements. Accelerometers can be attached to only limited sites on the body. They measure acceleration and velocity in one plane and therefore do not represent the movements in three dimensions, as would be necessary for akathisic movements.

Strain-gauge platform

The technical principles used are similar to those for accelerometers. A method we have adapted for the measurement of akathisia is the use of an akathisia platform. The patient sits in a chair which has strain-gauge transducers attached to the arms and legs, and keeps his or her feet on a footplate, again fitted with two transducers. The feet and arms are firmly but comfortably apposed to the footplate and arms of the chair, respectively. Any movement by the legs, arms, or trunk results in the deflection of a steel bar which is measured by foil strain-gauge elements circuited into a bridge form, the resultant signal being amplified by a bridge amplifier. Figure 9.1 gives the tracings from a patient with akathisia. Our preliminary work suggests that the platform

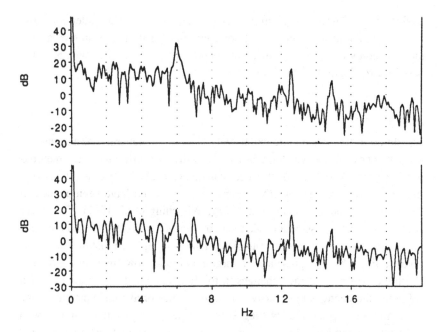

Fig. 9.1. The record of right and left leg movement from a patient with akathisia using a strain-gauge platform. The tracing is a mean of six 30-second epochs of data.

can provide a reliable and objective assessment of the motor restlessness of the patient. The system, however, suffers from the general limitations already alluded to. It imposes an artificial environment for the patient in which the akathisia may not manifest, thus underestimating the disorder. The transducers again record movement only in one plane, limiting their representativeness.

Ultrasound transducers

A number of authors (Haines and Sainsbury, 1972; Leonard et al, 1974; May et al, 1983) have reported the use of ultrasound transducers for the measurement of whole body movement in affective disorder, Huntington's chorea, TD, etc. The system works like the navigational system of a bat. The transducer emits and receives ultrasound waves, with any movement disturbing the pattern of the reflected waves, the frequency of which disturbance is digitally recorded. May et al (1983) demonstrated that the system provided activity counts proportional to the average velocity of all movements and was reasonably linear over a range from 6 to 60 counts per second but did not provide a frequency analysis of the signal. With this method, low-frequency, small-amplitude movements produce low counts, and large-amplitude, high-frequency movements very high counts. Small continuous movements therefore produce the same result as brief large movements, thus limiting the assessment (Bartzokis et al, 1989). These authors examined patients with Huntington's chorea in three positions and demonstrated that the system was sensitive in recording movements in the low-frequency range, with most movements being less than 2 Hz. High test–retest reliability was demonstrated by Resek et al (1981), and the results were valid in comparison with time-sampled scores from simultaneous videorecordings. The system is therefore adaptable to akathisia.

Three-dimensional motion analysis systems

Since limb movements are the most characteristic features of akathisia, a system that provides quantitative kinematics of several limb segments with high resolution in both the temporal and spatial domains would be extremely useful. Several systems are available that will accomplish this. One system described by Lee (1989) (WATSMART motion analysis system) uses infrared-emitting diodes that can be attached to the joints with two infrared cameras recording the position of each diode at a rate of 200/second. The results are then converted into three-dimensional coordinates that are used to compute movement path and velocity. It allows a fairly detailed analysis of movement if it is considered necessary.

Electromyography and polysomnography

The EMG activity in selected muscles will provide a map of the activity in those muscles. While this has been utilized to study the movements of dyskinesia (Haines and Sainsbury, 1972; Gardos and Cole, 1980), its general application to akathisia is limited by the nature of the movements being studied. Polysomnography, which relies on EMG as the measure of muscle activity and relates it to other measures such as EEG, electrocardiogram (ECG), respiration, etc, has been utilized in the assessment of RLS and in one study to investigate nocturnal leg movements and sleep in akathisia (Lipinski et al, 1991). EMG recordings from over the tibialis anterior were used to assess leg movements, a positive score being suggested by an abrupt increase in amplitude of at least 25 μV, duration of 0.5–3 seconds, and a ≥4-second interval from a previous movement. If five or more movements occurred in an interval of 90 seconds, it was recorded as an episode of periodic movements. If the episode was accompanied by a K-complex, EEG arousal or awakening, then leg movements with arousal were scored. The number of leg movements with arousal per hour of sleep gave the nocturnal myoclonus index. The authors did not find significant differences in the patterns of leg movement activity in sleep between akathisic patients and control subjects (healthy individuals and depressed patients). Akathisia patients were noted to exhibit 10- to 40-second bursts of increased leg muscle tone before sleep onset, the significance of which was unclear.

Microvibration

Microvibration has been suggested as an indicator of muscle tonus. Nishikawa et al (1992) proposed that its study could help differentiate AA from TA. However, the difference may have more to do with drug-induced rigidity than akathisia, and the claim does not seem to be based on firm theoretical reasons.

Activity monitoring (actigraph)

Some of the limitations of the preceding techniques (eg, the constraint of the laboratory and the brevity of the measurement) can be overcome by using a device that can be worn by the patient and allows ambulatory monitoring of movements. One such device is a microprocessor-controlled portable piezo-electric monitor that comes with many kilobytes of solid state memory and can record movements over days when worn continuously. The commercial varieties available (eg, the Mini-Motionlogger distributed by Ambulatory Monitoring, Inc.) are usually in the form of a small wrist-watch-sized accelerometer/recorder to be worn on the arm or leg. The device is sensitive enough to detect an acceleration of 0.01g/rad-sec. The epoch interval can be selected by the operator, and the sensitivity and gain can be varied. The data can be down-loaded to a microcomputer and read using customized software.

Actigraphy has been used in the assessment of both akathisia and RLS. Gardos et al (1992) collected 24-hour activity data in 29 neuroleptic-treated hospitalized patients and 9 normal controls. They found that this was a reliable and valid method, with highly significant correlations with clinical ratings. The depressed patients, even though being treated with smaller dosages of neuroleptics, had higher rates of akathisia than manic and schizophrenic patients. The authors also concluded that the measurement of akathisia was complicated by the patient's psychiatric disorder.

This technique shows great promise for determining factors that affect the manifestation of akathisia, eg, posture, time of day, stressful situations. It can also be adapted to provide objective outcome measures for treatment trials. Figures 6.2 and 6.3 give actigraphy tracings for an akathisic patient from our clinic over 4 and 24 hours. Each subject wore actigraphs on the left wrist and ankle over 3 days. The epoch interval used was for 1 second. The data are reported in arbitrary units. All movements higher than 3 Hz were filtered out.

Frequency counts of movements

Some authors have suggested the simple counting of movements in a prede-termined epoch as a measure of the severity of the movement disorder (Branchey et al, 1979). The method is ostensibly simple and reasonably pre-cise, and akathisia, with its large movements, would lend itself to such a mea-surement. There are, however, a number of disadvantages. The procedure is time-consuming and laborious, and usually depends on a videotape analysis. One can reliably count only one type of movement affecting one part of the body at one time, thus limiting the data set unless multiple measurements are done on the same subject. Counting does not take into account the amplitude of the movements and may therefore not have a high correlation with the overall severity of the disorder, as was reported by Richardson et al (1982) in the case of TD. No reports have been published in which this method of assessment has been used for akathisia. Its validity in the case of akathisia, therefore, remains to be established.

Videotape assessments

The idea of a videotape assessment of akathisia is attractive as a clinical record as well as for research. Serial assessments on videotape can be readily compared with each other and lend themselves to blind ratings. Not only are the motor symptoms adequately recorded, but the patient's subjective report is also captured and is available for later review. For case conferences and multiple ratings, videotapes present a less intrusive method of assessment, and many patients are less likely to freeze before a camera than before a large group of investigators or clinicians. Some patients may suppress their move-ments, deliberately or involuntarily, when under observation, but a properly conducted videotaped interview, giving the patient some time to 'forget' the presence of the camera, can usually overcome the problem. Videotape inter-views permit standardization of the assessment procedure. They can be used for training other raters and to establish interrater reliability. Subtle movements can sometimes be observed on videotapes that may be overlooked during clinical assessments. Videotapes also permit the observation of the same movement repeatedly in case of doubt about any ratings.

A number of investigators have used videotaped interviews for the assessment of TD (Asnis et al, 1977; Fann et al, 1977; Barnes and Trauer, 1982; Gerlach and Korsgaard, 1983), and the reliability and validity of at least two scales have been published (Barnes and Trauer, 1982; Gerlach et al, 1993). The St. Hans Rating Scale (Gerlach et al, 1993) incorporated a global rating of psychic and motor akathisia, each on a severity scale of 0–6. The intrarater reliability of the ratings over three occasions was generally good, although both experienced and inexperienced raters tended to vary slightly in their ratings of the motor component over sessions ($p < .05$). The interrater reliability was high (unbiased intraclass correlation coefficients were .82 and .76, respectively, for psychic and motor components on the first rating) but tended to fall over the three ratings (.63 and .60, respectively, for third rating). Divergent validity was demonstrated for akathisia, in that this rating had its own domain of information, with low correlations with the ratings for 'hyperkinesia' (essentially dyskinesia), parkinsonism and dystonia. This scale has been used successfully in a multicentre study (Nordic Dyskinesia Study Group, 1986).

Videotape ratings have a few limitations. First, they are dependent on the technical quality of the recordings, which may be compromised by poor equipment or an inexperienced recordist. Second, the need to produce good-quality recordings limits the portability of the assessment. Third, the patient may suppress the movements when under the scrutiny of the videocamera. The artificial lighting in the recording room may also adversely affect the 'naturalness' of the setting. Fourth, if the recording is being performed to rate other drug-induced movements as well, close-ups are necessary to focus on fine movements, with consequent loss of the full profile for brief periods. Overall, our impression is that videotape rating scales are likely to be extremely useful in the assessment of akathisia and their full potential has not been exploited.

Multi-item rating scales

Multi-item rating scales have been the most popular, with different scales being developed by different groups for use in their own investigations. These scales are generally simple to use, and the different characteristics of the disorders can be comprehensively rated. The assessment can be standardized, and even naive raters can be trained to perform reliable assessments. The scales generate ordinal or interval data which are suitable for manipulation by standard statistical techniques (Gardos et al, 1977). They are relatively inexpensive to use and do not rely on sophisticated and expensive equipment. They are therefore very portable and are excellent for screening purposes.

These scales have some disadvantages. Since subjective judgement is involved in the ratings, proper training and regular monitoring of the ratings are necessary. Even the same rater may show a drift during repeated ratings, with the thresholds used for the ratings falling or rising depending on circumstances and experience. The concurrent validity of rating scales is often examined in comparison with preexisting scales, with the potential to perpetuate errors. Rating scales are not generally designed to arrive at diagnoses, but rather to document the phenomena present and quantify their severity. They can, nevertheless, aid the diagnostic process. Investigators are often tempted to use a certain cut-off score on a scale to determine entry into a research study. For this reason, the issue of diagnosis using a particular scale must be generally addressed. In the case of akathisia, the relevant questions to ask are: Is there a certain score above which the diagnosis of akathisia is beyond doubt? Is a certain score on both the subjective and objective items necessary for a definitive diagnosis? Are there certain items that best characterize the disorder, and would a positive rating on them receive greater weighting? Is the scale useful for the assessment of all subtypes of akathisia? If global judgements are being made, are suitable anchor points present? Most scales used to assess akathisia have failed to address these questions.

An overview of published rating scales

A number of rating scales for akathisia have been used by investigators in the past, and these are summarized in Table 9.1.

The Extrapyramidal Rating Scale of Chouinard et al (1980) was developed to rate TD but also rates akathisia, parkinsonism and dystonia. The motor component of akathisia is rated on a scale of 6 (0 = *absent, 6 = constant movement*). It also rates the patient's complaints of being 'restless, nervous, unable to sit still' from 0 (*none*) to 3 (*unable to sit down*). Some investigators have used the sum of the objective and subjective items of this scale to obtain an overall akathisia rating on a scale of 0–9 (Lipinski et al, 1984).

Bartels et al (1981, 1987) used a 3-point scale for akathisia based on subjective and objective symptoms, but these were not rated separately. No reliability or validity data were published.

Table 9.1. *Synopsis of akathisia rating scales*

Scale	Specific for akathisia?	Global ratings range	Subjective features considered	Subjective/objective ratings separately	Reliability data published	Reference
Chouinard Extrapyramidal Rating Scale	No	0–9 (0–6 and 0–3)	Yes	Yes	Yes	Chouinard et al (1980)
Akathisia Rating Scale	Yes	0–3	Yes	No	No	Bartels et al (1981)
Extrapyramidal Side-Effects Rating Scale	No	0–3	No	No	No	Kabes et al (1982)
Akathisia Rating Scale	Yes	0–3	Yes	No	No	Friis et al (1983)
Involuntary Movement and Extrapyramidal Scale	No	0–6	Yes	No	No	Van Putten, May and Marder (unpublished)
Akathisia Questionnaire and Examination	Yes	0–3	Yes	Yes	No	Braude et al (1983)
Hillside-LIJ modification of Simpson and Angus Extrapyramidal Symptom Scale	Yes	0–4	No	No	No	Adler et al (1985, 1986)
Analogue Scale for Akathisia	Yes	100-mm line	No	No	No	Adler et al (1985)
Rating Scale for Drug-Induced Akathisia	Yes	0–5	Yes	Yes	Yes	Barnes (1989)
The Hillside Akathisia Scale	Yes	0–8	Yes	Yes	Yes	Fleischhacker et al (1989)
Visual Analogue Scale	Yes	100-mm line	Yes	No	No	Sachdev and Chee (1990)
PHH Akathisia Scale	Yes	0–3	Yes	Yes	Yes	Sachdev (1994c)

Kabes et al (1982) used a global (0 = *none*, 3 = *unable to sit down*) objective rating of akathisia for a pharmacological study. The subjective features were not rated, and the authors did not publish reliability and validity data.

Friis et al (1983) described a 4-point rating scale for both subjective and objective items, along with definitions of each rating.

Van Putten et al (1984b,c) used a 7-point rating of akathisia, based on subjective report and observed movements, as part of the Involuntary Movement and Extrapyramidal Scale.

Adler et al (1985, 1986) used the Hillside-LIJ modification of the Extrapyramidal Symptoms Scale of Simpson and Angus (1970), which rates the movement (objective) component of akathisia on a scale of 0–4 (0 = *absent*, 4 = *extreme, heightened activity*).

Kramer et al (1988) used a 10-item rating scale which had four subscales, and each item was rated on a 6-point (0–5) scale. Reliability and validity data on this scale have not been presented. The following items were used:

Subscale I, subjective symptoms of akathisia: item 1 (need to move), item 2 (need to move legs), item 3 (uncomfortable skin sensations), item 4 (internal restlessness)

Subscale II, patient's subjective global response

Subscale III, objective signs of akathisia: item 1 (shifting posture while seated), item 2 (movements of feet or legs while seated), item 3 (rocking while standing), item 4 (frank pacing)

Subscale IV, rater's global assessment of subjective and objective findings

Total score, sum of all subscale scores

Visual analogue ratings have been used by some investigators (Adler et al, 1986; Sachdev and Chee, 1990). The ratings performed by Sachdev and Chee were anchored on a 100-mm line based on perceived leg and toe movements: 0 = *none; 25 = sometimes and a little; 50 = sometimes and severe, or most of the time and a little; 75 = most of the time and severe; 100 = as severe as is possible and continuous.* Two investigators separately rated the patient, and an intraclass correlation coefficient of .82 was observed.

The Akathisia Questionnaire and Examination published by Braude et al (1983) was developed for the investigation of the clinical characteristics of akathisia. The authors used a 4-point scale to rate four subjective measures (questionnaire) and 14 objective measures (examination). Severity was judged by the proportion of observation time that a particular movement was present. A global rating into absent, mild, moderate and severe was also made. Although the authors described the procedure of assessment in detail, it was never developed into the form of a rating scale. Nevertheless, it was adapted to serve that function by Brown et al (1987) in a subsequent investigation, without any published data on its reliability and validity. It has been subsequently used by other investigators (Barton et al, 1990; Nemes et al, 1991; O'Loughlin et al, 1991).

Most of these scales have some common characteristics: the ratings are global, using either objective alone or both subjective and objective features; the scales were developed by groups for their own particular investigations; the akathisia ratings often form a part of larger scales for rating extrapyramidal symptoms; and the psychometric properties of the scales have not generally been published. In the past few years, three scales have been published for which reliability and validity data have been presented. These will be briefly discussed and their relative merits highlighted.

Barnes Akathisia Rating Scale

The clinical characteristics of akathisia reported by Braude et al (1983) and subsequently by Barnes and Braude (1985) were the basis for the Barnes Akathisia Rating Scale (BARS) derived by Barnes (1989). Observable movements and the subjectively experienced restlessness are rated on a scale of 0–3, with subjective distress also separately rated. Patients are observed while sitting and standing for a minimum of 2 minutes in each position, while they engage in neutral conversation. The author states that patients with akathisia would typically experience a desire to move, an awareness that they are unable to keep their legs still or a compulsion to move with a particular reference to the legs. This constituted the 'awareness of restlessness' aspect of the rating. The author distinguished this from the distress generated by the akathisia, arguing that this had significant practical implications, and in some cases, especially in CA, restlessness may be present without any subjective distress. This scale is thus unique in separating the experience of restlessness from the distress due to this experience. In addition, the scale rates akathisia globally on a scale of 0–5 (absent, nil, mild, moderate, marked, severe). The ratings take into consideration observations in the ward outside the time of the formal rating procedure. Special emphasis is placed on certain movements considered to be characteristic of akathisia, and these are included in the descriptors for the various ratings. A rating of 0 is given if subjective symptoms are absent. If only the motor features of akathisia are present, the author recommends the use of the term *pseudoakathisia* (see Chapters 4 and 7 for a detailed discussion of this concept). Mild distress and fidgetiness which cannot be easily distinguished from anxiety and agitation are rated as 'questionable'. The scale, therefore, yields four scores: objective, subjective awareness of restlessness, subjective distress related to restlessness and global.

The author demonstrated a high interrater reliability for all four scores between two raters who rated 42 chronically ill, hospitalized schizophrenic patients during the same examination (Barnes and Halstead, 1988). The scale has face and construct validity, but concurrent validity with other measures of akathisia has not been examined. The author argues that the scale is applicable to both acutely ill and long-term-medicated patients, but the application of the scale to different subtypes of akathisia has not been empirically examined. The scale is simple and easy to use. One difficulty in the ratings is the need to decide whether movements are present for less or greater than half the observation period, which can be a difficult clinical decision. In the objective ratings, the duration of characteristic movements, rather than their amplitude and frequency, is used for the ratings. The descriptive guidelines provided for the global ratings suggest some kind of hierarchy in the symptoms, but the empirical basis of this hierarchy is not presented. In spite of these limitations, the scale has been widely used by other investigators (eg, Sachdev and Loneragan, 1991b; McCreadie et al, 1992). A full description of the scale is presented in Appendix C.

The Hillside Akathisia Scale

Fleischhacker et al (1991) published the Hillside Akathisia Scale (HAS) primarily for use in clinical psychopharmacology. This scale comprises two subjective items ('a sensation of inner restlessness' and 'the urge to move') and three objective items ('akathisia present in the head and trunk', 'akathisia present in hands and arms' and 'akathisia present in feet and legs'), with anchor points provided for the ratings taking both amplitude and frequency of the movements into consideration. The authors did not attempt to characterize and rate the different phenomena separately, finding their inclusive approach more reliable. A judgement that the movements being rated are akathisic therefore needs to precede the actual rating of these movements. Patients are observed in sitting, standing and lying positions, and two manoeuvres (serial sevens and finger tapping) are performed. A global rating is performed using a scale of 0–7 adapted from the Clinical Global Impression (CGI) Scale (National Institute of Mental Health, 1985). Since this scale was designed primarily to measure severity of akathisia in psychopharmacological research, it incorporates a global measure of improvement on a scale of 0–7, along with a judgement of whether the improvement is entirely due to drug treatment. The reliability of this scale was examined by having four raters (two 'expert')

simultaneously rate 37 patients with NIA. The authors reported intraclass correlation coefficients of .94 for the HAS total score, .84 for the CGI Scale,
.97–.99 for the total subjective scores and .76 for the total objective scores.
The reliability of the total scores for arm (.55) and trunk (.66) movements was
relatively low, but for the legs (.82) was high (Fleischhacker et al, 1989).

A German version of this scale has also been published (Fleischhacker et
al, 1991) and its reliability demonstrated. The authors commented on the
higher correlation between the global and the objective scores, arguing that
the raters were more likely to place emphasis on observable rather than
reported features. In a pilot study investigating the effects of ritanserin on
akathisia, this scale has been demonstrated to be sensitive to change. The
HAS is presented in Appendix D.

The Prince Henry Hospital Akathisia Scale

Development and reliability. We recently reported the development, reliability and validity of the PHH Akathisia Scale (Sachdev, 1994c). Previously
reported clinical characteristics of akathisia (Braude et al, 1983) were used to
initially construct the Long Scale, which comprised 16 items listed in Table
6.2. Each item was rated on a scale of 0–3, which, however, was different
from the one used by Braude et al. The subjective items were rated as absent,
mild, moderate and severe on the basis of the patient's response to specific
questions. The objective items were rated on the basis of both intensity and
duration, unlike Braude et al, who rated these solely on the basis of the proportion of observation time for which these were present. We found the
Braude et al ratings of 'present for less than half the observation time' and
'more than half the time' difficult to apply in practice. Movements that were
otherwise judged to be severe in intensity often occurred intermittently for a
few seconds at a time, thus making their total duration of occurrence only a
small proportion of the actual period of observation. Furthermore, precise
timing of the movements proved to be difficult when multiple movements
were being observed simultaneously, and could be done only if the videotapes
of the ratings were rated on multiple occasions. Our decision to use both
intensity and duration in the ratings is in agreement with the practice adopted
in the HAS.

Our ratings were conservative, and when there was doubt about the presence of a particular item, it was rated as 0. There was, therefore, a categorical
shift from 0 to 1 denoting absence or presence, and the rating of 1, 2 or 3 was
then a decision regarding severity.

A standardized procedure was followed for the examinations. Subjects were seated in a comfortable chair with the full body visible to the examiner, with arms and legs partially unclothed. They were engaged in neutral conversation for the first 5 minutes, without the movements being rated in this period. The objective ratings were performed in the next 8 minutes, 4 minutes in the sitting and 2 each in the standing and lying positions. A mental task, counting from 30 backwards, and a motor task, tapping the fingers of both hands for 15 seconds each, were performed in each position. The subjects also listened to an audiotape recording of a passage for 2 minutes while sitting. They were then rated on their subjective report. Observations outside the period of the rating were not used for the ratings, although these were noted separately.

The Long Scale was administered to 100 consecutive psychiatric inpatients, recently started on neuroleptic medication, on days 7 and 14 of the study. The study's criteria allowed only AA patients to be included, while excluding TA subjects. Patients were also assessed on a global rating with overall ratings on a scale of 0–3 (absent, mild, moderate, severe) for akathisia based on the clinical judgement of the investigators.

It became clear from the examination of the mean scores for the three positions that the 'lying' items were scoring very low (range of means, day 7 = 0.05–0.24, day 14 = 0.03–0.16). We then examined the cases with a rating of 2 or more on any of the lying items. There were five such cases on day 7 and three on day 14. All these subjects had been simultaneously rated 2 or more on at least two other objective items (sitting or standing), thereby suggesting that the lying items were not providing further information. Deletion of the lying items did not considerably alter the Cronbach's alpha (day 7 = .9008, day 14 = .9053), and for the item 'coarse tremor of legs/feet', deletion actually increased the alpha. We concluded from these results that the lying items could be omitted without affecting the ability of the scale to assess the presence of akathisia or rate its severity accurately. The omission, however, would result in a considerable saving in assessment time.

Two other items were noted to have low mean values and a negative impact on Cronbach's alpha: Sub-1, 'distressing sensations in the legs'; and sit-3, 'inability to keep toes still'. These symptoms were not considered critical to the diagnosis of akathisia, and the items were, therefore deleted. Three more items rated low: sit-1, 'inability to remain seated'; sit-5, 'semipurposeful hand/arm movements'; stand-3, 'inability to remain standing on one spot'. Since these features were considered to be fairly characteristic of moderate to severe akathisia and exclusion of these items lowered the alpha, these were retained for the final version of the scale.

The new version of the scale had three subjective and seven objective items and required an examination of the subject in sitting and standing positions only. The ratings on this 10-item scale ('New Scale') were then subjected to a reliability analysis using the same data set as previously with the following results:

Day 7 assessment: item mean 0.33 (variance 0.02); interitem correlation mean .49 (range .17–.79, variance .02); Cronbach's alpha .9001; standardized item alpha .9053

Day 14 assessment: item mean 0.32 (variance 0.03); interitem correlation mean .41 (range .13–.66; variance .01); Cronbach's alpha .8674; standardized item alpha .8739

Split-half statistics were computed for the 10-item scale with the following results:

Day 7: alpha for part 1 = .87, part 2 = .89; correlation between forms = .62; equal-length Spearman–Brown coefficient = .77

Day 14: alpha for part 1 = .77, part 2 = .81; correlation between forms = .70; equal-length Spearman–Brown coefficient = .82

The Spearman rank-order correlation coefficients between the subjective and objective items of the 10-item scale and their sums (Sum-Sub and Sum-Obj, respectively) are presented in Table 9.2. Most correlations were significant, suggesting an internal consistency in the scale. The Sum-Sub and Sum-Obj scores had a modest but significant correlation ($r = .54$).

The Long Scale ratings were subjected to a factor analysis. The day 7 analysis extracted four factors, with the majority of the items loading highly on factors 1 and 2. Only two items (sit-3 and lie-1) had high loadings on factor 3 (factor score coefficient > .3) and one item (Sub-1) on factor 4. Day 14 data yielded three factors with somewhat similar loadings on factors 1 and 2. Since the items loading on factors 3 and 4 had been tentatively excluded after the reliability analysis, the principal components analysis was then repeated on the 10-item scale. Both days' data yielded two factors, the score coefficients for which are presented in Table 9.3. As is apparent, the subjective items loaded highly on factor 2, on which only one objective item had a high loading. A varimax rotation of the matrix suggested the 'objective' factor first and the 'subjective' factor second. Oblique rotations produced similar factor solutions, with the correlations between the factors being .45 for both days 7 and 14 data. The results of this analysis were interpreted as supporting the decision to rate the subjective and objective features of akathisia separately.

The sums of the subjective and objective items were considered to represent the total subjective (Sum-Sub) and objective (Sum-Obj) scores, respec-

Table 9.2. *Spearman's correlation coefficients between scores on different akathisia scale items on day 7 (n = 100)*

Items	Sub-2	Sub-3	Sub-4	Sit-1	Sit-2	Sit-4	Sit-5	Stand-1	Stand-2	Stand-3	Sum-Sub	Sum-Obj	Sum
Sub-2	1.00												
Sub-3	.51***	1.00											
Sub-4	.39***	.53***	1.00										
Sit-1	.42***	.40***	.40***	1.00									
Sit-2	.44***	.43***	.32**	.54***	1.00								
Sit-4	.33***	.31**	.31**	.51***	.46***	1.00							
Sit-5	.21*	.18*	.22*	.30**	.36***	.57***	1.00						
Stand-1	.37***	.37***	.43***	.55***	.58***	.66***	.54***	1.00					
Stand-2	.30**	.25**	.33***	.52***	.46***	.66***	.54***	.72***	1.00				
Stand-3	.30**	.30**	.36***	.53***	.41***	.41***	.51***	.46***	.50***	1.00			
Sum-Sub	.85***	.78***	.68***	.48***	.48***	.41***	.27**	.44***	.35***	.38***	1.00		
Sum-Obj	.46***	.43***	.37***	.59***	.77***	.76***	.58***	.78***	.75***	.54***	.54***	1.00	
Sum	.70***	.65***	.57***	.57***	.69***	.68***	.52***	.72***	.67***	.52***	.83***	.88***	1.00

Note: Sum-Sub and Sum-Obj are sums of three subjective and seven objective items, respectively, and Sum is total of all items. 2-tailed, $*p < .05$; $**p < .01$; $***p < .001$.

Table 9.3. *Factor analysis of the 10-item New Scale on days 7 and 14: the factor loadings on the unrotated and varimax rotated factor matrices*

| | Day 7 (n = 100) | | | | | Day 14 (n = 88) | | | | |
| | Mean score (SD) | Unrotated factors | | Rotated factors | | Mean score (SD) | Unrotated factors | | Rotated factors | |
Item		1	2	1	2		1	2	1	2
Sub-2	.59 (.8)	.62	.54	.14	.81	.71 (.8)	.64	.47	.20	.77
Sub-3	.41 (.7)	.59	.64	.06	.86	.33 (.5)	.60	.54	.13	.80
Sub-4	.26 (.5)	.68	.37	.30	.71	.30 (.5)	.62	.36	.26	.67
Sit-1	.19 (.5)	.75	.21	.45	.63	.10 (.3)	.61	−.11	.55	.50
Sit-2	.43 (.73)	.82	.10	.57	.59	.56 (.7)	.82	−.01	.65	.50
Sit-4	.33 (.68)	.79	−.24	.76	.31	.37 (.6)	.73	−.05	.61	.37
Sit-5	.19 (.5)	.61	−.50	.85	.05	.19 (.4)	.75	−.05	.61	.43
Stand-1	.39 (.7)	.89	−.13	.78	.46	.28 (.6)	.80	−.13	.70	.40
Stand-2	.34 (.6)	.79	−.38	.85	.20	.27 (.3)	.65	−.32	.70	.16
Stand-3	.16 (.4)	.73	−.33	.77	.20	.14 (.4)	.62	−.57	.84	−.05

tively. The sum of all the items gave an overall 'Sum' score, which represented a global rating for the severity of akathisia.

Validity. Since the items were drawn from those recognized to be characteristic of acute DIA, the scale has face validity. Construct validation was examined by calculating the Spearman correlation coefficients of the Sum-Sub, Sum-Obj and Sum scores of days 7 and 14 with the global scores. The correlations with the global score were modest (range .42–.59) but highly significant ($p < .001$). The relatively low correlations may reflect the fact that many subjects with a 0 global rating scored on at least some items of the 10-item scale.

The factorial separation of subjective and objective features has been alluded to. We were interested in examining whether the subjective items were rating something different from anxiety as rated on the Spielberger et al (1967) scale and the Brief Psychiatric Rating Scale (BPRS) (Overall and Gorham, 1962), and depression as rated on Zung's (1965) scale. Similarly, we wanted to know how the objective ratings correlated with the ratings of hyperactivity on the BPRS. The Spearman correlation coefficients are presented in Table 9.4. Of note is the fact that Sum-Sub had a low correlation with the anxiety and depression scores, suggesting that it was measuring a

Table 9.4. *Spearman correlation coefficients between akathisia scores and other ratings*

	Anxiety rating		Depression rating (Zung)	Motor hyperactivity (BPRS)
	Spielberger	BPRS		
Day 7				
Total group (*n* = 100)				
Sub-Sub	.17	.05	.20*	−.02
Sub-Obj	.01	.09	.09	.26**
Akathisia group (*n* = 23)				
Sum-Sub	.10	.12	.40	.22
Sum-Obj	−.10	.12	.05	.27
Day 14 (n = 88)				
Sum-Sub	.11	−.03	.04	.06
Sub-Obj	−.04	.02	−.02	.18

Note: 2-tailed, *p < .05; **p < .01.

different construct. The objective akathisia ratings correlated poorly with the BPRS ratings of motor activity. This further supported the contention that akathisia, as a syndrome, was distinguishable from anxiety, depression and agitation.

Interrater reliability and concurrent validity. The reliability of the PHH Scale was examined by administering it to a new group of 50 patients treated with neuroleptic drugs. Its concurrent validity was examined in relation to the BARS. The subjects were rated by two investigators experienced in diagnosing and rating akathisia, with one interviewing the patient while the other observed. Forty-three of the 50 patients were also simultaneous rated on the Barnes (1989) scale. The interrater reliability for the PHH Scale was determined by calculating the kappa coefficient for each item and for the global ratings by the two raters. The Sum-Sub, Sum-Obj and global ratings by each rater were correlated with the subjective, objective and global scores, respectively, on the BARS to examine the concurrent validity. Table 9.5 gives the kappa coefficients for each item and the global akathisia ratings. All correlations were highly significant ($p < .01$), with kappa ranging from .42 to .81. The Pearson correlations with the ratings on the BARS were high: (i) the sum of subjective items of the PHH Scale, when correlated with the subjective (awareness) and subjective (distress) scores of the BARS had $r = .84, .86$ (rater 1) and .75, .82 (rater 2), respectively; (ii) the sum of the objective items

Table 9.5. *Interrater reliability of the new akathisia scale: mean (SD)*
ratings by two investigators, kappa coefficients and t *score on 50 subjects*

Scale item	Rater 1	Rater 2	Kappa	t Score
Sub-1	.40	.48	.65	6.75
	(.73)	(.81)		
Sub-2	.38	.32	.80	7.54
	(.40)	(.68)		
Sub-3	.20	.26	.63	5.28
	(.45)	(.56)		
Sit-1	.44	.36	.81	8.18
	(.76)	(.75)		
Sit-2	.14	.18	.48	4.08
	(.76)	(.75)		
Sit-3	.06	.18	.42	4.67
	(.31)	(.48)		
Sit-4	.02	.04	.66	4.95
	(.14)	(.20)		
Stand-1	.15	.17	.55	5.12
	(.57)	(.59)		
Stand-2	.15	.22	.53	.37
	(.53)	(.49)		
Stand-3	.00	.05	—	—
	(.00)	(.22)		
Global	.36	.36	.70	6.75
	(.72)	(.75)		

Note: All correlations were highly significant ($p < .01$).

correlated with the objective rating on the BARS as $r = .91$ (rater 1) and .94 (rater 2). The global akathisia ratings on the two scales had correlations of .84 (rater 1) and .86 (rater 2). All correlations were significant (*t* test, two-tailed $p < .01$).

Comments. Some deficiencies in the data must be highlighted. Ideally, the PHH Scale and the global ratings should have been performed by independent raters for the validity analysis to be adequate. This condition was not met in the study, thus making further investigations necessary to establish fully the validity of the scale. The scale was developed for AA; its suitability for TA is not known and warrants empirical investigation. The scale is clearly not a diagnostic instrument and should not be used solely for this purpose. For research purposes, however, if it is indeed used to establish the inclusion criteria of akathisia, we propose that the ratings used should be as discussed in Chapter 4 on the diagnostic criteria.

Conclusions

The measurement of akathisia, important as it is for clinical research, presents a number of difficulties owing to the complex manifestations of the disorder, the lack of a well-accepted definition and its variability. The efforts at its quantification have been far from satisfactory. Methods that have been used include instrumental methods, frequency counts, videotape measures and rating scales. All have limitations, but multi-item rating scales have been the most popular. While different rating scales have been adapted by different investigators for their own purposes, at least three rating scales are now available whose psychometric properties have been studied. These scales need to be examined further for their relative merits. Videotape measures have been insufficiently studied but hold the potential for providing excellent records. There is no instrumental method that is totally satisfactory, but a combination of strain-gauge measurement and actigraphy may provide an accurate measure of the motor component of akathisia.

10

Aetiology and pathogenesis of akathisia

Out of the air a voice without a face
Proved by statistics that some cause was just
In tones as dry and level as the place
  W. H. Auden, *Shield of Achilles* (1955)

In this chapter, the various factors of importance in the aetiology of akathisia, and the proposed pathogenetic mechanisms, will be discussed. For this purpose, we will consider AA in the first part of the chapter and TA and WA in the second. The aetiology of akathisia must be understood in terms of the drugs that are directly causative and a number of background variables that are likely to increase the risk of its development. The pathogenesis of akathisia is incompletely understood, and many competing hypothesis exists. Some animal literature will be reviewed that provides some insights into the pathogenetic mechanisms. In addition, a model will be presented that attempts to synthesize the diverse information on pathogenesis. This model takes into consideration our preliminary understanding of the neurophysiological basis of movement disorders and the role of parallel, segregated neuronal circuits that involve the basal ganglia and the cortex.

Acute akathisia

Aetiology

Drug-related variables

Nature of drugs causing akathisia. The various drugs reported to cause akathisia are listed in Table 10.1. In summary, akathisia is typically associated with the classical neuroleptics, but many newer antipsychotics and a

Table 10.1. *Drugs reported to cause acute akathisia*

Antipsychotic drugs
Conventional neuroleptics
  Phenothiazines
  Butyrophenones
  Thioxanthenes
  Dibenzoxazepines
  Indolic derivative
  Rauwolfia alkaloid
Newer antipsychotics
  Benzamides – sulpiride, remoxipride, raclopride, metoclopramide
  Clozapine and related drugs
  Benzisoxazoles – risperidone
  Other drugs – savoxepine, sertindole

Antidepressant drugs
  5HT reuptake inhibitors – fluoxetine, paroxetine, fluvoxamine
  Heterocyclic antidepressants – amoxapine, mianserin, TCAs ±
    conjugated oestrogen

Catecholamine-depleting drugs
  Tetrabenazine

5HT antagonists
  Methysergide
  Buspirone

Anticonvulsants
  Carbamazepine
  Ethosuximide

Calcium channel antagonists
  Diltiazem, flunarizine, cinnarizine

Mood-stabilizing drugs
  Lithium carbonate

---

number of other drugs have been reported to cause akathisia. In addition, as discussed in the chapters on restlessness and dysphoria, many drugs produce side-effects closely resembling akathisia, which could also provide some insights into its pathophysiology.

A study of the pharmacology of these drugs does not directly provide insights into the pathogenesis of akathisia, largely because these drugs manifest a variety of actions in the CNS. The classical neuroleptics affect many neurotransmitter systems in the brain, in particular DA, ACh, histamine (H), α-adrenergic (αA) and 5HT, and less importantly βA, opiate and GABA, receptors (Richelson, 1984). Neuroleptic drugs distribute favourably to the brain, with brain concentrations 2–40 times those in the blood (Sunderland,

Cohen, 1987), where they are preferentially associated with the cell membranes (Seeman, 1977), in proximity to the receptors at which they are antagonists (Carlsson, 1978). By concentrating near their sites of action, even small amounts can produce significant effects (Cohen et al, 1992).

Interaction with the DA receptors has received the greatest attention in the understanding of the mechanism of action of neuroleptic drugs. It has been recognized for 10–15 years that there were two subtypes of DA receptors, the so-called D_1 and D_2 receptors (Kebabian and Caine, 1979). In this schema, based on pharmacological and biochemical data, the D_1 receptor was responsible for the stimulation of adenyl cyclase (AC) and had low affinity for butyrophenone neuroleptics, whereas the D_2 receptors had no effect or mediated the inhibition of AC and possessed high affinity for the butyrophenones and substituted benzamides (Strange, 1990). An excellent correlation was demonstrated between the affinities of neuroleptic drugs for D_2 receptors and the average daily dose used to treat schizophrenia (Creese et al, 1976; Seeman et al, 1976). DA receptors are present in several parts of the CNS, and antagonism of these receptors is responsible for certain endocrinological and extrapyramidal side-effects of the drugs as well. However, it is no longer tenable to attribute all antipsychotic action to the antagonism of D_2 receptors. Recent advances in molecular biology have provided evidence for a larger family of DA receptors (see later), and there is emerging evidence that many of the newer 'atypical' antipsychotics may not be potent D_2 antagonists and may act through other mechanisms. For example, clozapine, a potent antipsychotic, has a high affinity for the D_4 receptor but is a less effective D_2 receptor antagonist than the classical neuroleptics (Meltzer, 1991). A number of new antipsychotic drugs have been developed that are selective D_1 and D_2/D_3 antagonists or partial D_2 agonists or antagonize D_2 along with other receptors (Gerlach, 1991). A study of the EPSE and akathisia associated with the newer agents provides some insights into the neurotransmitter systems involved in their pathogenesis.

Table 10.2 gives the relative affinities of various neuroleptics for different receptors, indicating the lack of specificity of these drugs for any particular receptor. The drugs have significant antimuscarinic, antihistaminergic, antiadrenergic and antiserotoninergic effects, some of which may be relevant to the understanding of akathisia.

The second group of drugs strongly associated with akathisia are the 5HT reuptake inhibitors that selectively enhance 5HT neurotransmission (Lipinski et al, 1989). Since 5HT inhibits DA cells in the VTA, the final pathway of akathisia may again be reduced DA neurotransmission. The issue of 5HT–DA interaction and akathisia will be discussed later.

Table 10.2. *Affinities of neuroleptics for human brain receptors*

Drug	Dopamine D_2	ACh muscarinic	Histamine H_1	Adrenergic α_1	α_2
Neuroleptic					
Chlorpromazine	5.3	1.4	11	38	0.13
Thioridazine	3.8	5.6	6.2	20	0.13
Trifluoperazine	38	0.15	1.6	4.2	0.38
Fluphenazine	125	0.053	4.8	11	0.064
Haloperidol	25	0.0042	0.053	16	0.026
cis-Thiothixene	222	0.034	17	9.1	0.50
Loxapine	1.4	0.22	20	3.6	0.042
Molindone	0.83	0.00026	0.00081	0.04	0.16
Clozapine	0.56	8.3	36	11	0.62
Reference drug					
Spiperone	625	—	—	—	—
Atropine	—	42	—	—	—
d-Chlorpheniramine	—	—	6.7	—	—
Phentolamine	—	—	—	6.7	—
Yohimbine	—	—	—	—	62

Note: Affinity $10^{-7} \times 1/K_D$, where K_D is the equilibrium dissociation constant in molarity.
Source: Richelson (1984).

Antidepressants that are generally recognized to produce akathisia (eg, amoxapine) have an intrinsic antidopaminergic activity (Ross et al, 1983). Mianserin, which enhances adrenergic activity but does not significantly affect DA function, has been reported to cause RLS rather than true akathisia (Paik et al, 1989). The evidence that other tricyclic antidepressants cause akathisia is less firmly established, with only one report in their favour (Zubenko et al, 1987). Oestrogens, when given in conjunction with tricyclics, possibly enhance the antidopaminergic effects of the latter (Krishnan et al, 1984).

Calcium channel antagonists have been demonstrated to have a significant role in DA function in the brain, with some antiserotonergic and antihistaminic activity as well (Micheli et al, 1987). Some calcium channel blockers have been shown to inhibit DA release (Ehlert et al, 1982) or directly compete with DA for D_2 receptor binding in the striatum (DeVries and Beart, 1985). They can cause a significant parkinsonian syndrome (Chouza et al, 1986). These drugs have a potential role in the treatment of movement disorders (Goldstein, 1984), mania (Giannini et al, 1984) and schizophrenia (Dustan and Jackson, 1976). Some neuroleptics, such as pimozide and penfluidol, that are structurally similar to verapamil are also relatively potent calcium channel blockers (DeVries and Beart, 1985). The association of akathisia with calcium channel antagonists may, therefore, be explained entirely on the basis of their antidopaminergic action.

The uncommon association of akathisia with lithium may again be explained on the basis of its mild antidopaminergic action (Friedman and Gershon, 1973). Lithium is known to cause mild parkinsonian side-effects or worsen NIP (Sachdev, 1986). In addition, lithium enhances noradrenergic functions (Terao et al, 1991) and has a physostigmine-like effect, which may also account for its action on the extrapyramidal system. Methysergide, a 5HT antagonist, with some vasoconstrictor and oxytocic activity, has been reported to cause akathisia in one case report (Bernick, 1988), but it also has mild DA antagonist properties.

In summary, the biochemical property that best links the various drugs that cause AA is their ability to reduce DA function in the CNS. The relative role of the different DA receptors and the brain areas that may be particularly responsible for this can, however, not be decided from this information. There are a few drugs occasionally reported to cause akathisia that may ostensibly challenge this hypothesis, but the evidence in their favour is weak. Anticonvulsants like carbamazepine and ethosuximide may rarely cause akathisia, but on a substratum of organic impairment.

Neuroleptic drug potency and akathisia. A systematic study examining the incidence of NIA with different drugs is lacking, but there is a general clinical impression that, of the classical neuroleptics, akathisia is more likely to occur with higher-potency drugs. Ayd (1961) commented that akathisia developed earlier and with smaller dosages as the potency of the drug increased. Van Putten et al (1984b) studied patients on oral haloperidol (5 mg) and thiothixene (0.22 mg/kg); 70% of the patients on the former drug and 28% on the latter developed akathisia by day 7. In the AA study, the effect of medication type was small, with higher potency associated with an increased risk of akathisia (Table 10.3 gives the results of a logistic regression analysis).

Drug dosage and rate of increment of dosage. The association of akathisia with drug dosage is generally accepted. In the McClelland et al (1976) study, the rate of akathisia was 22% in the high- and 9% in the standard-dosage groups. In the Van Putten et al (1990) study, the 20-mg haloperidol group had a higher overall rate of akathisia. In the AA study, drug dosage made a significant contribution to the day 14, but not the day 7 akathisia rates, but this was

Table 10.3. *Results of a logistic regression analysis using presence/absence of akathisia (Criterion 1) as the dependent variable and 12 independent variables in a forward stepwise procedure*

N	Variable	B	SE	Exp(B)	p	−2LL[a]	Percent correctly classified	
							Overall	Akathisia group
Entire sample								
Day 7								
97	EPSE	0.302	0.18	1.652	.01	123.0	76.3	37.5
	Rate of dosage increment	0.001	0.00	1.001	.09			
	Age	0.337	0.23	1.034	.15			
Day 14								
87	EPSE	0.209	0.09	1.232	.02	109.3	77.0	42.9
	Current dosage (CPZE)	0.003	0.00	1.003	.04			
	Rate of dose increment	−0.002	0.00	0.998	.14			
Half-sample								
Day 7								
42	EPSE	1.602	0.67	4.963	.02	56.6	88.1	76.57
	Medication type	−4.581	2.07	0.010	.03			
	Serum iron level	−0.472	0.22	0.624	.03			
	Duration of illness	0.250	0.13	1.285	.05			
Day 14								
37	EPSE	0.341	0.18	1.410	.05	50.6	75.7	62.5
	Current dosage (CPZE)	0.002	0.00	1.002	.09			
	Serum iron level	−0.157	0.10	0.855	.13			

Note: Analyses were performed on the whole sample as well as the first half, the latter including iron status parameters; $p = .05$ for inclusion; $p = .20$ for removal.
[a] −2LL is the −2 log likelihood.
Source: AA study (Sachdev and Kruk, 1994).

after the EPSE scores had been included as an independent variable. Only the study by Rifkin et al (1991) was at variance, not finding a significant difference between 10-, 30- and 80-mg haloperidol groups.

The rate of dosage increment is another variable of some significance. Braude et al (1983) reported that in patients with a large dosage increase in the first 10 days after admission (log ratio of increase > 3.0), akathisia rates increased considerably. This variable was significant in the AA study as well (Table 10.3).

Clinical experience would also suggest that parenteral administration of the neuroleptic is more likely to cause akathisia. This is not supported by any research evidence that we are aware of, and if true may be because of any of the following possibilities: (i) neuroleptics administered parenterally are usually of high potency; (ii) parenteral drugs are often given during acute management, thus rapidly increasing the plasma levels from nil or low baseline levels; and (iii) bypassing the first-pass metabolism leads to a rapid increment of levels.

Plasma levels of drugs. Patients on the same dosage are known to have an enormous variation in plasma drug levels, which may be up to a hundredfold in some cases (Dahl, 1986). This observation raised hopes that aberrant plasma levels could explain the occurrence of side-effects in some patients. Overall, this promise has not been fulfilled. Much of the past research on plasma drug levels has been difficult to interpret because of shortcomings with the assays or design deficiencies, and specific examination of akathisia and plasma levels has been lacking. Van Putten et al (1991) studied the relationship between plasma haloperidol levels and drug effects in 61 patients and found that patients with levels greater than 12 ng/ml tended not to do so well; they felt this was due to adverse effects of the drug. Objectively rated akathisia and akinesia did not, however, show a significant relationship with plasma haloperidol levels. When side-effects were rated on a clinical global impression scale, there was a powerful relationship between plasma levels and what the patient experienced as 'disabling side effects' (p. 204). The same authors demonstrated a significant relationship ($p < .001$) between disabling side-effects and plasma levels of fluphenazine. The disabling side-effects ratings were significantly correlated with the ratings of akathisia ($r = .6$) and akinesia ($r = .44$). There is, therefore, some evidence that increasing plasma levels are related with more side-effects, in particular for akathisia and akinesia, but more systematic examination of this relationship is necessary.

Past exposure to neuroleptic drugs and the duration of such exposure. It has been suggested that patients may be more likely to develop akathisia at the time of first exposure to the drug, which tendency may decrease with repeated or chronic exposures. The AA study supported this contention but suggested that the effect was probably small. In this study, the duration of illness before the current episode made a positive contribution.

Sociodemographic factors and primary psychiatric diagnosis

The role of age and sex has already been discussed in Chapter 6. Most studies do not report such a role, but a few suggest that increasing age and female sex may make a small contribution to the vulnerability to akathisia. Primary psychiatric diagnosis is discussed in detail in Chapter 6.

Iron status

Background. Iron has received increasing attention for its possible role in the development of neuroleptic-induced movement disorders, in particular akathisia, for a number of reasons (Sachdev, 1993a). Iron is the most abundant metal in the human body (Pollitt and Leibel, 1982), and its concentration in the brain is relatively high, being about one-quarter that in the liver, the principal storage organ (Hallgren and Sourander, 1958; Hoeck et al, 1975). It is unevenly distributed in the brain, being highest in the globus pallidus, followed by the red nucleus, substantia nigra pars reticulata, putamen and dentate nucleus (Hallgren and Sourander, 1958). Its concentration in the globus pallidus is comparable to that in the liver. This morphological distribution is important for two reasons: (i) the organs with high concentrations have a demonstrated role in the pathogenesis of movement disorders, and (ii) these areas of the brain have a high content of DA, GABA, 5HT and neuropeptides (Hill, 1988), neurotransmitters important in movement disorders and psychiatric illnesses. The association between DA and iron has been repeatedly emphasized (Youdim et al, 1989). This needs to be qualified in light of recent findings. Some areas of the brain that are important for dopaminergic transmission, such as nucleus accumbens and the caudate, are relatively poor in stored iron. On the other hand, they have a high density of transferrin receptors (Hill et al, 1985). The iron-rich globus pallidus and substantia nigra, themselves low in transferrin receptors, receive input from the nucleus accumbens and the caudate-putamen. These findings suggest that iron is taken up by the brain in some areas and transported to, and accumulated in, some other areas. The iron-rich areas are also the sites of termination of GABA neurones, thus suggesting a role for iron in GABA utilization (Hill et al, 1985).

Recent findings on the biological role of iron in the body suggest that this morphological distribution of iron may not be without a reason. Iron is associated with many enzymes involved in the metabolism of neurotransmitters. Monoamine oxidase is associated with iron, although the exact nature of the association is now uncertain (Oreland, 1971). Iron deficiency (ID) leads to an increased concentration of brain 5HT and other 5-hydroxyindole compounds in animals studies (Mackler and Finch, 1982), while the concentrations of GABA and the excitatory glutamate are decreased (Oreland, 1971). In addition to its metabolic role, iron is important for the D_2 receptor function. Evidence from a number of sources suggests that ID leads to a subsensitivity of D_2 receptors (Ashkenazi et al, 1982; Youdim et al, 1983). Iron may be part of the receptor site or alternatively important for the formation of the D_2 protein or the confirmation of the membrane (Youdim et al, 1983). Increased iron, on the other hand, due to a direct injection of $FeCl_3$ into the brain, leads to the development of D_2 receptor supersensitivity. Iron deficiency can disrupt the blood–brain barrier (BBB) and, in addition, alter the content of proteins in some areas of the brain. A further important role for iron is as a catalyst in oxidation, hydroxylation and peroxidation reactions. The basal ganglia and the hippocampus are particularly susceptible to iron-mediated lipid peroxidation (Csernansky et al, 1983). Iron also promotes the generation of hydroxyl radicals, with their associated toxicity, from hydrogen peroxide. Some biological functions of brain iron are presented in Table 10.4.

Alongside the increased knowledge of the biological functions of brain iron, it has become known that ID is not uncommon even in developed countries (Hallberg et al, 1979). It is also recognized that ID may affect tissue functions before or in concert with decrease in haemoglobin production (Pollitt and Leibel, 1982). Since the turnover of brain iron is low, the brain resists iron depletion, matched by a reduced rate of repletion upon therapy (Dallman et al, 1975). The BBB protects the brain against the acquisition of excess iron (Youdim et al, 1989). Iron overloading of the body, as occurs in haematochromatosis, does not lead to iron overloading of the brain. For the preceding reasons, serum iron status may not be an accurate reflection of brain iron levels. Several studies have suggested that magnetic resonance imaging (MRI) may be useful in the evaluation of brain iron in vivo. Particles of iron and iron storage compounds (ferritin and haemosiderin) reduce T_2 relaxation times of the surrounding tissues, while producing little effect on T_1 (Drayer et al, 1986). While there is controversy regarding which form of iron is responsible for T_2 shortening (Chen et al, 1989), most reports point to the potential for the use of MRI to study brain iron.

Table 10.4. *Biological functions of brain iron*

I. Catalytic role in enzymatic processes
  A. Tricarboxylic cycle enzymes
    1. Succinate dehydrogenase[a]
    2. Aconitase[a]
  B. Oxidative phosphorylation enzymes, eg, cytochrome oxidase C^a
  C. Amino acid and neurotransmitter metabolism enzymes
    1. Phenylalanine hydroxylase[a]
    2. Monoamine oxidase
    3. Aminobutyric acid transaminase
    4. Glutamate dehydrogenase
II. Effect on D_2 receptor function
III. Effect on other transmitters
  A. GABA
  B. 5HT
  C. Opiate peptides
IV. Role in peroxidation, oxidation and hydroxylation reactions
V. Other functions (not established)
  A. Role in protein synthesis
  B. Role in maintenance of blood–brain barrier

---

[a]Brain enzyme levels remain unchanged in iron deficiency (Galan et al, 1984; Gerber and Connor, 1989).

Iron and akathisia. The role of ID in the pathogenesis of akathisia has been examined in a number of studies, involving both AA and TA. These studies were prompted by the observations that ID can cause motor restlessness in rats (Weinberg et al, 1980) and may contribute to hyperactivity in children (Webb and Oski, 1974). The symptoms of akathisia resemble those of RLS, a disorder that is more common in individuals with ID (Ekbom, 1960). Our study did not reveal a significant relationship between serum iron status and the propensity to develop AA in 50 short-term-medicated patients (Sachdev and Loneragan, 1991b). A logistic regression analysis did suggest, however, that ID made a small contribution to the development of akathisia. Fornazzari et al (1991) reported a patient, also suffering from acute intermittent porphyria, who developed akathisia in the setting of ID but who responded to propranolol without correction of the ID. The study by O'Loughlin et al (1991) is of interest because they examined serum iron and transferrin levels at admission and at follow-up 2–3 weeks later, and related these to the development of AA. The baseline iron and transferrin levels did not have a significant relationship with akathisia. In the akathisia group, the transferrin levels were significantly lower at follow-up and there was an inverse correlation between akathisia scores and transferrin levels at follow-up. The authors acknowledged the preliminary nature of the findings (only 6 subjects had akathisia and the definition of akathisia was not clearly stated) but went on to speculate on the possible significance. Since serum transferrin concentrations are regulated in vitro in choroid plexus epithelial cells by 5HT, and many neuroleptics are $5HT_2$ antagonists, it is possible that intrinsic differences in the regulation mechanisms in different subjects may be related to the likelihood of the development of akathisia. Considering the importance of transferrin as a transporter protein and its role in the regulation of iron in the brain (Gerber and Connor, 1989), reduced transferrin will result in the reduced availability of iron in the brain, which, in combination with neuroleptics, possibly leads to akathisia.

Since only two studies have systematically examined the iron status in AA, more work is needed before a definitive conclusion can be reached. Further, haematological and serum biochemical measures are inadequate in assessing iron function in the brain in vivo. MRI shows promise in this area, but further delineation of appropriate measures is necessary.

Organic brain disease

In the preceding chapter, we discussed EL, PD, traumatic brain lesions and brain abscess involving the subthalamus and basal ganglia as possible causes of akathisia.

Other putative risk factors

Alcohol. Case reports have appeared in which the ingestion of alcohol was temporally associated with the development of akathisia in patients being treated with neuroleptics (Lutz, 1976) or amoxapine (Shen, 1984). The exact mechanism is not known, but the finding is not inconsistent with the DA hypothesis of akathisia. Alcohol affects numerous neurotransmitters in the brain, including DA, GABA and enkephalins. Its effect on DA transmission is complex. In experimental animals, it decreases striatal DA release and DA-induced adenylate cyclase activity (Lai et al, 1978). Prolonged use of alcohol, or withdrawal from it, may induce DA receptor supersensitivity in animals (Liljequist, 1978) and humans (Balldin et al, 1985).

Smoking. There has been a recent interest in the relationship between movement disorders and smoking for a number of reasons: (i) Patients with PD have a lower lifetime exposure to smoking (Godwin-Austen et al, 1982). (ii)

There may be a relationship between smoking and the development of TD (Binder et al, 1987; Yassa et al, 1987), although the evidence is divided (Youssef and Waddington, 1987; Menza et al, 1991). (iii) Nicotine has a complex interaction with DA neurotransmission. Smoking promotes the short-term release of DA (Balfour, 1982), and increases the firing rate of dopaminergic neurones (Mukherjee et al, 1985). In both human and animal studies, nicotine is effective in reinforcing drug self-administration paradigms known to be mediated by mesolimbic dopaminergic systems (Henningfield and Goldberg, 1983). The effect of long-term smoking is more variable, with both continued increase and a decrease reported (Kirch et al, 1987; Weiner et al, 1989). (iv) Cigarette smoking lowers neuroleptic levels by stimulating hepatic microsomal enzymes and increasing the clearance of the drugs (Jann et al, 1985). (v) Nicotine withdrawal is a recognized cause of restlessness (Chapter 2). Based on this information, one would hypothesize that smoking would have an ameliorating effect on AA. The results of a study by Menza et al (1991) were at variance with this. These authors reported that in their patients with chronic psychiatric illness, female smokers had more objective, but not subjective akathisia. One possible interpretation of their finding is that their patients had TA rather than AA, and one can predict that the finding for TA would be similar to that for TD. Of course, the study is an isolated one and needs replication. Further, the smokers in this study had higher levels of neuroleptics, which could account for the higher rates of akathisia quite independently of the status of smoking.

Diabetes mellitus. The reported association between glucose intolerance and TD (Mukherjee et al, 1985), as well as the effect of glucose on striatal dopaminergic activity (Saller and Chiodo, 1980), prompted Sandyk et al (1991) to examine 68 chronically ill schizophrenic patients referred to the movement disorder clinic of a large urban psychiatric hospital for an association between diabetes mellitus and akathisia. Sixteen (23.5%) of their patients had diabetes on retrospective chart review, and the akathisia ratings in the diabetics were more than twice those in the nondiabetics. This study had many methodological limitations, which we will not discuss in detail, but does draw attention to a hitherto unexplored risk factor.

Figure 10.1 presents a model of AA based on the data from the AA study. As is apparent, a significant proportion of the variability is unexplained and can be best regarded as 'individual susceptibility'. Furthermore, the development of parkinsonism also predicts the development of akathisia, although akathisia may occur first or concurrently in many cases. This may be another indicator of susceptibility, thereby emphasizing that it is still, to a large

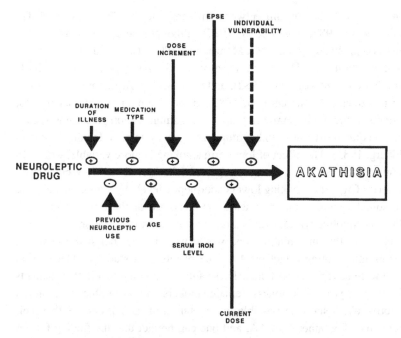

Fig. 10.1. Proposed model for the development of acute akathisia indicating its risk factors. The size of the arrows represents the strength of the association each variable has with akathisia, as determined by the correlation of the variable with the presence or absence of akathisia in the 2 weeks of treatment. The dashed line represents unexplained variance. Data from Sachdev and Kruk (1994).

extent, unclear why some individuals develop akathisia when exposed to neuroleptics whereas others don't. An examination of the likely pathophysiology does not greatly illuminate this mystery.

Pathogenesis

An animal model for akathisia?

The difficulty in conducting research in acutely ill psychiatric patients suffering from a distressing and poorly defined disorder like akathisia is obvious to any researcher. There have therefore been a number of efforts to establish a suitable animal model for the disorder. The principles used in the construction of these models are those of symptom similarity, pharmacological isomorphism and cross-species biochemical processes (Matthysse, 1986).

The principle of symptom similarity, while important, leads to the first difficulties in finding a suitable model. As we well recognize, two features of akathisia – increased motor activity and subjective distress (or emotionality) – have to be targeted. The motor activity of akathisia has some particular characteristics, is mostly recognized by the subject as voluntary and is partly suppressible. Even if an animal model of increased locomotion is produced, its similarity with the particular motor activity of akathisia can be questioned. The aspect of subjective distress fares even worse since indirect methods have to be utilized in the animal to ascertain a negative emotional-cognitive response, and its finer subjective points cannot be dissected. Further, as already discussed in Chapter 3, an animal model may demonstrate the motor or the emotional–cognitive features, but not both. The most common spontaneous effect of neuroleptic drugs is immobility, usually measured by the catalepsy test – measuring the time during which an animal (usually a rat) maintains an unnatural position (Sanberg et al, 1980). Hyperlocomotoric behaviour is not a usual response. Further, it has been demonstrated that neuroleptics reduce the indices of emotionality in rats tested in a novel environment (Allain and Lechat, 1970; Nakama et al, 1972). Thus, both features of akathisia are not spontaneously duplicated, at least in the rat. Arguably, the complex phenomena of akathisia may be more readily duplicated in primates, but no such research is currently available, and the difficulty and prohibitive expense of such research makes it unlikely that it will provide a workable model in the near future. Not all akathisia is, however, drug induced and models of akathisia that rely on brain lesions or other methods used to produce similar symptoms may have some relevance to our understanding of the brain mechanisms involved.

Instead of, or in addition to, symptom similarity, some investigators have attempted to produce biochemical abnormalities in animals that ostensibly are responsible for the occurrence of akathisia in humans. The most obvious target is reduced DA transmission in certain parts of the brain, with emphasis on the mesocortical and mesolimbic pathways. Another approach has been to increase 5HT activity, akin to the 'akathisia' caused by SRI drugs.

The principle of pharmacological isomorphism argues that all the relationships within and between the drugs known to produce akathisia in man should have a parallel relationship in the animal model (Matthysse, 1986). Some examples are as follows: (i) Drugs with higher potency should tend to produce more akathisia in the animal model. (ii) The model akathisia should demonstrate a relationship with drug dosage. (iii) The model akathisia should certainly be an acute effect, but may also be a chronic or tardive effect. (iv) At least in some animals, the akathisia equivalent should respond to ACh or βA antagonists. (v) Drugs not known to produce akathisia in humans, such as the benzodiazepines, opiates and TCAs, should not produce it in the animal model.

Models of the subjective aspects of akathisia. The models that parallel the dysphoric response produced by neuroleptics were discussed in Chapter 3 and are again listed here: (i) neuroleptics as aversive stimuli in a rat model of conditioned suppression (Berger, 1972); (ii) avoidance of neuroleptic administration by the monkey (Hoffmeister, 1975, 1977); (iii) neuroleptics as effective unconditioned stimuli in a conditioned taste-aversion paradigm (Giardini, 1985; Bignami, 1991); and (iv) neuroleptic-induced defecation in a well-habituated environment (Russell et al, 1987a,b; Sanberg et al, 1989; Sachdev et al, 1993). The defecation model has been most extensively investigated, and some of its advantages and limitations are recognized, as discussed in Chapter 3.

The advantages are as follows. Defecation index is considered to be an 'emotionality index of choice in the rat' (Broadhurst, 1957). Neuroleptic-induced defecation is a central rather than a peripheral effect (Russell et al, 1987a). The effect occurs rapidly, within minutes of the injection, akin to AA. The effect is modified by the arousal state of the animal (Russell et al, 1987b), and in the home cage is different from that in the open field environment. Morphine-induced catalepsy does not result in increased defecation (Sanberg et al, 1989). Scopolamine reduces neuroleptic-induced defecation (Sanberg et al, 1989). However, *n*-scopolamine produces a response similar to scopolamine, suggesting that it is because of a peripheral rather than a central action. There is evidence that fecal pellet scores show a significant correspondence with striatal DA levels (Pradhan and Arunasmitha, 1991).

The disadvantages of this model are as follows. While increased emotionality or dysphoria is recognized, the motor component of akathisia is not produced by the model (Sachdev et al, 1993). The response can be attenuated by pretreatment of the rat with antianxiety drugs, but akathisia does not generally respond to these drugs (Russell et al, 1987b). The effect of antiadrenergic and other drugs on the model has not been demonstrated.

Lesions of the mesocortical dopaminergic pathway. The VTA of the rat contains cell bodies of the mesocortical and mesolimbic DA systems, as well as 5HT fibres originating from the raphe nuclei and innervating the forebrain. In 1969, Le Moal et al described what came to be known as the *VTA syndrome* – a complex behavioural syndrome produced by bilateral lesions of the VTA. This syndrome was characterized by (i) hyperactivity, or increased daytime exploratory activity, nocturnal activity, Skinner box activity, hyperreactivity to external stimuli and reduced threshold of arousal by electrical stimulus of the lateral hypothalamus; (ii) difficulty in suppressing previously learned responses or in tolerating frustrating situations; (iii) disappearance of the freezing reaction; (iv) disturbance of organized behaviours (eg, hoarding and eating; and (v) hypoemotivity, or quietness, absence of fear reactions, reduced defecation and reduced effect of penalties in avoidance conditioning (Le Moal et al, 1969, 1975, 1976).

The hyperactivity of the VTA syndrome is of long duration and may remain for the whole life of the animal. This is in contrast with drug-induced hyperactivity in rats, which is generally of short duration (see later). Parallels have been drawn between this hyperactivity and the akathisia syndrome produced by organic disorders and perhaps by drugs. However, the hyperactivity is associated with decreased exploratory capacity, ongoing behaviour and attention span, suggesting a hypoarousal state which is different from the akathisia syndrome in humans. In other words, the VTA model of akathisia is the reverse of the defecation model discussed earlier, in that it produces increased motor activity but not emotionality.

Nevertheless, an understanding of the biochemical basis of the lesion-induced hyperlocomotion is of interest. Tassin et al (1978) demonstrated that it could not be explained on the basis of changes in brain NE or 5HT. The average level of NE in the frontal cortices of lesioned rats with increased activity was never reduced by more than 25% in their study. The activity levels also did not correspond with changes in the 5HT levels in structures innervated by the mesolimbic (B8) and mesostriatal (B7) 5HT neurones. A good correlation was observed between the increase in locomotor activity and the decrease in DA content in the frontal cortex ($r = .82$, $n = 20$, $p < .01$). The correlation with the reduction of DA in the nucleus accumbens was also significant ($r = .47$, $n = 24$, $p < .05$). These changes can be attributed to lesions in the A10 area of the VTA (Dahlstrom and Fuxe, 1965). Hyperlocomotion could therefore be related to the destruction of both mesocortical and mesolimbic DA neurones, but the mesocortical pathway was considered to be crucial. When the levels of DA in the frontal cortex decreased by more than 80%, the hyperactivity levels were 3–8 times those of sham-operated rats. A similar reduction of DA in the nucleus accumbens produced only a twofold increase. Lesions in the A9 area lead to the nigrostriatal syndrome with hypoactivity, difficulty in initiation and alimentary disorders. In addition to electrolytic lesions produced by Tassin et al, a similar syndrome has been described if lesions are created in the A10 area by local injections of 6-hydroxydopamine (Le Moal et al, 1975; Galey et al, 1977). The administration of small dosages of apomorphine and sustained dosages of amphetamine

(1–2 mg/kg) abolishes the locomotor hyperactivity in lesioned rats (Gualtieri et al, 1980).

The VTA model is the only one in which reduced DA transmission leads to increased motor activity. This is important in our understanding of DIA, since neuroleptics uniformly reduce DA transmission. Many investigators have demonstrated psychomotor activation in association with increased DA in the nucleus accumbens, produced by the direct injection of DA agonists into this nucleus (Costall and Naylor, 1975; Pijnenburg et al, 1975). Similar injections into the striatum or the amygdala do not produce the same response.

Serotonergic function and animal models of akathisia. The locomotor activity of the rat has been related to serotonergic mechanisms by a number of authors. The results from lesion studies have been somewhat controversial. Earlier reports suggested that a reduction in 5HT, induced by *p*-chlorophenylalanine-induced inhibition of synthesis, increased locomotor activity in the rat (Sheard, 1969). Destruction of the median raphe nucleus, which reduced 5HT levels in the hippocampus, produced similar results (Kostowski et al, 1968; Jacobs et al, 1974). Lesions of the dorsal raphe nuclei did not affect motor activity (Jacobs et al, 1974), and simultaneous lesions of the median and dorsal raphe by local injections of 5,7-dihydroxytryptamine also did not modify locomotor activity (Lorens et al, 1976).

Much work has been published on a hyperactivity syndrome in rats due to increased 5HT levels induced pharmacologically. The simultaneous administration of tryptophan and tranylcypromine, a monoamine oxidase inhibitor, leads to intense locomotor activity in the rat (Grahame-Smith, 1971; Green and Grahame-Smith, 1974), which is abolished by pretreatment with α-methyl-*p*-tyrosine. This motor activity is part of what has been described as the rodent 5HT syndrome, which also includes salivation, piloerection, hyperthermia, tremor, stereotypic behaviours, seizures and death. This syndrome has also been described after the coadministration of fluoxetine and phenelzine or tranylcypromine (Holman et al, 1976; Marley, Wozniak, 1984). It has been suggested that the 5HT syndrome results from the stimulation of both $5HT_{1A}$ and $5HT_2$ receptors (Peroutka, 1988). A dopaminergic link has been suggested in the 5HT-induced locomotor response. The preventative effect of α-methyl-*p*-tyrosine could be reversed by L-dopa alone or in combination with disulfiram, an inhibitor of dopamine β-hydroxylase (Green and Grahame-Smith, 1974). 5HT is known to reduce dopaminergic transmission via presynaptic inhibition of DA release (Meltzer et al, 1979). Both clinical and preclinical data have been presented to support this (Meltzer et al, 1979;

Martensson et al, 1989; Baldessarini and Marsh, 1990), but not all reports have been consistent (Martensson et al, 1989; Perry and Fuller, 1992).

In summary, while lesion studies are inconsistent, pharmacological manipulation to increase brain 5HT levels leads to increased locomotion in the rat, along with a number of other features. This knowledge may be applied to our understanding of the pathomechanism of akathisia, in particular that induced by SRIs. It must be acknowledged, however, that there are many determinants of increased locomotion in the rat, and its analogy with akathisia in humans is at best tentative. For example, facilitation of DA transmission in the ventral striatum (Le Moal and Simon, 1991) leads to locomotor activity. Similarly, blocking glutamatergic transmission at the *N*-methyl D-aspartate (NMDA) receptor complex with MK-801 leads to a robust, dose-dependent increase in motor activity (Ouagazzal et al, 1993). A locomotor hyperactivity model in the rat can, therefore, provide only limited insight into the pathophysiology of akathisia.

Serotonin also has an effect on defecation behaviour in the rat, and this effect seems to be different in the open field (OF) and home cage (HC) environments. In the OF environment, 5-hydroxytryptophan (5HTP) and intraventricular 5HT decrease fecal boluses, while pretreatment with *p*-chlorophenylalanine (pCPA) and 5,6-dihydroxytryptamine (5,6DHT) leads to a slight increase. In the HC environment, defecation increases with 5HTP administration and decreases under pretreatment with pCPA (Kameyama et al, 1980). Arguably, increased 5HT activity induced by pharmacological challenge in the HC could induce both hyperactivity and increased emotionality, possibly representing an adequate model of akathisia. This assertion remains to be empirically tested.

The dopaminergic hypothesis of acute akathisia

These are several reasons why DA has been implicated in the pathogenesis of AA. As we discussed in reference to the aetiology of DIA, most (perhaps all) drugs that cause AA directly or indirectly reduce DA function in the brain. Even drugs like the calcium channel antagonists and SRIs with no direct effect on DA receptors alter DA function, as discussed previously. Reduced DA transmission can, therefore, be considered to be importantly associated with akathisia.

The particular focus, in trying to understand the pathophysiology of akathisia, is on neuroleptics. These drugs are potent DA antagonists, with varying effects on the different subtypes of receptors and different brain regions. In the case of classical neuroleptics, the antipsychotic property best relates to the antagonism of D_2 receptors (Creese et al, 1977). High-potency drugs, that are more likely to cause akathisia, are more potent antagonists of D_2 receptors. The relationship of akathisia to drug dosage and the route of administration is consistent with this. Nordstrom et al (1992), using PET, demonstrated that the occupancy of D_2 receptors in humans was 73% and 92% 3 hours after single 4- and 7.5-mg oral doses of haloperidol, respectively. Akathisia developed about 2–5 hours after the drug challenge in three of four subjects and was worst at the time when the D_2 receptor occupancy was maximal. In a PET study of recently treated schizophrenic patients, EPSE, which included parkinsonism and akathisia, related again with D_2 and not D_1 receptor occupancy (Farde et al, 1992). The authors, in fact, argued that there was a threshold for EPSE between 74% and 82% D_2 occupancy.

There are a number of difficulties with a D_2 antagonism hypothesis of akathisia:

1. D_2 receptors are most prevalent in the nigrostriatal pathway, and their antagonism leads to parkinsonian side-effects. The correlation between these side-effects and akathisia is modest at best (see Chapter 6). Typically, D_2 antagonism in the corpus striatum leads to reduced rather than increased activity (Salamone, 1992), and parkinsonian side-effects relate best to this action.
2. In the rodent model, D_2 antagonists produce motoric inhibition in the form of catalepsy, as discussed previously.
3. The association of D_2 antagonism and akathisia demonstrated in the PET studies cannot be considered more than an association. The authors did not examine the simultaneous effects of the drugs on the other DA receptors or, indeed, other neurotransmitters, nor did they study the antagonism in different brain regions to determine if it was the nigrostriatal or some other (mesocortical or mesolimbic) DA system that was implicated.
4. The nigrostriatal D_2 antagonism hypothesis does not explain why ACh antagonists, which are very effective in DIP and dystonia, are only partially effective in akathisia. Nor does it explain the efficacy of βA antagonists in some cases (see treatment review in Chapter 11). It is possible, however, that akathisia is a consequence of downstream effects of D_2 antagonism, some of which can be reversed by these drugs, leading to amelioration.
5. The occurrence of akathisia, or akathisia-like syndromes, secondary to SRIs or with no known cause, is again difficult to reconcile with a high degree of D_2 antagonism.
6. The heterogeneity of the DA receptors in the brain is only now beginning to be understood. Thus far, five different genes for functional DA recep-

tors have been characterized using modern molecular biological techniques, but this probably does not represent the full extent of the family (Gingrich and Caron, 1993). More mRNA variants are known, for example those arising from alternate splicing of exons in the D_2 receptor family or the pseudogenes found in the D_1 receptor family. The receptors may be broadly classified into D_2-like and D_1-like, but important molecular differences exist in the various subtypes. A summary of the receptors is presented in Table 10.5. The level of complexity is increased when one considers the regional distribution of the subtypes and the relative affinity of different drugs for the various receptors (Meltzer, 1991). For example, the limbic and frontal cortices, which may be of significance in the pathogenesis of akathisia, are particularly rich in D_3 and D_4 subtypes. The physiological and pharmacological roles of the various subtypes is not known, but some differences are emerging. For example, unlike the D_2 and D_3 receptors, D_4 has a relatively low affinity for the classical neuroleptics like raclopride (30- to 165-fold lower) and high affinity for clozapine (6- to 20-fold higher) (Van Tol et al, 1991). The affinities of DA agonists are often higher at D_3 than D_2 receptors, whereas most antagonists have affinities in the reverse (Sokoloff et al, 1990). Typical antipsychotic drugs show a 10- to 20-fold preference for D_2 over D_3 receptors, whereas atypical antipsychotics show a 2- to 3-fold preference (Sokoloff et al, 1990). The relative propensity of the neuroleptics to produce akathisia may, therefore, provide some insight into its pathogenesis.

In summary, the hypothesis that akathisia is produced by the antagonism of the D_2 receptors in the nigrostriatal areas is weak. The role of the various subtypes of DA receptors must be further investigated.

Is akathisia due to dopamine receptor antagonism in the mesocortical and mesolimbic areas? This attractive hypothesis was initially suggested by Marsden and Jenner (1980). The study of the dopaminergic projections to the forebrain areas is relatively new in the investigation of brain DA (Thierry et al, 1973). The DA projections to the limbic cortex (medial prefrontal, cingulate and entorhinal areas) and other limbic areas (regions of the septum, olfactory tubercle, nucleus accumbens septi, and amygdaloid complex, and piriform cortex) originate from a large band of neurones, the A10 and A9 cell complex, located in the ventral mesencephalon. The mesocortical and mesolimbic DA projections have been studied in rodents, but recent primate work has shown some important distinctions. In primates, the cortical DA innervation is more extensive and includes dense innervation of the motor, premotor and supplementary motor areas, as well as modest innervation of parietal, temporal and anterior cingulate cortices. Other differences between

Table 10.5. *Summary characteristics of the dopamine receptor subtypes*

Subtype	D_1A	D_5/D_1B	D_{2S}	D_{2L}	D_3	D_4
No. of amino acids	446	475, 477	415	444	446, 400	387
Exons	1	1	6	7	6	5
				?		
Introns	0	0	5	6	5	4
				?		
Gene localization	5q35.1	4p15.1–16.1	11q22–23	3p13.3	11p	—
Species	Human, rat	Rat, human	Human, rat	Bovine, *Xenopus*	Rat, human	Human
2nd messenger	AC↑	AC↑	↓AC, ↑K⁺	—	—	—
G-Protein coupling	Yes	Yes	Yes	—	—	Yes
Affinity (nM) for						
DA	10^3	10^3	10^3	—	10^1	10^2
SCH 23390	10^{-1}	10^{-1}	10^3	—	10^3	10^3
Spiperone	10^2	—	10^{-2}	—	10^{-1}	10^{-2}
Haloperidol	10^2	10^2	10^{-1}	—	10^1	10^1
Clozapine	—	10^2	10^2	—	10^2	10^0
Distribution in CNS						
Caudate	+++	—	+++	+++	++	++
Putamen	+++	—	+++	+++	++	++
Frontal cortex	++	—	—	—	—	+++
VTA	+	+	++	++	++	—
SN	+	+	++	++	—	—
Amygdala	++	—	—	—	++	+++
Olfactory tubercle	+++	—	+++	+++	+++	+
Hypothalamus	++	—	—	—	++	+
Nucleus accumbens	+++	—	+++	+++	+++	—

Note: + denotes mild; ++, moderate; +++, high; —, unknown.
Source: Data from Gingrich and Caron (1993); Grandy and Civelli (1992).

primates and rodents include those in the laminar distribution of DA terminals, the co-localization of neuropeptides and the early prenatal development (Berger et al, 1991).

Cortical DA plays a role in higher integrative cortical functions involving movement and cognition, as well as the processing of sensorimotor information (Bannon and Roth, 1983). The direct effect of DA on cortical targets complements the indirect effect on the long subcorticocortical loops through the basal ganglia (Albin et al, 1989). DA inhibits the various excitatory responses to internal or external stimuli demonstrated in the rodent prefrontal cortex, and this could be true of the association and somatosensory areas in the primates. As discussed in the animal models, lesions of the mesocortical DA neurones in the rodent lead to increased locomotor activity that cannot be attributed to changes in 5HT or NE (Tassin et al, 1978). It is possible that the human equivalent of VTA-lesioned hyperactivity in the rat is akathisia.

In addition to support from the rat model, there is some clinical and theoretical support for the mesocortical DA antagonism hypothesis. The lesions in traumatic brain damage that produce akathisia were reported to be in the prefrontal cortex (Stewart, 1989). Because of the role of DA in the somatosensory and association cortices, this model may explain both the subjective and motor aspects of akathisia. It has previously been demonstrated that stimulation of the supplementary motor area (SMA) can lead to an urge to move (Penfield and Welch, 1951). Recent unpublished data (Kit-Yun Chee and colleagues, personal communication) using [^{15}O]PET suggests that the sensory urge preceding motor or vocal tics, which resembles the subjective aspect of akathisia, is temporally associated with increased blood flow to the SMA, among other areas. Since subtypes other than D_2 are relatively more dense in the cortical areas, it may help explain the low correspondence between parkinsonian symptoms and akathisia. Yet it is consistent with the PET findings of the temporal association between D_2 antagonism and akathisia, as one can presume a good correspondence between the antagonism of nigrostriatal and cortical DA receptors.

There are some further aspects of the mesocortical DA systems that need to be considered. DA cells that project to the prefrontal and cingulate cortices appear to have a greatly diminished number of autoreceptors, or to lack them entirely. They differ from the DA neurones possessing autoreceptors in a number of important ways, which may have some relevance to our understanding of akathisia. They have a higher turnover rate and metabolism of dopamine, and correspondingly have a higher rate of physiological activity (firing) and a different pattern of activity (more bursting). They have a diminished biochemical and electrophysiological responsiveness to DA agonists and antagonists. Drugs like haloperidol, therefore, produce large increases in synthesis and accumulation of DA metabolites in the nigrostriatal, mesolimbic and mesopiriform DA neurones but only modest increases in the mesoprefrontal and mesocingulate pathways (Randrup and Munkvad, 1966, p. 318). This may further explain the low correlation between parkinsonian side-effects and akathisia. The DA projections to the prefrontal and cingulate areas also do not seem to develop depolarization deactivation after repeated administration of neuroleptics. This may explain the frequent development of CA, and the usual absence of tolerance to the side-effect. Stress (eg, foot shock, swim stress or conditioned fear) in the rat produces a selective (benzodiazepine-reversible) metabolic activation of the mesoprefrontal DA neurones, without significantly affecting other DA systems. This would explain the worsening of akathisia in relation to stress.

The mesocortical DA antagonism model of akathisia has some weaknesses: (i) It is largely speculative and without empirical support. (ii) The rat model with increased locomotor activity is only a partial representation. (iii) The partial, but sometimes dramatic response of akathisia to ACh or βA antagonists is not easily explained. However, it can be argued that ACh and NE, without being important in the aetiology, may have a modulatory role and may thus influence the manifestation of the symptoms of akathisia. This will be discussed later.

Noradrenergic mechanisms in akathisia

The reasons why noradrenergic mechanisms have been implicated in the pathophysiology of akathisia are as follows. First, neuroleptics are known to affect adrenergic function. They competitively antagonize α_1- and α_2-receptors, with classical neuroleptics being much more potent at α_1, and the newer atypical neuroleptics like clozapine at α_2. Their direct effect on β-receptors is weak (Richelson, 1985). Patients being treated with neuroleptics have significantly higher levels of NE in the cerebrospinal fluid (CSF) than patients not on drugs or healthy controls (Gattaz et al, 1983). Neuroleptics increase the level of brain NE in animals (Bartholini et al, 1976). The mechanism may be the blockade of presynaptic DA receptors on NE pathways, which have been demonstrated in the rat hypothalamus to regulate the release of NE (Misu et al, 1985).

Second, the locus coeruleus sends NEergic projections widely to the limbic system (Cooper et al, 1991), and the ventral limbic system projects to the basal ganglia. Noradrenergic mechanisms may, by this pathway, influence motor expression. Increased NE activity is associated with a higher level of behavioural vigilance and hyperactivity (Cooper et al, 1991).

Third, βA antagonists are effective in the treatment of some (but not all) patients with akathisia, suggesting an overactive βA state in the expression of akathisia (Lipinski et al, 1983; Adler et al, 1986). Some preliminary reports of the use of clonidine, an α_2-adrenergic agonist that reduces noradrenergic activity, in the treatment of akathisia have also appeared (Zubenko et al, 1984; Adler et al, 1987a; 1989b), but βA antagonists seem to be more efficacious. The importance of central vs peripheral β-receptors, or β_1 vs β_2 in the treatment response has been investigated in a number of studies reviewed by Adler et al (1989). Hydrophilic β-antagonists, such as atenolol (Reiter et al, 1987a), sotalol (Dupuis et al, 1987) and nadolol (Lipinski et al, 1984), were noted to be less efficacious than lipophilic drugs like propranolol and betaxolol, thereby suggesting a central mechanism of action. The relative importance of β_1- and β_2-receptor antagonism cannot be decided from the literature. The role of β-antagonists and α_2-agonists in the treatment of akathisia will be reviewed in Chapter 11. Wilbur et al (1988) propose that propranolol and similar drugs act by blocking β-receptors on limbic nuclei, thereby interfering with the noradrenergic outflow.

The treatment efficacy of β-antagonists should be considered in light of the fact that these drugs have additional properties that may be relevant. Propranolol is known to facilitate DA neurotransmission in the VTA but not in the substantia nigra (Wiesel, 1976), and this could be the mechanism of its antiakathisia effect (Lipinski et al, 1988). There is some evidence that NE has inhibitory effects on DA projections, and the VTA receives a more dense noradrenergic innervation than the substantia nigra (Dahlstrom and Fuxe, 1965). This accords well with the mesocortical DA antagonism hypothesis for akathisia. Since both the D- and L-isomers of propranolol are effective in increasing DA turnover in the VTA (Fuxe et al, 1976), and D-propranolol has little β-antagonist activity, the mechanism of action may be because of some other property of the drug. Drugs like propranolol and metoprolol have a membrane-stabilizing property (Connolly et al, 1976) that could also have a role in their mechanism of action. The relevance of the alternative properties of propranolol may explain why it failed to benefit akathisia in an iv challenge study (Sachdev and Loneragan, 1993a,b).

Fourth, Bartels et al (1981) suggested that akathisia could be the result of neuroleptic-induced supersensitivity of spinal noradrenergic receptors innervated by the 'mesencephalic locomotor region' (MLMR). They cited evidence (Hinsey et al, 1930; Bard and Macht, 1958; Orlovsky, 1969) that mesencephalic structures were important in the initiation of locomotion and that these were NE neurones that exerted a tonic descending brainstem control for locomotion (Grillner, 1973). In the decerebrate preparation, stimulation of the MLMR electrically or by the iv administration of dopa (a precursor of NE) or high-dosage clonidine (which stimulates α-receptors at this dosage) leads to walking movements. This effect is also achieved in the spinal preparation, arguing that it is dependent on postsynaptic NE receptors in the spinal cord. Bartels et al demonstrated reduced night-time urinary excretion of 3-methoxy-4-hydroxyphenyl glycol (MHPG) in 10 schizophrenic patients suffering from moderate to severe akathisia, compared with nonakathisic schizophrenic patients on neuroleptics and normal controls. They did state that the akathisic patients had been treated with neuroleptics 'for a long period of time' (1981, p. 37) but did not clarify whether they suffered from AA or TA. The authors argued that reduced MHPG could be explained by chronic blocking of postsynaptic α-receptors with subsequent supersensitivity of receptors. This supersensitivity was responsible for the increased spontaneous activity of the spinal locomotor centres.

The Bartels et al hypothesis does not explain the development of akathisia within minutes or hours of the administration of neuroleptics. It also does not explain the development of akathisia from a number of drugs which have no effect on the α-adrenergic receptor or the treatment effects of βA or nonadrenergic drugs. Drugs like thioridazine and chloropromazine, which produce less akathisia, are much more potent α-antagonists than haloperidol and trifluoperazine. Moreover, no further support for this hypothesis has been forthcoming, although this may be due to insufficient research.

Fifth, Zubenko et al (1987), in their report of akathisia induced by antidepressants (trazodone, desipramine, imipramine and tranylcypromine), suggested that akathisia was produced by the enhancement of βA transmission. However, antidepressant-induced akathisia is uncommon, making it unlikely that NE mechanisms are paramount in the pathogenesis. Increased noradrenergic activity was also considered to be the basis of the jitteriness syndrome, which has similarities to akathisia (Pohl et al, 1988). The latter hypothesis was based on the observation that the syndrome tends to occur in panic disorder patients who have a baseline of increased noradrenergic activity and is most common with desipramine, which is a potent noradrenergic reuptake inhibitor. The pharmacological response of jitteriness to benzodiazepines and phenothiazines argues against the hypothesis.

In summary, the noradrenergic hypothesis of akathisia has only partial support and has a number of limitations. It is possible that these mechanisms play a partial and perhaps indirect role in the pathogenesis of akathisia, and that the effect of NE receptor function on DA transmission may be the final common pathway.

Serotonergic mechanisms in akathisia

The role of 5HT in the pathogenesis of akathisia is suggested by the following observations. Many neuroleptic drugs, especially the atypical ones such as clozapine and thioridazine, which produce less akathisia, are potent 5HT receptor antagonists, in particular at the $5HT_2$ receptor (Peroutka and Snyder, 1980). The $5HT_2$ receptor is particularly dense in the cortex, which may have relevance to its behavioural effects. However, antipsychotics have effects on a number of other neurotransmitters, and the role of 5HT in the pathogenesis of akathisia cannot, therefore, be deduced from this observation. It is possible that $5HT_2$ antagonism, in addition to the D_2 antagonism, may reduce the propensity of a drug to produce EPSE, including akathisia (Meltzer et al, 1989). This hypothesis suggests that a favourable $5HT_2/D_2$ ratio of a neuroleptic drug will reduce or prevent acute EPSE. There is some evidence to support this hypothesis using catalepsy in rodents as a model (Balsara et al, 1979; Waldmeier and Delini-Stula, 1979), but the evidence is not totally consistent (Arnt et al, 1986). In nonhuman primates, Casey (1993) demonstrated that various antipsychotic drugs, with different $5HT_2/D_2$ ratios, produced clinically indistinguishable dosage-related akathisia, with the exception of clozapine. He argued that a high ratio did not necessarily explain a low incidence of EPSE. In humans, the prevalence of akathisia secondary to clozapine is still uncertain, as discussed in Chapter 5. Risperidone, with a favourable ratio, reportedly produces less akathisia (Heylen and Gelders, 1992). Remoxipride and sulpiride, both potent D_2 antagonists, possibly produce less akathisia (this is by no means established) and yet do not have $5HT_2$ antagonist properties (Lepola et al, 1989; Lindstrom et al, 1990; Andersen et al, 1990).

In support of this hypothesis, Fleischhacker et al (1990) reported improvement in akathisia in response to ritanserin, a potent and specific $5HT_2$ antagonist (Leysen et al, 1985). Therefore, overall evidence is in favour of the hypothesis that antagonism of $5HT_2$ receptors may be useful in reducing the development of akathisia or in ameliorating it.

A number of reports have appeared implicating SRI drugs in the aetiology of akathisia, as discussed previously. Fluoxetine, for example, is a relatively selective antagonist of 5HT reuptake and thereby increases 5HT transmission without directly affecting other neurotransmitters. While a number of authors have reported akathisia with this drug, a systematic comparison of fluoxetine- and neuroleptic-induced akathisias has not been carried out. The evidence with regard to increased 5HT transmission is conflicting, however. A case report of akathisia due to methysergide, a $5HT_{1c}$ antagonist, has appeared, although this would need further corroboration. Some anecdotal reports of improvement of NIA with L-tryptophan, a precursor of 5HT, have appeared (Sandyk, 1986; Kramer et al, 1990). These reports are difficult to reconcile, but an examination of the literature suggests that increased 5HT levels are more often associated with akathisia-like symptoms.

The animal data supporting increased hyperactivity, and defecation in the HC environment, that is secondary to increased 5HT activity have been discussed previously, although the evidence is again not totally consistent.

In conclusion, the majority of evidence suggests that increased 5HT transmission leads to akathisia-like symptoms, and antagonism of 5HT receptors leads to reduction or prevention of akathisia. The exact mechanism of this action is uncertain. The 5HT-containing neurones in the brain are restricted to clusters of cells in or near the midline or raphe regions of the pons and upper brain stem, with widespread projections. The median raphe nucleus (B8 group) contributes a large component of the 5HT innervation of the limbic system. The dorsal raphe nucleus (B7) projects to the neostriatum, cerebral and cerebellar cortices and the thalamus (Cooper et al, 1991). Serotonin has direct and indirect effects on complex sensory and motor patterns of behaviour. Its activity is highest during states of arousal. A descending projection to the ventral horn of the spinal cord serves to enhance motor neurone excitability. Serotonin is known to modulate DA transmission, and this may be the crucial link responsible for its role in akathisia. For this, the subtypes $5HT_2$ and $5HT_3$ seem to be the most significant. It is relevant that ritanserin, a specific $5HT_2$ antagonist with no affinity for D_2 receptors, increases the rates of firing and bursts in the A9 and A10 DA neurones (Ugedo et al, 1989). Other receptor subtypes may have different effects. There has been recent interest in $5HT_3$ receptors, the stimulation of which leads to increased DA release in the mesolimbic and mesocortical areas (Blandina et al, 1988). Ondansetron, a selective $5HT_3$ antagonist, inhibits hyperactivity caused by the release of endogenous DA in the nucleus accumbens by amphetamine or stimulation of VTA, and by exogenous DA infusion (Hagan et al, 1987), without influencing nigrostriatal DA-mediated responses. 5HT may therefore also influence akathisia by its effects on DA transmission in the mesocortical and mesolimbic areas.

Cholinergic mechanisms in akathisia

The main evidence implicating cholinergic mechanisms in the pathogenesis of akathisia comes from studies attesting to the usefulness of ACh antagonists in the treatment or prophylaxis of akathisia. These studies will be reviewed in Chapter 11, but one can conclude that while many authors have reported positive results, and ACh antagonists are commonly used to treat akathisia, their efficacy in well-controlled studies is not completely established. Further, the suggestion that it is the akathisic patients who also have DIP that responds to these drugs (Braude et al, 1983) has received only inconsistent support. Our recent iv challenge study of akathisia with benztropine found a significant improvement in NIA, more apparent in the subjective component (Sachdev and Loneragan, 1993b). The debate is therefore alive and warrants further investigation. Some further support for the role of cholinergic mechanisms comes from an examination of the relative propensity of different neuroleptics to antagonize the muscarinic receptors and the relationship this may have with their likelihood to cause akathisia. Table 10.2 presents the dissociation equilibrium constants for muscarinic receptors for some neuroleptics and, in comparison, some anticholinergic drugs. The relationship of anticholinergic property and parkinsonian side-effects is much more clearly established (Miller and Hiley, 1974), but there is some evidence that the more anticholinergic drugs may produce less akathisia.

There is no direct evidence that cholinergic mechanisms are involved in AA. The few polysomnographic studies of akathisia have not reported disturbances in rapid eye movement (REM) or slow-wave sleep that could be associated with cholinergic hyperactivity. There is no evidence that schizophrenics who develop AA have more or fewer negative symptoms. No cholinergic animal model of akathisia has been proposed.

The mechanism by which ACh antagonists benefit akathisia may be through the interaction of cholinergic and monoaminergic function in the brain. There is recent evidence of a number of cholinergic tracts in the brain. In addition to the basal forebrain cholinergic complex that projects to the entire nonstriatal telencephalon (Woolf and Butcher, 1989), there are local circuit cholinergic cells as interneurones of the caudate-putamen, nucleus accumbens, olfactory tubercle and islands of Calleja complex (Cooper et al, 1991). Indeed, as Dilsaver and Greden (1984) argued, neurotransmitter systems do not, and cannot, exist in isolation. There is evidence of interaction in the regulation of receptor density, synthesis of enzymes involved in neurotransmitter synthesis and the synthesis, turnover and release of neurotransmitters. Cholinergic mechanisms regulate the activity of tyrosine hydroxylase, the synthesis and release of monoamines and monoamine receptor binding (Dilsaver and Greden, 1984). Cholinergic agonists can increase the turnover of DA (Anderson et al, 1981) and vice versa (Beani and Bianchi, 1973). Cholinergic receptor stimulation produces a significant drop in hypothalamic and brain stem NE (Kazic, 1973). Further, the DA–ACh balance in striatal function has much heuristic support (Strange, 1992).

In conclusion, while clinical and research evidence points to lower rates of akathisia in relation to drugs that reduce cholinergic function, the effects may well be explained by the interaction of cholinergic and dopaminergic systems in the brain, and this evidence does not challenge the notion that DA mechanisms are primary in the aetiopathogenesis of akathisia.

GABAergic mechanisms

There are at least two reasons why GABA may have a role in the pathogenesis of AA: (i) The symptoms of akathisia superficially resemble anxiety and are influenced by arousal, both of which involve GABA in the pathogenesis. (ii) Benzodiazepines are effective antiakathisia drugs in some patients, although their precise mechanism of action in this context is unclear. On the other hand, sodium valproate, another GABAergic drug, was not shown to be effective in one study, even though it proved useful for TD in the same study (Friis et al, 1983). The precise role possibly played by GABA in the pathogenetic pathways will be discussed later in this chapter, but the evidence for its involvement is only indirect.

The endogenous opioids and akathisia

The endogenous opioid system has been implicated in the causation of restlessness, especially in opiate withdrawal syndrome and RLS (Walters et al, 1986). This is not surprising when we consider the modulating role of neuropeptides (enkephalin, dynorphin, neurokinin B, substance P, substance K, somatostatin and galanin) in the basal ganglia and the fact that expression of many of the peptides may be under the control of DA (Graybiel, 1990). The exact role of the opioid system in DIA, however, is unclear.

The glutamatergic system and akathisia

More recently, glutamatergic neurotransmission in the striatum has been suggested to have a primary role in the regulation of psychomotor function (Carlsson and Carlsson, 1990), giving prominence to the corticostriatal glutamatergic system. It has been shown that the noncompetitive NMDA antagonist MK-801 causes a pronounced locomotor stimulation in mice depleted of monoaminergic stores (Carlsson and Carlsson, 1989). This may explain the restlessness induced by phencyclidine and related compounds. NMDA antagonism reduces dopaminergic tone, and it is therefore unclear whether the locomotor effects are mediated by catecholaminergic pathways or by independent mechanisms, even though evidence for the latter is now emerging

(Carlsson and Carlsson, 1990). Glutamatergic drugs have not been directly implicated in the pathogenesis of DIA.

The pathophysiology of akathisia: a synthesis

In the preceding section, we discussed the neurotransmitter systems that possibly have a role in the pathogenesis or expression of AA. It is clear that disturbance in no one transmitter system can exclusively account for all the features of AA; the disorder is the consequence of the interaction of a number of systems. Dopaminergic mechanisms seem to be most significant, but they possibly interact with NE, 5HT, ACh, GABA, Glu and opioid systems to produce both the motor and subjective components of akathisia. In this section, we will present a simple model that will synthesize some of the information presented. The model takes into consideration our preliminary understanding of the neurophysiological basis of movement disorders and the role of parallel, segregated neuronal circuits that involve the basal ganglia and the cortex.

The only hyperkinetic movement disorder with an established neuroanatomic basis is ballismus, which results in humans and nonhuman primates from destruction of the subthalamic nucleus (STN) (Albin et al, 1989). The STN receives inhibitory GABAergic input from the globus pallidus externa (GPe) and sends excitatory glutamatergic output to the globus pallidus interna (GPi) and the substantia nigra pars reticulata (SNr). STN lesions therefore result in disinhibition of the thalamus due to reduced tonic, and perhaps phasic, inhibitory (GABA) output from the GPi and SNr to the thalamus. The thalamocortical neurones are disinhibited, becoming increasingly responsive to cortical inputs or tending to discharge spontaneously, thus leading to hyperkinesia. The movements of hemiballismus are different from those seen in akathisia. They are usually wild, rapidly flinging movements that occur at irregular intervals, originating proximally in a limb. Abnormal facial movements may also occur. Movements of hemiballismus are exacerbated by stress and reduced by relaxation, disappearing in sleep, which is similar to akathisia. The movements can be controlled for seconds with great effort on the part of the patient. As discussed in Chapter 8, the patient reported by Carrazana et al developed akathisia-like movements rather than a ballism due to a subthalamic abscess, and this may be due to the fact that their patient had oedematous lesions of the basal ganglia as well, and the lesion was not localized to the subthalamic nucleus.

In Huntington's chorea, another disorder with hyperkinesia, there is evidence of early loss of striatal GABA/enkephalin neurones that provide inhibitory input into the GPe, thereby increasing the inhibition of the STN

(DeLong, 1990). The loss of the striatal neurones in Huntington's chorea is selective, and the STN is importantly involved, explaining the hyperkinetic movements of this disorder. The movements of Huntington's chorea are unlike those of akathisia, being clearly involuntary. However, both are hyper-kinesias and arguably involve similar brain structures.

These findings suggest that abnormalities in the basal ganglia, and their connections with the cortex and the brainstem, are central to the pathophysiol-ogy of hyperkinesia and, by inference, akathisia. One may be able to extend this further to explain restlessness in general. The brain structures within the neuronal circuit involved in a particular disorder, and the relative involvement of different structures, may explain the pattern of disturbance seen. For exam-ple, involvement of the supplementary motor and premotor areas may be responsible for the urge to move that one typically sees in akathisia. The extent to which prefrontal cortical areas can exert inhibitory influences on the movements will determine the degree to which 'involuntariness' of a move-ment is recognized. This issue will be taken up further.

The model

In Fig. 10.2, we present a model for the production of akathisia along the pre-ceding lines. This model holds that akathisia is the result of disturbances in the segregated parallel neuronal pathways that pass through the limbic and sensorimotor limbs of the striatum. The cerebral cortex projects into the dor-sal striatum (caudate, putamen and dorsal pallidum) and the limbic-related ventral striatum (nucleus accumbens, ventral pallidum and SNr) in a stri-atic–pallidic–thalamic–cortical doubly inhibitory loop. The cortical projec-tions of the circuit are predominantly to the prefrontal and sensorimotor cor-tex and are excitatory, thus suggesting that the striatum promotes arousal of the system (Chevalier and Deniau, 1990). In addition to this principal circuit, there is a pallidal side-loop that connects the pallidum to the STN and back. The major transmitter of the striatal, pallidal and SNr projections is GABA, which coexists with a number of neuropeptides in various combinations. The GABAergic fast transmission in the basal ganglia is modulated by neuropep-tides, DA, ACh and Glu in the interneurones (Graybiel, 1990). In addition, the striatum receives dopaminergic input from the SNc and the VTA, and serotonergic input from the dorsal raphe nuclei. The VTA projects DA fibres to the prefrontal cortex as well as the limbic striatum, and these mesocortical DA neurones have inhibitory effects on the cortical neuronal system and the dopaminergic network (Le Moal and Simon, 1991). The prefrontomesen-cephalic neurones in turn influence the midbrain projections to the septum,

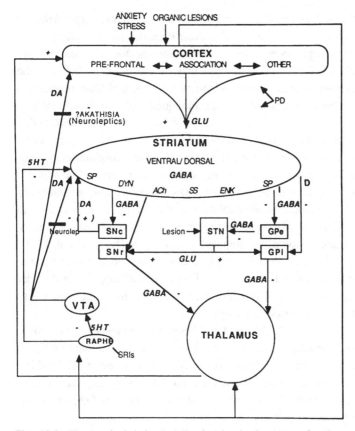

Fig. 10.2. The cortical–striatal–thalamic circuits important for the pathogenesis of restlessness (see description of the model in the text). STN denotes subthalamic nucleus; GPe/GPi, global pallidus externa/interna; SNc/SNr, substantia nigra pars compacta/pars reticulata; VTA, ventral tegmental area; RAPHE, median raphe nuclei; GABA, γ-aminobutyric acid; GLU, glutamate; DA, dopamine; 5HT, serotonin; SP, substance P; DYN, dynorphin; ACh, acetylcholine; SS, somatostatin; ENK, enkephalin; +, excitatory; –, inhibitory.

nucleus accumbens and the frontal cortex itself. The functional target of the mesostriatal DA neurone is the striatal medium spiny cell. DA reduces the basal firing rate of these cells, making them more responsive to cortical inputs. At the same time, it inhibits the cortical inputs to these cells, resulting in the facilitation of the transmission in some medium spiny cells and inhibiting others.

Even though the dorsal and ventral cortical–striatal–thalamic circuits are largely parallel, there are prominent connections between the two, involving striatal interneurones principally using ACh, GABA or somatostatin (Graybiel, 1990). Nauta et al (1978) also described a monosynaptic output from the nucleus accumbens to SNc, by which information the limbic system could influence dopaminergic modulation of information the dorsal striatum. Nauta and Domesick (1978) proposed this pathway as the interface between the emotional and motivational aspects and the motor aspects of brain function.

According to the model, akathisia is the consequence of disturbances in these circuits that finally lead to the loss of excitatory drive to the GPi/SNr and/or disinhibition of the thalamocortical and brainstem neurones. This result can be brought about in a number of ways. The most important mechanism, as suggested previously, is the antagonism of mesocortical DA receptors. There is evidence from diverse sources that prefrontal DA neurones exert an inhibitory influence on locomotion. Bilateral ablation of the prefrontal cortex leads to increased locomotor activity in the rat and other animals (Le Moal and Simon, 1991) and an exaggeration of the amphetamine response (Iversen et al, 1971). Such lesions also produce altered social behaviour, impaired learning of strategies and other behavioural disturbances, indicating that a 'pure' motor disorder is not to be expected. The case report of akathisia due to traumatic brain injury also involved bilateral prefrontal damage.

As depicted in Fig. 10.2, this model explains the influences of NE, 5HT, ACh and GABA on akathisia, as these neurotransmitters have important roles to play in the circuits or exert other influences. The influence of 5HT and NE on the VTA affects mesocortical DA function. ACh is an important neurotransmitter in the cortical interneurones and interacts with DA, as do the endogenous opiates.

This model can be extended to explain restlessness due to other causes. For example, increased dopaminergic stimulation of the striatum (eg, by amphetamine, L-dopa) leads to reduced excitation (by the indirect pathway) or inhibition (by the direct pathway) of the GPi/SNr (DeLong, 1990), explaining the motor hyperactivity induced by stimulants. The different mechanism may explain why the restlessness produced by stimulants is qualitatively different from that due to DA antagonists, the former often being pleasurable and purposive while the latter are uniformly dysphoric. Since the pathogenesis of depression, schizophrenia or delirium is poorly understood, the underlying basis for agitation in these disorders is not known. A number of neurotransmitter disturbances – NE, 5HT and DA in depression, DA and Glu in schizophrenia and DA, NE and ACh in delirium (Lipowski, 1990) – may account for the agitation or restlessness seen in some patients. Recent imaging studies have provided evidence for a prefrontal hypoactivity in both depression (Baxter et al, 1989) and schizophrenia (Weinberger et al, 1992), which again could lead to a disinhibition of striatal pathways and therefore agitation. The prefrontal DA systems have been implicated in anxiety, stress and integrative functions (Le Moal and Simon, 1991), and this may explain not only why emotional distress is such an important feature of DIA, but also why restlessness is often brought on by anxiety and stress, both of which increase DA utilization.

Why is there a particular reference to the legs in akathisia? There is no satisfactory explanation for the particular symptoms of akathisia, especially the inability to maintain a posture and the reference of the distress and restlessness to the legs. Some possible explanations are as follows: (i) Since the disturbance is in locomotion, it is perhaps understandable that the lower limbs and muscles involved in posture are preferentially affected. (ii) There are animal data to suggest that DA receptors in the spinal cord may modulate motor output (Carp and Anderson, 1982). Antagonism of these receptors by neuroleptics may contribute to the distinctive symptoms of NIA. However, the subjective distress associated with akathisia and the urge to move that precedes the movements suggest that the disturbance is primarily central in origin.

Conclusion

The pathophysiology of AA is unknown, and various mechanisms have been suggested, none of which explains all observed facts relating to the disorder. The antagonism of mesocortical and mesolimbic DA pathways is an attractive hypothesis for the development of neuroleptic-induced AA, but it is not completely satisfactory. An examination of the neuronal pathways suggests that there may be multiple possibilities by which the same outcome is achieved. Therefore, a single transmitter hypothesis may be insufficient to account for the complex characteristics of the disorder, and the interaction of the various neurotransmitter systems at various levels in the CNS must be examined to understand it fully. The study of in vivo brain metabolism and receptor function by newer imaging techniques, such as PET, may be one way to achieve this. More suitable animal models may be another.

Tardive and withdrawal akathisia

Aetiology

Drug-related variables

TA and WA have not been reported with nonneuroleptic drugs, suggesting that, unlike AA, they may be pure neuroleptic-related syndromes. This makes them potentially important syndromes to examine with regard to pathophysi-ology. Other drug-related variables (eg, drug type, single/multiple drugs, cur-rent drug dosage, duration of use, cumulative drug exposure, and continuous/ intermittent exposure) have not been examined systematically. The only available information is from our unpublished TA/CA study (see Table 10.6 for a summary of the regression analysis), which indicated a small effect of current neuroleptic dosage, with the TA/CA group being on a nonsignifi-cantly higher mean neuroleptic dosage in chlorpromazine equivalents (608.1 vs 570.3 mg for nonakathisia controls). Since the akathisia in this study was a mixture of TA and CA, the relevance of this small dosage difference is diffi-cult to interpret. None of the other drug-related variables emerged to be sig-nificant in this study.

Patient-related variables

Age and sex. The role of age and sex as risk factors for TA was discussed in Chapter 7. As was concluded, the information is very preliminary and no definitive statement can be made, except to state that, unlike TD, old age and female sex have not emerged to be important risk factors in the published studies thus far. Our TA/CA study supported age and sex as risk factors for TD, especially the OBLF syndrome, but not for TA (Table 10.3).

Iron status. The possible significance of iron status as a vulnerability factor for akathisia was discussed earlier in this chapter. At least six studies have examined the relationship between serum iron status and TA or CA (although the subtype was not always specified), with conflicting results. The report by Brown et al (1987) demonstrated reduced serum iron and percentage satura-tion, as well as increased total iron-binding capacity, in 13 akathisic patients compared with nonakathisic controls. A negative correlation ($-.42$, $p < .1$) between akathisia rating and serum iron levels was also demonstrated. Paradoxically, the serum ferritin was higher in the akathisics, which was attributed to one outlier. Barton et al (1990) investigated 15 akathisia patients who had been on stable neuroleptic medication for at least 1 month and found that they had lower ferritin levels than matched controls but did not differ on plasma iron levels and percentage saturation. However, the severity of akathisia correlated inversely with the plasma iron level ($r = .49$, $p < .05$). Horiguchi (1991) found that serum iron levels were lower in 10 CA patients vs nonakathisic nondystonic controls, but the groups did not differ on any other biochemical or haematological parameter. Their dystonia (tardive?)

Table 10.6. *Hierarchy of variables significantly related by stepwise multiple regression analysis to severity of tardive akathisia and tardive dyskinesia using different dependent variables (N = 88)*

Variable	B	SE B	β	t	p
Sum of all akathisia items					
EPSE score	.77	.22	.37	3.51	<.001
Negative symptoms (affect)	−.81	.32	−.38	−2.56	<.05
Negative symptoms (volition)	.43	.23	.28	1.87	<.1
Negative symptoms (thought)	.57	.37	.23	1.69	<.1
Socioeconomic status (current)	−.49	.29	−.18	−1.73	<.2
Current neuroleptic dose (CPZE)	.15	−.16	.12	−1.38	<.2
FTT score	−.15	−.16	.12	−1.38	<.2
Sum of objective akathisia items					
EPSE score	.50	.13	.38	3.80	<.001
Negative symptoms (thought)	.36	.16	.22	2.23	<.05
Negative symptoms (affect)	−.20	−.18	−.18	−1.60	<.15
SDMT	−.18	−.16	.13	−1.41	<.2
Sum of subjective akathisia items					
Current neuroleptic dose (CPZE)	1.1 E-3	4.7 E-4	.26	2.40	<.05
Socioeconomic status (current)	−.41	.17	−.27	−2.50	<.05
SDMT	−.15	−.16	.13	−1.43	<.2
Negative symptoms (cognition)	.15	.16	.12	1.41	<.2
Sum of seven AIMS items					
Age	.11	.03	.38	3.61	<.001
EPSE score	.30	.16	.20	1.88	<.1
Sex	−.94	.67	−.15	−1.41	<.2
Global AIMS					
Age	.02	.01	.22	2.01	<.05
Sex	−.35	.21	−.18	−1.66	<.15
Trail B	.003	.002	.22	1.91	<.1
Negative symptoms (cognition)	−.07	.04	−.18	−1.54	<.15
Sum of four AIMS items (OBLF syndrome)					
Age	.07	.02	.36	3.47	<.001
Sex	−.77	.44	−.19	−1.76	<.1
Negative symptoms (affect)	−.21	.11	−.21	−1.86	<.1
Trail B	.004	.003	.16	1.38	<.2
Sum of three AIMS items (LT dyskinesia)					
EPSE score	.21	.10	.24	2.21	<.05
Age	.04	.02	.23	2.21	<.05
SDMT	−.03	.02	−.18	−1.66	<.15

Abbreviations: EPSE, Extrapyramidal Symptom Scale (Simpson and Angus, 1970); FTT, Finger Tapping Test (Reitan and Davison, 1974); CPZE, chlorpromazine equivalents (mg) (Davis, 1976); SDMT, Symbol Digits Modalities Test (Smith, 1973).

patients also had lower serum iron levels. Nemes et al (1991) found no significant differences between 25 CA patients and nonakathisic schizophrenic and normal controls on any of the biochemical or haematological parameters. Barnes et al (1990) found no difference in iron levels between CA and non-akathisia patients. Interestingly, their 'pseudoakathisia' patients had higher serum iron levels and percentage saturation than the CA group. Sachdev (1994b) found no difference in iron status between 30 TA patients and controls. Overall, the discrepant findings are difficult to reconcile. We suggest that the positive findings of the Brown et al and Barton et al studies are not robust, and the weight of the evidence is against iron deficiency being a vulnerability factor for TA.

Psychiatric diagnosis. TA is not exclusively seen in schizophrenia and has been reported in individuals treated with neuroleptics for other causes, eg, affective disorder and behavioural disturbance. We have observed the syndrome develop in a patient with Tourette's syndrome. There is no information, however, that different diagnoses pose different risks, although Burke et al (1989), from their tertiary referral case series, pointed out the frequency with which depressed patients were referred.

Alcohol, smoking and diabetes mellitus. Earlier in this chapter, we examined these three factors in relation to AA. As discussed, some of the arguments presented there apply more appropriately to TA than AA. Further discussion must await empirical investigation.

Negative symptoms and cognitive dysfunction. Brown and White (1991a) reported that patients with objective akathisia (the so-called pseudoakathisia syndrome) had significantly more negative symptoms than nonakathisia controls. Sachdev et al (TA/CA study) examined the relationship of neuropsychological deficits and negative symptoms with TA/CA in 100 chronically ill schizophrenic patients. Multiple criteria were used for the diagnosis of TA/CA, and group comparisons and multiple and logistic regression analyses were performed to test the robustness of the findings. TA/CA ratings showed a robust association with the Negative Symptom Rating Scale scores and a consistent association with some neuropsychological test scores (Symbol Digits Modalities Test and, to a lesser extent, Trail Making Test and Finger Tapping Test), suggesting that neuropsychological function may be a risk factor for TA/CA. The association was greater with TA than TD in this study. Prospective studies are necessary to establish whether organicity is a vulnerability factor for TA/CA.

Pathogenesis

The pathogenesis of TA is unknown, and the discussion that follows is largely speculative. Any proposed model must account for the following facts: (i) the delay in the onset of symptoms in relation to neuroleptic drugs, as well as onset upon withdrawal; (ii) the persistence of symptoms for months or years after discontinuation of the drugs; (iii) the similarity of the clinical features with AA, even though the relative emphasis on subjective and objective features in the two disorders may be different; (iv) the strong overlap with TD; (v) the efficacy of catecholamine-depleting and perhaps anticholinergic drugs in some cases.

No one model can be proposed to account for all these observations. It is possible that this reflects the heterogeneity of the syndrome. For example, CA of acute onset is not easily separable from TA but may be pharmacologically distinct. One can speculate that TA that responds to anticholinergic drugs may, in fact, be CA of acute onset. The similarity in the clinical features between TA and AA suggests that the same neuronal pathways are likely to be involved, and the neurotransmitter basis may be the same.

Dopaminergic mechanisms

Dopaminergic mechanisms are strong contenders for the pathogenesis of TA. Tardive or withdrawal onset, persistence after the cessation of neuroleptic drugs, overlap with TD, suppression with neuroleptics and response to DA-depleting drugs all support the contention that the DA supersensitivity hypothesis, which has been suggested for TD (Klawans, 1973), may also apply to TA. The recent report by Sachdev and Loneragan (1993c) of the improvement of the objective manifestations of TA in some patients with a low-dosage apomorphine (0.01 mg/kg sc) challenge lends support to this hypothesis. This hypothesis, however, has a number of limitations: (i) We have previously discussed the proposal that AA may result from DA receptor antagonism in the mesolimbic and mesocortical areas. The DA supersensitivity hypothesis of TA argues that the same symptoms can paradoxically be produced by increased dopaminergic transmission. This paradox is sustainable if evidence is presented that the supersensitivity in TA is striatal rather than mesocortical and that different subtypes of DA receptors, or their mix, are involved in TA and AA. Thus far, no such evidence is available. The striatal, rather than mesocortical or mesolimbic, DA receptor involvement in TA may explain the relative emphasis on the movement disorder rather than on the distress, in comparison with AA, although admittedly, the evidence for this is still tentative. (ii) The animal models on which the DA supersensitivity hypothesis is based cannot be applied to TA, and even their explanation of TD is weak (see, eg, Smith, 1988, for this argument). (iii) There is no direct evidence that DA supersensitivity actually occurs in TA. No studies examining DA receptors in brains, neuroendocrine response to dopaminergic challenges and DA metabolites in the blood and CSF have been conducted. (iv) Sachdev and Chee (1990) reported improvement in a TA patient with an oral bromocriptine challenge and no change with metoclopramide, thus arguing against the DA hypothesis. The same patient, on the other hand, responded to anticholinergic and βA antagonist drugs.

The persistence of AA in some patients leading to chronicity may be explained on the basis of continuing DA receptor antagonism, especially in the mesocortical and mesolimbic areas. It has been shown that the DA projections to the prefrontal and cingulate areas do not seem to develop depolarization deactivation after repeated administration of neuroleptics, unlike the striatal DA receptors (Cooper et al, 1991). This does not, however, explain tardive and withdrawal onset or persistence beyond the cessation and elimination of the drug. Moreover, the pharmacological status of CA, acute onset, should be similar to AA, and this remains to be demonstrated.

Noradrenergic mechanisms

Some of the arguments regarding NE mechanisms that were discussed for AA can also be applied to TA. In particular, the hypothesis of NE supersensitivity is as appealing as the DA supersensitivity hypothesis. Long-term administration of neuroleptics results in the supersensitivity of brain adrenergic receptors, which has been demonstrated at the biochemical (Lai et al, 1978) and behavioural levels (Dustan and Jackson, 1976). The Bartels et al (1981) study discussed earlier is consistent with this hypothesis, although these authors argued for the involvement of spinal NE receptors innervated by the 'mesencephalic locomotor region'. The results of treatment studies of adrenergic antagonists in TA are summarized in Chapter 11 and provide inconsistent support to the hypothesis. Treatment with fusaric acid, an inhibitor of dopamine β-hydroxylase, was unsuccessful in one study (Viukari and Linnoila, 1977), which does not support the NE hypothesis. The attractiveness of the NE hypothesis for akathisia, if more evidence can be presented for it, is that increased noradrenergic transmission can be argued to be the basis for AA as well as TA, which is not possible with a simple DA hypothesis. It must, however, be stated that these neurotransmitters do not act in isolation, and considerable functional interaction between the two exists.

Cholinergic mechanisms

The importance of cholinergic mechanisms in TA is suggested mainly by the efficacy of anticholinergic drugs in some cases (see Chapter 11 for details). In this aspect, TA differs from TD as the latter is reported to worsen with ACh antagonists (Klawans and Rubovits, 1974). It is possible that the patients with TA who improve with these drugs are, in fact, suffering from CA, acute onset, and therefore have the pharmacological properties of AA. If this is the case (empirical evidence is lacking), then the discrepant observations are reconcilable. More investigation of the cholinergic mechanisms in akathisia is necessary.

GABAergic mechanisms

The possible role of GABA in the pathogenesis of TA is suggested by the following: (i) GABAergic drugs (eg, benzodiazepines) are effective in the treatment of some cases of TA, at least partially. It is not certain, however, whether this is a direct effect on akathisia or an indirect result of a reduction in the level of arousal. (ii) The role of GABA in the neuronal circuits is putatively important in the pathogenesis of akathisia. (iii) The evidence implicates GABA in the pathogenesis of TD (Gunne et al, 1984).

Endogenous opioids

The role of opioids, either alone or in interaction with DA, is suggested by some treatment studies (eg, Walters et al, 1985, 1986, 1989) and the similarities with RLS.

An organic hypothesis

In addition to disturbances in neurotransmitters, it is possible to argue that the development of TA may be related to organic brain dysfunction. That persistent akathisia can be produced by organic lesions was documented in Chapter 8. However, there is no direct evidence that patients who develop TA have some subtle brain abnormality that other similarly ill but nonakathisic patients do not. The putative association between negative symptoms, cognitive dysfunction and TA is difficult to interpret, as is the case for a similar association with TD (Waddington et al, 1987). Even if the association is shown to be robust, it would remain to be determined whether the cognitive dysfunction represents an organic vulnerability or a state marker. If the former, its overall contribution to the development of the disorder would have to be studied. Neuroimaging and postmortem studies of TA are lacking, except for one CT scan case report of cortical atrophy (Sandyk and Kay, 1990a), and suggest a direction for future research.

11

Treatment of drug-induced akathisia

The studies that have examined the treatment of akathisia will be reviewed in this chapter. Since the various subtypes of akathisia have different pathomechanisms, different treatment approaches will apply. On the other hand, the efferent limb of the neuronal pathway involved in akathisia is possibly shared by the various subtypes. Drugs that work on this aspect of the pathophysiology should, therefore, be effective in all subtypes. The published literature is not always explicit on the subtype of the akathisia syndrome being studied; this makes it necessary to draw inferences from the clinical descriptions, which in some cases are incomplete. Overall, the treatment of AA has been examined in some well-controlled studies, but the information on the treatment of TA is preliminary. I will discuss AA and TA separately.

The studies reported vary in the rigour of their methodology. Many of the earlier reports are anecdotes of individual cases, often published to highlight a promising treatment. Only some of the larger studies are controlled, and fewer still have a double-blind design and the appropriate methodology. The results of each study will, therefore, be examined in light of the methodology used, so that appropriate weight can be placed on its findings. Most studies report changes in only a proportion of patients. I will list the percent change in the studies and calculate the effect sizes for the studies with an acceptable methodology. Conclusions will be drawn from groups of studies.

Many authors describe the use of a particular drug based on some rationale about the mechanisms of action of the drug. Most drugs, however, have multiple actions, one or more of which may be relevant to their effects on akathisia. In this chapter, the drugs have been grouped according to the major property that is ostensibly the rationale for their use. A summary is presented at the end of each section, and guidelines for the treatment and prevention of akathisia at the end of the chapter.

Acute akathisia

The principal treatments that have been tried in AA are as follows:

1. modification of the offending drug: cessation, reduction in dosage, change to another type, reduced rate of increment;
2. modification of risk factors;
3. anticholinergic agents;
4. antiadrenergic agents: β-antagonists, α_2-agonists
5. benzodiazepines;
6. other agents: ritanserin, amantadine, piracetam, TCAs and sodium valproate

Modification of the offending drug

One or more drugs, most often antipsychotics, are necessary, if not sufficient, causes of akathisia. Good clinical practice dictates that the side-effect of a drug be managed by the optimal use of that drug rather than the introduction of another drug. With regard to the development of akathisia secondary to neuroleptics, we have previously discussed the following in the chapters on epidemiology and aetiopathogenesis.

The association of akathisia with drug dosage is generally accepted. In the Braude et al (1983) study, all 10 patients who had a significant reduction in the antipsychotic drug dosage showed improvement in akathisia. Smaller dosages of neuroleptics are therefore recommended, without, of course, compromising antipsychotic efficacy. Recent reviews (eg, Baldessarini et al, 1988) have suggested that high dosages of neuroleptics do not offer any distinct advantage over smaller dosages in the management of acute psychosis, but produce more toxicity. These authors also observed that clinicians tended to use high-potency drugs at relatively higher dosages than the low-potency ones.

The rate of dosage increment may be of some significance. It is advisable to increase the neuroleptic dosage gradually, especially in drug-naive subjects. In some patients who develop akathisia, a temporary reduction in dosage and then a gradual increment may not produce a recurrence. The parenteral administration of large amounts of high-potency drugs is often responsible for a sharp rise in neuroleptic levels in hospital patients. There is emerging evidence that this practice to produce rapid tranquillization in acutely psychotic individuals can be replaced by the use of benzodiazepines in conjunction with neuroleptics, thereby reducing the total neuroleptic exposure (see review by Dubin, 1988).

The type of neuroleptic is important. Of the classical neuroleptics, akathisia is more likely to occur with higher-potency drugs, and this should be borne in mind when treating a patient with a known propensity for the development of akathisia. Sometimes a switch to a lower-potency drug is appropriate. Occasionally, the use of an atypical or newer antipsychotic drug may be necessary. We have profitably used pimozide in patients who could not tolerate other high-potency drugs. If the conventional antipsychotics are not tolerated, sulpiride (or other substituted benzamide) or risperidone should be tried. The status of clozapine with regard to AA is still uncertain, but it may be worthy of consideration in the extreme cases.

A dosage–incidence relationship has been demonstrated in relation to some other drugs (eg, SRIs and calcium channel antagonists), and a reduction of dosage, if clinically permissible, is appropriate.

Modification of risk factors

Unfortunately, not a great deal is known about risk factors to make any significant recommendations. In general, it is advisable to be cautious in the use of neuroleptics in patients with a past history of severe akathisia or EPSE. The issue of iron deficiency as a risk factor is far from established, and no study has examined the consequences of correcting iron deficiency in a patient population. Correcting iron deficiency is a worthwhile clinical endeavour, in any event. The question is whether every patient with akathisia, or at risk of developing it, should be investigated for iron deficiency. We feel that the evidence is too ambiguous to advocate incurring such an expense. We measure the iron status of a patient only if the patient has haematological indices of iron deficiency anaemia or evidence of chronic blood loss, or if significant akathisia resistant to treatment is present.

Anticholinergic drugs

ACh antagonists are one of two classes of drugs used most commonly to treat akathisia or for its prophylaxis. There was an enthusiasm for these drugs in the earlier literature. Ayd (1961) stated, 'The fastest relief can be achieved by the intramuscular injection of 2 mg of benztropine methanesulfonate or by biperiden. It may also be allayed by oral doses of any antiparkinsonian drug, often without lowering the dose of the phenothiazine' (p. 1060). This is further reflected in the use of a positive response to these drugs as a diagnostic test for akathisia by at least one group of investigators (Van Putten et al, 1984c), although other authors acknowledged that this response was variable

(Marsden et al, 1975; Sovner and DiMascio, 1978). Subsequent literature has been less than enthusiastic, and we feel that the pendulum may lately have swung too far against these drugs (see, eg, Adler et al, 1989b), as this review will suggest. A summary of the studies that have examined the use of anticholinergic drugs in the treatment of AA is presented in Table 11.1.

Anecdotal case reports have been published intermittently that attest to the benefit of ACh antagonists in at least some patients (Harris et al, 1981; Shen, 1981; Nishikawa et al, 1992). A few open studies have been published, the earliest by Kruse (1960), who treated 112 patients with EPSE for 3 months each with benztropine or procyclidine. About half of these patients predominantly had akathisia, the rest rigidity and/or tremor. In the benztropine group, 21% of the akathisic and 86% of the other group improved. The comparable figures for procyclidine were 57% and 86%, respectively. Braude et al (1983) reported that of their 20 patients who were treated with an anticholinergic drug, 6 (30%) improved. They do not state the type and dosages of the drugs used, the duration of the treatment and whether other measures had been tried prior to the use of ACh antagonists. Van Putten et al (1984c), in their study of akathisia secondary to haloperidol and thiothixene, reported the proportion of patients with akathisia who responded to an anticholinergic drug (up to 8 mg/day of benztropine or 15 mg/day of benzhexol). In the haloperidol group, of the 32 patients so treated, 14 (44%) showed complete alleviation of their akathisia. All but 3 of the thiothixene patients treated with ACh antagonists ($n = 27$?) also showed complete alleviation. The authors do not present details about the treatment methodology, thereby reducing the significance of the study. Adler et al (1987c, 1988) treated 8 patients with benztropine (1.5–4 mg/day) for 2–5 days in an open, parallel, nonrandom design comparison with propranolol ($n = 9$). The benztropine-treated patients showed no change in the objective and a nonsignificant decrease in the subjective ratings of akathisia. The akathisia group was heterogeneous; other drugs (eg, benzodiazepines) were used concurrently; the raters were not blind to the diagnosis of akathisia; and most patients did not tolerate more than 2 mg/day of benztropine. Therefore, the results of this preliminary study cannot be generalized. In general, little more information can be drawn from the open studies but to say that a proportion of patients with AA benefit from ACh antagonists.

Only a few controlled studies have been published. DiMascio et al (1976) conducted a double-blind study to compare the efficacy of amantadine with that of benztropine for EPSE, including akathisia, in schizophrenic patients. The criteria for diagnosis were not explicitly stated, and it is not possible to say whether all suffered from AA. The akathisia patients ($n = 24$) had a mean rating of 1.71 on a scale of 0 (*nil*) to 3 (*severe*). Eleven were given

Table 11.1. *Anticholinergic drugs in the treatment of acute akathisia*

Drug (mg/day)	N	Duration	Results[a]				Comment[b]	Reference
			Overall effect (%)	Percent change	Effect size	Adjusted effect size		
Open studies								
• Benztropine	112	3 months	21					Kruse (1960b)
Procyclidine	20		57					Braude et al (1983)
• Not specified			30					
• Benztropine (≤8)	14		44					Van Putten et al (1984b,c)
Benzhexhol (≤15)	27							
• Benztropine (1.5–4)	8	2–5 days	No change				Parallel design, nonrandom	Adler et al (1987c, 1988)
Propranolol (40–80)	9	3–7 days		50				
Controlled studies								
• Benztropine (2)	11 (9)[c]	4 weeks	Marked improvement	94.2			DB, no placebo	DiMascio et al (1976)
Amantadine (100)	13 (9)[c]	4 weeks		100				
• Biperiden (6–18)	15	4 weeks	73	57.4	−1.94	−1.41	DB, crossover, no placebo	Friis et al (1983)
Sodium valproate (1,700)			26	14.3	−0.37	−0.34		
• Benztropine (6)	7	3 days	42.8	37.5			DB, placebo, parallel design, preliminary analysis	Adler et al (1993)
Propranolol (80)	11		37.5	29.2				
• Benztropine (2)	6	Single iv challenge	50		−1.80	−0.36	DB, placebo, crossover, single challenge	Sachdev and Loneragan (1993b)
Propranolol (1)			15		−0.39	−0.36		
Prophylactic study								
• ACh antagonists	80	2 weeks	$p < .01$[d]				Retrospective chart review	Keepers et al (1983)
Nil	135							

[a] Overall effect indicates the percentage of patients who improved; percent change reflects the change in akathisia score from baseline; effect size reflects the change from baseline in relation to control drug; adjusted effect size is corrected for sample size.

[b] DB denotes double blind study.

[c] Nine of 11 and 9 of 13 patients completed the benztropine and amantadine trials, respectively.

[d] Significantly less akathisia in the ACh antagonists' group.

benztropine and 9 completed the 4-week trial (cf 13 and 9 for the amantadine group, respectively). At 4 weeks, the mean rating dropped to 0.10 (94.2% improvement) (cf 0.0 for the amantadine group). The majority of the patients received 4 mg/day benztropine. The antipsychotic drug dosage was not controlled, and the lack of placebo control compromised the value of the study. Nevertheless, the study was a good endorsement of both benztropine and amantadine. Benztropine produced more side-effects than did amantadine.

Friis et al (1983) performed a double-blind, placebo-controlled, crossover study to compare biperiden and sodium valproate in 15 psychiatric inpatients with akathisia (diagnosed as having a score of greater than 1 on both subjective and objective features on a scale of 0–3). All patients received 4 weeks each of both active drugs and placebo and were randomly assigned. Eleven patients additionally had parkinsonism. Biperiden (6–18 mg/day, median 12) significantly reduced the akathisia score (from 1.4 to 0.6, $p < .01$) and the parkinsonism score (from 2.0 to 0.6, $p < .01$) and increased the TD score ($p < .05$). In all, 11 of the 15 patients improved with the drug. The effect size was −1.44 (corrected −1.41). The antipsychotic drug dosages were kept relatively constant over the period of the study. This is one of the better treatment studies reported. One criticism that can be levelled against it is that it was not specified whether the patients had AA or CA (possibly TA) and the fact that the akathisia persisted over 3 months suggests that it may not have been AA.

Sachdev and Loneragan (1993b) challenged six patients with well-defined AA using iv benztropine (2 mg), propranolol (1 mg) and placebo (saline) using a random, double-blind, crossover design and reported that benztropine produced a significant ($p < .05$) amelioration of NIA, more apparent in the subjective component. Four patients improved significantly on the subjective score, and two on the objective score. Three of the four who responded to benztropine also had tremor, and two had rigidity. The effect size of the change was −1.80 (corrected −1.66).

Adler et al (1993) published the interim analysis of an ongoing placebo-controlled, double-blind comparisons of benztropine and propranolol. In the six patients treated with benztropine (6 mg/day) in the double-blind phase, there was a 37.5% improvement in akathisia (a significant result). An interim analysis of both the single- and double-blind phases of the study suggested that three of seven improved with benztropine, and zero of nine with placebo. All patients who entered the double-blind phase of the study had not responded initially to 1–2 days of placebo given in a single-blind fashion. Three of eight patients developed confusion or forgetfulness requiring the cessation of benztropine. This was a well-designed study, and the results of the completed study are keenly awaited. There are a few deficiencies: the population was heterogeneous, with both AA and CA being included, and several patients were concomitantly on benzodiazpines or amantadine, although the dosages of these drugs were kept constant.

Gagrat et al (1978) compared iv diphenhydramine (an antihistaminic drug with some central ACh antagonist properties which are responsible for its antiparkinsonian effects) with iv diazepam in a double-blind study, but without placebo control. Patients did better on the former, although the difference was not statistically significant. The acute effect was evident 5 minutes after the infusion and was still present 2 hours later.

A number of studies have examined the benefits of prophylactic use of anticholinergics during short-term treatment with antipsychotic drugs. Most of these studies have examined EPSE in general without special reference to akathisia. A significant study was by Keepers et al (1983). The authors reviewed the records of 215 patients for the first 21 days of neuroleptic treatment to determine whether anticholinergic drugs influenced EPSE rates. Eighty (37%) patients received these drugs prophylactically, and 135 not. Prophylaxis reduced the incidence of akathisia in the first 2 weeks of treatment ($p < .01$), and this effect was more prominent in women than men.

In summary, the controlled studies support the contention of the open trials and studies of prophylactic use that anticholinergic drugs are effective in the treatment of a large number of akathisia patients. The only largely negative report (Adler et al, 1988) was preliminary and methodologically flawed as discussed earlier, and the same authors have reported positive results in a subsequent better, yet incomplete, study. It is at present not clear why some patients do not respond. A suggestion that was put forward by Braude et al (1983) was that the akathisic patients who additionally have parkinsonian symptoms are the ones who do best on ACh antagonists. This has not been systematically studied. The patients in the Friis et al and the Gagrat et al studies had a high incidence of concomitant parkinsonism, but the relationship between the improvements in parkinsonism and akathisia was not examined. In the Kruse (1960b) study, the patients with akathisia alone had a slightly lower response than those with akathisia and rigidity/tremor. The negative Adler et al report had patients with little or no parkinsonism, but its methodology was weak. The Sachdev and Loneragan study had too small a sample to make a definitive comment. This hypothesis therefore warrants further examination.

Another issue of importance is the relative effect of different ACh antagonists. Some of the drugs commonly used to treat PD and EPSE are listed in Table 11.2, along with their relative potency. There is no evidence that any one drug is superior, although claims on behalf of benzhexol and procyclidine

Table 11.2. *Anticholinergic drugs used in the treatment of akathisia and EPSE*

Generic drug	Trade name	Dose forms[a]	Range of daily dosage (mg)
Benztropine mesylate	Cogentin	O, I[b]	0.5–8
Trihexyphenidyl HCl (benzhexol)	Artane	O, I	1–15
Procyclidine	Kemadrin	O	7.5–20
Biperiden HCl	Akineton	O, I[c]	2–8
Orphenadrine HCl	Disipal	O	100–400
Diphenhydramine HCl[d]	Benadryl	O, I	75–400

[a]O denotes oral; I, injection.
[b]Benztropine maleate.
[c]Biperiden lactate.
[d]Antihistamine with significant ACh antagonist property.

have been made. The recent discovery of subclasses of muscarinic receptors makes it possible that patterns of muscarinic selectivity of each of the drugs will emerge with implications for their use in akathisia or parkinsonism. At least four receptor subtypes are recognized (M_1 to M_4), and a fifth, mRNA, has been found in the CNS, but a translation product has not been found in vivo (TiPS Receptor Nomenclature Supplement, 1992). Most available information is on M_1 and M_2 subtypes, and it has been shown that M_1 receptors predominate in the cortex, striatum and hippocampus, while M_2 receptors predominate in the cerebellum, ventricles, heart and intestinal smooth muscle (Hammer and Giachetti, 1982; Cortes and Palacios, 1986; Cortes et al, 1986). While no drug is available that is totally selective for any receptor subtype, they vary in their affinities. Biperiden is 15 times more selective for M_1 receptors, and benztropine, benzhexol and procyclidine are 2, 5 and 10 times more selective, respectively. Methixen shows no selective binding to any of the tissues studied. One advantage of the M_1-selective drugs is the sparsity of peripheral antimuscarinic side-effects (Schreiber et al, 1988). At present, there are no drugs with a preferential binding for cortical ACh receptors, which would theoretically be important for the antiakathisia effect. As more information about the relative binding of these drugs becomes available, it is likely that improved usage will result.

Pharmacokinetic data on these drugs are meagre. For benzhexol, procyclidine and biperiden, peak plasma concentrations are reached in 1–2 hours, and terminal elimination $t/2$'s are 10–12 hours. A twice-daily schedule should therefore be appropriate for most patients, although some benefit from more frequent administration. The optimal dosage for a patient should be titrated, starting with a small initial dose. Prominent peripheral and central anticholinergic side-effects should be monitored, especially in the elderly, who are more vulnerable. The measurement of serum anticholinergic activity has been recommended by some authors since it fluctuates markedly in different individuals given the same oral dosage (Harris et al, 1981; Tune and Coyle, 1981), but the facility for such measurements is not readily available. Some of Van Putten's patients needed high dosages (benztropine 8 mg/day), and one of our patients (Sachdev and Loneragan, 1993b) responded to benztropine 10 mg/day. The published studies are usually of short duration, studying the effect over the first few days or weeks of treatment. The utility of longer-term anticholinergic drug use for akathisia has not been examined, but it is well recognized that akathisia may become apparent in patients on long-term neuroleptic use whose anticholinergic drugs are stopped (Sachdev, 1994a). Whether tolerance to the antiakathisia effect develops is worthy of examination.

β-Adrenergic antagonists

Ever since the Lipinski et al (1983) and Wilbur and Kulik (1983) reports of the use of propranolol in akathisia, there has been a spate of studies of β-antagonists in the treatment of NIA. The initial studies examined propranolol as a lipophilic, nonspecific antagonist, and this has been the most extensively studied treatment of akathisia. Later studies attempted to characterize the antiakathisia effect of hydrophilic drugs, as well as specific β_1- and β_2-antagonists, not only to find a safer drug but also to probe the pathophysiology of the disorder being treated. The studies have been previously reviewed by Adler et al (1989b) and Fleischhacker et al (1990).

Propranolol

We will first examine the studies that have used propranolol (summarized in Table 11.3). The original suggestion for the use of propranolol came from a report by Strang (1967), who found this drug to be useful in the treatment of RLS. Wilbur and Kulik (1983) reported a single case of successful treatment of akathisia with propranolol. Lipinski et al (1983) reported an open study involving 12 patients with akathisia, of whom 9 had a complete remission, 2 showed about 70% improvement and 1 showed 50% improvement. The dosage most commonly used was 30 mg/day, and the response was typically

Table 11.3. *Propranolol in the treatment of acute akathisia*

N	Daily dosage (mg)	Duration	Results[a] Overall effect (%)	Percent change	Effect size	Adjusted effect size	Comment[b]	Reference
Open studies								
12	30	2 days	100	90	—	—	Patients resistant to ACh antagonists	Lipinski et al (1983)
1	160	—	100		—	—	Single case report	Wilbur and Kulik (1983)
14	42 (15–60)	1 day	100	88.6	−4.70	−4.40	Subjects possibly common with earlier study	Lipinski et al (1984)
9	56 (40–80)	3–7 days	—	50	—	—	Parallel nonrandom comparison with benztropine	Adler et al (1987c, 1988)
16	20–40	4 days	50	—	—	—	Only objective ratings; 7 patients treated for 6 months	Dupuis et al (1987)
4	40–100	4–13 months	100	—	—	—	Patients resistant to trihexiphenidyl and diazepam	Hermesh et al (1988)
Controlled studies								
5	45 (30–80)	2–3 days	—	86.8	—	—	DB, crossover with metoprolol (300 mg/day)	Zubenko et al (1984c)
6	20–30	3–4 days	—	50	—	—	DB, crossover with lorazepam (2 mg/day)	Adler et al (1986)

12	51 (40–60)	6–10 days	83	50	—	—	DB, placebo, crossover	Adler et al (1986)
7	20–60	2–7 days	—	50	—	—	DB, placebo, with atenolol	Reiter et al (1987a)
6 (placebos)	60–80	2 days	Nil	—	0.18	0.17	Negative study; propranolol as primary treatment	Irwin et al (1988)
20	60	5 days	—	—	1.18	1.13	DB, placebo, crossover; effect at 2 days was not significant	Kramer et al (1988)
6	120	5 days	—	—	−3.88	−3.58	DB, placebo, crossover; effect at 2 days was not significant	Kramer et al (1989)
19	20–40	10 days	100	—	−4.17	−4.06	DB, crossover comparison with betaxolol; 2 parts	Dumon et al (1992)
11	80	3 days	37.5	29.2	—	—	DB, placebo, parallel design, preliminary analysis	Adler et al (1993)
6	1 (iv)	1 hour	15	—	−0.39	−0.36	DB, placebo, crossover single challenge	Sachdev and Loneragan (1993b)

[a]Overall effect indicates the percentage of patients who improved; percent change reflects the change in akathisia score from baseline; effect size reflects the change from baseline in relation to control drug; adjusted effect size is corrected for sample size.
[b]DB denotes double-blind study.

seen within an hour of the first dose and was maximal in 24–48 hours. Parkinsonian side-effects were unaffected. In a further report, which ostensibly was an extension of the preceding study, Lipinski et al (1984) reported 14 patients (which probably included the 12 patients reported earlier by the authors) with akathisia, most of whom suffered from bipolar disorder. Eleven were on lithium and had a lithium-induced tremor. Ten had parkinsonian side-effects and were being treated with benztropine. Nine of the 14 showed complete remission. Hypotension and bradycardia were not observed, and 1 patient had an exacerbation of asthma. The largest dosage used was 80 mg/day. The open study comparing propranolol and benztropine reported by Adler et al (1987c, 1988) was mentioned in the preceding section, in which its deficiencies were also highlighted. In this study, 9 patients were treated with 40–80 mg/day (mean 56 mg) for 3–5 days and showed 50% improvement in both subjective and objective ratings of akathisia. Hermesh et al (1988) reported 4 patients with AA resistant to trihexyphenidyl (10–15 mg/day) for 3 days and this, along with diazepam (20–30 mg/day), for another 3 days. They were treated with propranolol (3 needed 100 mg/day) with significant improvement (a drop in mean akathisia rating from 20.25 to 2.5 [$p < .01$]). The assessment of the akathisia was not different when the anticholinergic drug was discontinued. The patients were followed up for 4–13 months while on continued neuroleptics. Three patients who were noncompliant with the propranolol had a reemergence of severe akathisia.

Dupuis et al (1987) reported an open trial of propranolol in 16 patients with akathisia (it is unclear whether this was acute or chronic). Patients were treated with 20 mg propranolol in a single daily dose for 2 days. If the patient responded, this dosage was continued for 6 months. In nonresponders the dosage was doubled for 2 days, and if they still did not respond, they were excluded from the study. After 6 months, responders went on to a 2-week washout and a trial of sotalol and betaxolol each. Propranolol was successful (disappearance of akathisia) in 7 patients at a dosage 20 mg and in one patient at 40 mg. The effect was maintained for 6 months in all except one, who had a recurrence after 9 weeks. Six patients had a 2-week wash-out period, all developing akathisia. The study is significant in that about half the patients had a rapid and impressive improvement in their akathisia which was maintained over 6 months, reappearing after the discontinuation of the drug. A number of questions about the study remain: the authors used only objective ratings of the akathisia; the nature of the akathisia is uncertain since its persistence over 6 months justifies the diagnosis of CA, and we are unaware of the duration prior to entry into the study; the dose used and duration of trial were both small; a once-a-day schedule for propranolol is unusual. This group of investigators has also published a controlled study which will be discussed later.

A number of controlled investigations have now been published. Zubenko et al (1984c) compared propranolol with metoprolol (a β_1-selective lipophilic drug) in five patients using an on-drug/off-drug crossover design. Propranolol was given first in four of the five patients. The drug dosage was increased until there were no additional benefits or side-effects. Once maximal improvement occurred (usually within 24–72 hours), medication was discontinued. The second drug was introduced after akathisia had returned to baseline (usually in 3–5 days). The authors reported good improvement with propranolol at dosages of 30–80 mg/day (mean 45 mg) with a drop in akathisia rating from 7.6 to 1.0. Cessation of propranolol results in reemergence of akathisia. The study had a number of limitations: small number of subjects, the simultaneous administration of lithium and benztropine in four subjects each, nonblind ratings and nonrandom allocation, the lack of placebo control, no definitive criteria for akathisia and short duration. Only limited significance can therefore be attached to this study. In general, the enthusiasm Lipinski and his colleagues have shown for propranolol in akathisia must be tempered by the inadequacy of the evidence they have presented. A number of other authors have taken these investigations further.

Adler and colleagues have published some studies presenting more convincing evidence. Adler et al (1985) compared propranolol (20–30 mg/day) with lorazepam (2 mg/day) in six patients using a single-blind crossover design, with 3–4 days of active treatment separated by 3–4 days of no treatment. Propranolol led to a reduction of 50% or more in both subjective and objective ratings, and the no-treatment ratings were no different from baseline. All patients were schizophrenic and on relatively high dosages of antipsychotics. Patients also showed an improvement in EPSE. In 1986, Adler and colleagues reported a double-blind, crossover, placebo-controlled study of propranolol in 12 subjects who received up to 60 mg/day of propranolol (mean 51 mg) for 6–10 days. The subjective rating for akathisia fell from 56.0 ± 5.0 to 22.8 ± 5.0, and the objective rating from 1.75 ± 0.13 to 0.75 ± 0.18 with propranolol, the placebo producing no change. Ten patients, while blind to the drug, indicated a preference for continuation with propranolol. Concomitant medication was nevertheless used in this study (anticholinergics 8 patients, amantadine 1, benzodiazepines as needed 3), making it possible that it was a subtype of akathisia not responsive to other drugs that was being treated. Reiter et al (1987a) compared propranolol with atenolol (a hydrophilic β_1-antagonist). Seven subjects (age 21–58 years) were first treated with atenolol for 3–4 days, and then crossed over to propranolol

20–60 mg/day for 2–7 days (mean 3.4 days). There was an approximately 50% drop in both subjective and objective ratings with propranolol ($p < .01$). All other medication was kept constant during the study, but 4 patients were concomitantly on benztropine. The ongoing study of Adler et al (1993) was mentioned earlier. In the 11 patients who entered the double-blind phase of the study, an overall 29.2% improvement in akathisia was seen. Including those treated in the follow-up phase, 6 (37.5%) of 16 patients had a positive response to propranolol (80 mg/day).

Kramer et al (1988) conducted a double-blind, placebo-controlled study of propranolol in 20 patients with schizophrenia and akathisia. All patients had previously failed a trial of benztropine (29 ± 8.8 days, mean 4.35 mg/day) for akathisia and were continued on this drug during the study. Akathisia was diagnosed if the patient had 'restless, adventitious movements of the lower extremities or frank pacing' (p. 823) or reported uncomfortable sensations that caused them to walk, pace or shift posture. They were divided into two treatment tracks: I ($n = 10$), 2 days of placebo followed by 5 days of propranolol (20 mg tid); II ($n = 10$), 2 days of propranolol followed by 5 days of placebo. A 10-item rating scale designed for this study was used. Overall, propranolol produced greater change than the placebo on 18 of the 26 measures of akathisia. The authors performed two-tailed t tests on the change scores between baseline and after drug treatment. The effect of the 2-day propranolol treatment did not differ from that of the placebo. After the 5-day treatment, propranolol was superior on the measures of 'inability to stay still (subjective)' and 'global subjective distress' ($p < .05$) (effect size 1.18, corrected 1.13). The design of this study is an improvement over those of most previous studies, but the lack of strict diagnostic criteria for akathisia and reliability data on the rating scale, as well as the possibility of carry-over effects, weaken it somewhat. While the study supported the use of propranolol, the demonstrated effect was not dramatic and took longer than that suggested by Lipinski and co-workers. Again, propranolol was not the primary drug used. Kramer et al (1989) reported a controlled replication study, with six subjects each in tracks I and II, this time with a higher dosage of propranolol (40 mg tid). A repeated measures analysis suggested no drug–placebo difference after the 2-day phase, but propranolol was significantly superior after 5 days of treatment (effect size −3.88, corrected −3.58). The authors demonstrated a significant 'time effect', highlighting the need for a placebo group in such studies, and argued that the effect of propranolol may be delayed beyond the 2 days suggested by Lipinski. They justified the continuation of benztropine on the basis of parkinsonian side-effects.

Irwin et al (1988) conducted a randomized, double-blind, placebo-controlled trial of propranolol on inpatients who developed AA. Eleven subjects entered the trial (all men, mean age 36.8 years), with 6 being given propranolol (60–80 mg/day) and 5 a placebo for 48 hours. Neither group showed a significant improvement over the 2 days. While it is possible that a longer duration of treatment or a larger dosage might have produced different results, the study is significant for using propranolol as a primary therapy for schizophrenic patients clearly suffering from AA. Eight subjects subsequently had an open trial of benztropine (6 mg/day), with significant improvement over 2 days.

Further to the Dupuis et al study mentioned earlier, Dumon et al (1992) conducted a two-period crossover clinical trial to compare propranolol with betaxolol. In the first phase of the study, 45 subjects with severe akathisia were treated with propranolol 20 mg/day; 19 (42%) were judged to have complete alleviation of symptoms. These 19 were then randomly assigned to propranolol (20 mg/day) or betaxolol (10 mg/day) for up to 10 days, the dosage being doubled in case of nonresponse. After a wash-out period of 3–10 days, the drugs were reversed. The two drugs were found to be comparable in their antiakathisia effect, and also significantly, propranolol consistently resulted in an akathisia rating of 0 in these patients.

The Sachdev and Loneragan (1993b) iv challenge study of six patients has been previously mentioned. Propranolol, in this double-blind, controlled study of well-selected AA patients, was no different from placebo in the 1 hour after the challenge. The small number of subjects increases the likelihood of type 2 error, but it does argue against a dramatic effect of the drug. The small dosage used may be a problem, which should be rectified in future studies of this kind, but the marked variability in the manifestations of akathisia make an iv challenge design appealing.

In summary, the large number of studies of propranolol in the treatment of AA cannot be easily collated because of the diverse methodologies used. While the weight of research evidence seems to suggest that propranolol may be a useful drug, its earlier promise is unlikely to be borne out. A balanced viewpoint should be based on the following placebo-controlled studies: Adler et al (1986, 1993), Kramer et al (1988, 1989), Irwin et al (1988) and Sachdev and Loneragan (1993b). The two former groups reported positive results, and latter two negative. It is significant that, in negative studies, propranolol was a primary treatment, ie, the patients were not on some antiparkinsonian or other ostensibly antiakathisia medication. Does it mean that propranolol is more likely to work in patients who are resistant to other medication? More research, using well-selected AA patients, properly validated instruments and placebo-controlled double-blind designs are necessary before the issue can be definitely settled.

The question of dosage and duration of treatment must remain open and dependent on first settling the issue of efficacy. Nevertheless, clinicians will continue to encounter and treat akathisia. The suggestion from the literature is that relatively small dosages of propranolol are sufficient, most researchers using dosages of the order of 60 mg/day, rarely above 120 mg/day. Most also agree that the benefit is seen fairly quickly, but it may take a few days. A trial of 5 days at the higher dosage would be justified before the drug is considered ineffective. The short half-life would suggest at least twice-a-day doses, but it is possible that once-a-day schedule may be effective (Dupuis et al, 1987). The relationships between the plasma concentrations of propranolol and its pharmacodynamic effects are complex, eg, the antihypertensive effect of pro-pranolol is sufficiently long to permit administration once or twice daily. A sustained-release formulation has been developed to maintain therapeutic concentrations throughout a 24-hour period (Nace and Wood, 1987). Propranolol seems to be well tolerated in this population and hypotension, bradycardia, sedation or depression have not generally been reported in appropriately selected individuals. Interestingly, a case of TD induced by pro-pranolol used to treat akathisia has been reported (Sandyk, 1985b). If benefit does occur, how long it will last is not known; the Dupuis et al and Hermesh et al studies suggest persistence of the benefit over several months, the other studies all being of short duration. The propranolol studies are summarized in Table 11.3.

Benztropine vs propranolol

What is the relative efficacy of these two most commonly used drugs in the treatment of akathisia? Only three studies have made a direct comparison (Adler et al, 1987b, 1993; Sachdev and Loneragan, 1993b), and all suffer from some deficiencies that have already been alluded to. In the Adler et al (1987c) study, propranolol was superior, but this was an open study in which low dosages of benztropine were used and the ratings were nonblind. In the Sachdev and Loneragan study, benztropine was superior, but the dosage of propranolol may have been too small, and the effect may not be as acute as anticipated by the authors. In the 1993 Adler et al study benztropine and pro-pranolol were about equally effective, although benztropine produced more side-effects necessitating cessation of the drug, but many of the patients had CA rather than AA. A review of these studies suggests that both drugs are useful. Benztropine (or other similar drug) has historical primacy, and the research evidence for its efficacy is convincing. Propranolol has evoked recent interest and a spate of publications, but the better studies are divided on its usefulness. In a number of studies, the two drugs have been used consecutively or concomitantly. Many studies of propranolol (Lipinski et al, 1983, 1984; Adler et al, 1986; Hermesh et al, 1988; Kramer et al, 1988, 1989) were of patients who had failed to respond to an anticholinergic drug and overall showed improvement. In one study (Irwin et al, 1988), patients responded to benztropine after having failed a trial of propranolol.

The only conclusion one can draw from this evidence is that both drugs are useful and have a place. Which one should be tried first cannot be decided from the research evidence, although only anticholinergics have been successfully used as primary agents in controlled studies. Perhaps the suggestion that akathisic patients with parkinsonism respond well to ACh antagonists should be taken up, with benztropine or similar drug used preferentially in these subjects. In others, either drug may be tried first; a therapeutic trial of 5–7 days should be adequate at dosages of up to 6 mg/day benztropine or 120 mg/day propranolol. While these drugs have been used concomitantly, no research evidence comparing combined with individual use has been published. This remains an area for further work.

Other β-antagonist drugs

A number of studies have examined the efficacy of β-antagonists other than propranolol in the treatment of akathisia. The rationale has been twofold: to determine if a more selective drug, with fewer side-effects, would be equally effective, and to investigate whether the antiakathisia effect of propranolol is central or peripheral, and whether β_1- or β_2-receptors are primarily involved. β-Antagonists can be classified according to their selectivity for receptor subtypes, lipophilicity (which determines how effectively they cross the BBB) and intrinsic sympathomimetic activity. Table 11.4 summarizes the properties of some of the important β-antagonists.

Hydrophilic drugs

The question of whether the antiakathisia effect of β-antagonists is a central or peripheral effect is answered by studying the effect of hydrophilic drugs. Nadolol and sotalol are two nonselective β-antagonists, and atenolol a selective β_1-antagonist, that are hydrophilic and have been examined in the treatment of akathisia. It must be emphasized that at higher dosages these drugs

Table 11.4. *Pharmacological characteristics of β-adrenergic antagonists*

Drug	β_1-Antagonism	β_2-Antagonism	ISA[a]	Lipid solubility	Oral bioavailability (percentage of dose)	Time/2 in plasma (hours)
Nonselective						
Propranolol	++	++	0	+++	~25	3–5
Nadolol	++	++	0	+	~35	10–20
Timolol	++	++	0	++	~50	3–5
Pindolol	++	++	++	++	~75	3–4
Sotalol	++	++	0	+/–	—	—
Selective β_1-antagonists						
Metoprolol	++	+/–	0	++	~40	3–4
Atenolol	++	0	0	0	~50	5–8
Betaxolol	++	0	0	++	—	—
Esmolol	++		0	–	—	0–13
Selective β_2-antagonist						
ICI 118,551[b]	0	++	0	+++	—	—

[a]ISA, intrinsic sympathomimetic activity.
[b]Investigational drug no longer available.

penetrate the BBB sufficiently to produce central effects. Lipinski et al (1984) anecdotally reported that nadolol was not effective, but no data were presented. Ratey et al (1985) reported the successful treatment of 3 patients with nadolol (40–80 mg/day). These patients showed immediate relief in motor restlessness and a more gradual improvement of the subjective distress during the second week of treatment. However, 2 of these patients had benzodiazepines added to the regimen. Wells et al (1991) examined nadolol in a placebo-controlled, double-blind study involving 20 patients with at least moderately severe akathisia. Patients were randomly assigned to receive 40–80 mg nadolol/day and were rated daily for 4 days and on alternate days for 15 days. No significant differences were found between nadolol and placebo in either the subjective or the objective rating of akathisia, while both groups showed an improvement in the objective manifestations on day 9 compared with day 1. The study convincingly demonstrated the lack of efficacy of nadolol. In their open trial previously mentioned, Dupuis et al (1987) treated 6 patients with sotalol (40 mg/day for 2 days followed by 80 mg/day for 2 days) and reported a lack of improvement. Atenolol was reported by Derom et al (1984) to be ineffective in a patient who improved with propranolol. Reiter et al (1987a) treated 7 patients with atenolol (25–100 mg/day) for 2–7 days and then crossed them over to propranolol. While propranolol was effective, atenolol produced no change in the objective ratings and significantly worsened the subjective ratings. The authors speculated on the possible reasons for the worsening: (i) direct effect, ie, peripheral β_1-receptor antagonism; (ii) indirect effect of the β_1-antagonism leading to a compensatory increase in central noradrenergic activity; and/or (iii) pharmacokinetic effect of the drug on neuroleptic levels, with reports that β-antagonists can increase plasma levels of neuroleptic drugs (Silver et al, 1986; Greendyke and Kanter, 1987). A report of akathisia-like symptoms in a hypertensive patient treated with atenolol supports the two latter possibilities (Patterson, 1986).

In conclusion, the published evidence suggests that hydrophilic β-antagonists are ineffective in the treatment of akathisia, and there is even a suggestion that atenolol may make it worse.

Lipophilic selective β_1-antagonists

Zubenko et al (1984c), as previously mentioned, compared metoprolol with propranolol and found that the former was less effective and required administration at high dosages (200–400 mg/day). The authors argued that, at these dosages, the selectivity of the drug for the β_1-receptor was lost, as suggested by the development of a wheeze in one patient. They concluded that the antagonism of the β_2-receptor was necessary for the antiakathisia effect. The findings of Kim et al (1989) were different. They treated nine patients with low-dosage metoprolol (25–100 mg/day) and found that seven patients showed significant improvement. The patients were directly crossed to treatment with propranolol (40–60 mg/day) and did not show any further improvement.

The efficacy of betaxolol, another selective β_1-antagonist, was examined in two studies by one group of investigators. In the Dupuis et al (1987) study, the four patients who went on to have a trial of betaxolol (10 or 20 mg/day) all had a good recovery in 2 days. Dumon et al (1992) reported a randomized, controlled trial comparing betaxolol with propranolol in 19 subjects and found that the antiakathisia effects of the two drugs were comparable.

In summary, the evidence is generally in favour of cardioselective drugs being effective in the treatment of akathisia.

Lipophilic selective β_2-antagonist

Adler et al (1989a) used an investigational drug, ICI 118,551, in a double-blind, placebo-controlled study on 10 subjects (6 drug, 4 placebo). Five of 6 drug-treated and 1 of 4 placebo-treated subjects improved ($p < .05$). The drug-treated patients did not show further treatment when they went on to open treatment with propranolol. The authors suggested that since there was evidence for both β_1- and β_2-antagonists being effective, there was possibly a redundancy of these receptors in the CNS. ICI 118,551 is the only β_2-receptor-selective drug studied in akathisia and is no longer available for investigation.

Lipophilic nonselective antagonist with intrinsic sympathomimetic activity

Pindolol is one such drug that, because of the intrinsic sympathomimetic activity (ISA), has less tendency to lower the heart rate. Reiter et al (1987b) reported the successful treatment of an akathisia patient with pindolol. In a further study, the same group of investigators (Adler et al, 1987b) treated nine patients with 5 mg/day pindolol for 2–4 days and reported improvement in four. Four of the remaining five patients improved with propranolol. Pindolol was therefore less effective either because of less lipophilicity or its partial agonist action, as the authors suggested.

The following conclusions can be drawn from this review of the studies investigating other β-antagonist drugs: (i) A centrally acting drug is necessary to be effective against akathisia. (ii) A lipophilic β_1-antagonist is effective. A specificity for the β_1-receptor in the manifestation of akathisia cannot be concluded from this since a β_2-antagonist drug was also demonstrated to be effective. (iii) A drug with ISA is less effective. The various studies are summarized in Table 11.5.

α-Adrenergic drug

Clonidine, an α_2-agonist that reduces central noradrenergic activity (Langer, 1980), has been investigated in two studies. Zubenko et al (1984b) treated six akathisia patients with clonidine (0.2–0.8 mg/day, mean 0.43), with improvement in all patients and complete remission in four. All improvement was seen within 48 hours of treatment. Concomitant medications included lithium carbonate in four patients and benztropine in three. Side-effects were prominent, and the increment of dosage had to be gradual. In the two patients with partial improvement, dosages were limited by hypotension and sedation. The authors therefore concluded that the improvement in akathisia was not a nonspecific effect of sedation. Adler et al (1987a) reported the results of clonidine treatment in six patients, who were started on a dosage of 0.05–0.20 mg/day, which was gradually increased to a maximally tolerated 0.15–0.40 mg/day over 3–15 days. The ratings were performed by a blind rater. In 2–4 days of treatment, four subjects showed improvement in subjective and one in objective ratings of akathisia. By the time of maximal dosage schedule, all patients had improved substantially, and their ratings on the Hamilton Anxiety Rating Scale were also reduced. Side-effects included hypotension in five patients, and sedation in four, which limited the dosage. The authors argued that their study could not resolve whether the beneficial effect of clonidine was a specific noradrenergic effect or a nonspecific effect of sedation.

In conclusion, the limited investigation (only two small, open studies) of the role of clonidine in the treatment of akathisia suggests that while clonidine may be beneficial, side-effects limit its practical use. Further studies are clearly necessary, including those utilizing the 'clonidine patch', ie, transdermal application.

Benzodiazepines

The rationale for the use of benzodiazepines in the treatment of akathisia stems from the following observations: (i) The subjective symptoms of akathisia resemble anxiety and are often mistaken for them by clinicians and patients. (ii) The level of anxiety influences the manifestations of akathisia.

Table 11.5. *Other β-adrenergic antagonists in the treatment of akathisia*

Drug	N	Daily dosage (mg)	Duration	Overall effect (%)	Results[a] Effect size	Results[a] Adjusted effect size	Comment[b]	Reference
Hydrophilic drugs								
Nadolol	3	40–80	2 weeks	100	—	—	Open	Ratey et al (1985)
Nadolol	20	40–80	2 weeks	Nil	−0.31	−0.30	DB, placebo, crossover	Wells et al (1991)
Sotalol	6	40–80	4 days	Nil	—	—	Open	Dupuis et al (1987)
Atenolol	1	—	—	Nil	—	—	Single case report	Derom et al (1984)
Atenolol	9	25–100	7 days	Worse subjectively	—	—	DB, crossover with propranolol	Reiter et al (1987a)
Lipophilic β₁-antagonists								
Metoprolol	5	300 (200–400)	2–3 days	47.4	—	—	DB, crossover with propranolol	Zubenko et al (1984)
Metoprolol	9	25–100	6 days	77.8	−1.81	−1.72	Crossover with propranolol	Kim et al (1989)
Betaxolol	4	10–20	2 days	100	—	—	Open	Dupuis et al (1987)
Betaxolol	19	10	2 days	—	−3.10	−3.01	Comparable to propranolol	Dumon et al (1992)
Lipophilic β₂-antagonist								
ICI 118,551	6 (placebo 4)			83 25			Drug no longer available	Adler et al (1989a)
Lipophilic nonselective antagonist with intrinsic sympathomimetic activity								
Pindolol	1	5	—	100	—	—	Single case report	Reiter et al (1987b)
Pindolol	9	5	2–4 days	44	—	—	—	Adler et al (1987b)

[a] Overall effect indicates the percentage who improved; effect size reflects the change from baseline in relation to control drug; adjusted effect size is controlled for sample size.
[b] DB denotes double-blind study.

(iii) RLS, which resembles akathisia, has been reported to respond to benzodiazepines (see Chapter 13). The drugs that have been investigated include diazepam, lorazepam and clonazepam, and a summary of the published studies is presented in Table 11.6. These drugs have similar mechanisms of action but different pharmacokinetic profiles, with their plasma half-lives being 30–60, 10–20 and 18–27 hours, respectively (Rall, 1990). In the early 1960s, the use of barbiturates was recommended by Ayd (1961), but these are no longer used for this purpose.

Diazepam

Donlon (1973) reported an open study of 13 outpatients (mean age 32.2 ± 8.6 years) with akathisia who were treated with diazepam 5 mg tid over 3 days. Ten patients effectively improved. The 3 who didn't complained of drowsiness and requested discontinuation, although it is not certain whether this did happen. Overall, a 38.5% improvement was noted. All patients had previously been unsuccessfully treated with diphenhydramine (75 mg/day), and 9 of the 10 responders were concurrently on anticholinergics. A case of akathisia that responded to diazepam 15 mg/day after having received no benefit from diphenhydramine and benztropine was reported by Director and Muniz (1982). This patient maintained the improvement over 6 months of follow-up. Braude et al (1983) reported that they treated 4 patients with diazepam (15–40 mg/day) but with no benefit. The single iv dose, double-blind comparison between diazepam and diphenhydramine by Gagrat et al (1978) was mentioned earlier. The diazepam (5 mg) challenge did produce a significant improvement, although somewhat less than that of diphenhydramine. Sedation was not different between the two groups.

Lorazepam

Bartels et al (1987) conducted an open trial of lorazepam (1.5–5 mg/day, mean 2.34) on 16 patients with AA and reported marked improvement in 9 and moderate in 5 over a 2-week period. The mean akathisia rating scale (0–3) before treatment was 1.81 and after treatment 0.32, indicating an 82.3% reduction (effect size −1.55, corrected −1.51). Five patients who improved were also on biperiden. The Adler et al (1985) single-blind, crossover comparison of lorazepam and propranolol has already been alluded to. Lorazepam (2 mg/day) produced improvement in the subjective but not the objective ratings and was therefore inferior to propranolol in this study.

Table 11.6. *Benzodiazepines in the treatment of acute akathisia*

Drug	N	Daily dosage (mg)	Duration	Results[a]				Comment[b]	Reference
				Overall effect (%)	Percent change	Effect size	Adjusted effect size		
Diazepam	13	15	3 days	75.4	38.5	—	—	Open study	Donlon et al (1973)
	20	5	Single iv dose	++	—	—	—	Less than diphenhydramine	Gagrat et al (1978)
	1	15	6 months	100	—	—	—	Single case	Director and Muniz (1982)
	4	15–40	—	Nil	—	—	—	No details given	Braude et al (1983)
Lorazepam	6	2	3–4 days	Sub[c] only	—	—	—	DB, crossover with propranolol	Adler et al (1985)
	16	2–3 (1.5–5)	2 weeks	100	82.3	−1.55	−1.55	Open study	Bartels et al (1987)
Clonazepam	10	0.5	1 week	100	61	—	—	Open study	Kutcher et al (1987)
	6	1.5	6 weeks	87	—	—	—	DB comparison with antiparkinsonian drug	Horiguchi and Nishimatsu (1992)

[a]Overall effect indicates the percentage of patients who improved; percent change reflects the change in akathisia score from baseline; effect size reflects the change in baseline from control drug; adjusted effect size is controlled in sample size.
[b]DB denotes double-blind study.
[c]Sub, subjective akathisia.

Clonazepam

Kutcher et al (1987) treated 10 adolescent (mean age 17.1 years) schizophrenic patients suffering from akathisia (both subjective and objective features) with clonazepam (0.5 mg/day) in an open study. The mean ratings on the objective Chouinard rating scale (0–6) dropped from 4.1 to 1.6 over 1 week (61% change), with all patients demonstrating at least a 1-point drop objectively and reporting subjective improvement. Nine patients received benztropine (mean 2.8 mg/day) concomitantly. Horiguchi and Nishimatsu (1992) published a double-blind comparison of clonazepam ($n = 8$) and antiparkinsonian drugs (trihexyphenidyl or promethazine) ($n = 6$). Clonazepam was 'effective' in 7 patients and 'slightly effective' in 1, while the antiparkinsonian drugs were 'effective' in 4 and 'slightly effective' in 1 and there was 'no change' in 1. The one patient who did not improve was subsequently given clonazepam in addition and improved considerably.

In conclusion, most published studies of benzodiazepines in akathisia have been positive. These results do not reflect the general lack of enthusiasm among clinicians about the utility of these drugs in akathisia. The studies are, of course, deficient in a number of ways: (i) They were not double-blind placebo-controlled studies. (ii) All studies include a small number of subjects. (iii) Benzodiazepines are often administered to patients already on antiparkinsonian (and possibly antiakathisia) drugs, which are often continued through the study. The Horiguchi and Nishimatsu (1992) study was an exception. (iv) The relative efficacy of different benzodiazepines is uncertain. Considering the obvious promise of these drugs, larger and better studies are indicated.

The mechanism by which benzodiazepines act in akathisia, if they are indeed effective, is uncertain. Benzodiazepines have direct and indirect effects at all levels of the neuraxis, leading to anxiolysis, sedation and hypnosis progressing to stupor. They induce muscle hypotonia and anterograde amnesia, and inhibit seizure activity. Most, if not all, actions of these drugs are a result of increased neural inhibition mediated by the GABA–benzodiazepine receptor complex (Rall, 1990). At very high dosages, they can cause neuromuscular blockade. While all benzodiazepines have a similar mode of action, they differ in their selectivity and, therefore, usefulness. Clonazepam has been particularly useful in movement disorders, including myoclonus, and is the logical drug to investigate further in akathisia.

Amantadine

Amantadine hydrochloride, originally introduced as an antiviral drug, has been demonstrated to have antiparkinsonian effects (Appleton et al, 1970;

Parkes et al, 1970). Its investigation in the treatment of akathisia has been limited. DiMascio et al (1976) published a double-blind controlled comparison of amantadine (200–400 mg/day) with benztropine (4–8 mg/day, 12 mg/day in 1 patient) for the treatment of neuroleptic-induced EPSE, including akathisia (the study has been mentioned previously). Both groups showed marked improvement by day 3 (benztropine > amantadine), and of the 13 patients treated with amantadine, 9 were still available at four weeks and were free of akathisia. The authors found the two drugs comparable, with benztropine performing better overall only in the first week, and reported fewer side-effects with amantadine. Four patients reported 'excitement' with amantadine. Some deficiencies of the study are the lack of both a placebo-controlled group and control of neuroleptic medication, no detailed description of the akathisia and too simple a global rating of akathisia. The findings of the study need to be confirmed in a better-designed study.

Two further reports of the use of amantadine in akathisia have been published, but they do not enhance the status of the drug. Gelenberg (1978) reported 14 cases with benztropine-refractory EPSE who were treated with this drug (200–300 mg/day) over 10 days. Three had akathisia, 2 in conjunction with parkinsonism. Of the latter, 1 improved substantially and 1 minimally. The patient with akathisia alone worsened. Details are lacking in this paper, so a reasoned judgement of it is not possible. Zubenko et al (1984a) studied 4 patients with akathisia who responded to amantadine but developed tolerance to the effect within a week. These patients suffered from an affective disorder and were on lithium as well as anticholinergics for their DIP. These reports further highlight the need for more investigation of amantadine in this disorder before it can be accepted or rejected.

Ritanserin

A theoretically promising approach to the treatment of akathisia is the use of drugs that act on the 5HT receptor. While investigations of 5HT receptor antagonists in PD have been disappointing, there is one previous report of improvement in EPSE with ritanserin, a specific $5HT_2$ antagonist (Bersani et al, 1986). Miller et al (1990) investigated ritanserin in 10 akathisic patients (mean age 26.4 years) in a single-blind open study. Concomitant medication was used with 8 patients (biperiden with 4, oxazepam with 3, propranolol with 2), but all drugs were kept constant during the study and for 1 week before. Ritanserin (5–20 mg/day, mean 13.5 mg/day) resulted in a significant ($p < .01$) drop in Hillside Akathisia Scale scores in 3 days of treatment: objective score from 8.6 ± 0.40 to 2.1 ± 2.0, and subjective from 7.8 ± 5.2 to 3.3 ±

3.7. Overall, the improvement was >50% in 6 and ~50% in 2. The effect was generally visible in the first day, and no side-effects were noted. Placebo-controlled discontinuation led to the recurrence of the akathisia. Miller et al (1992) reported 3 patients of NIA resistant to first-line treatment who responded rapidly and substantially to ritanserin 20 mg/day, with relapse of the akathisia upon discontinuation. Only one case was placebo-controlled. This and similarly acting drugs clearly deserve further study.

Tricyclic antidepressants

Danel et al (1988) published a case report of a 26-year-old patient with AA who failed to respond to trihexyphenidyl (6 mg/day) but had a dramatic improvement within a few days of the addition of amitryptiline (100 mg/day). The authors argued that this was due to the β-postsynaptic desensitization produced by the drug (Vetulani and Suster, 1975), but the additive anticholinergic effect of amitryptiline and trihexyphenidyl cannot be ruled out. This promising finding has not been taken up further.

Sodium valproate

The only study that examined valproate (Friis et al, 1983) was alluded to earlier. In this double-blind, placebo-controlled study on 15 patients, valproate (900–2,400 mg/day, median 1,700) did not produce any significant effect on akathisia compared with placebo, even though it benefited dyskinesia. In 7 patients, it induced or aggravated parkinsonism. Understandably, this study did not prompt further investigation.

Piracetam

Piracetam is an unusual drug in that, even though related to GABA, it does not affect the known neurotransmitter functions. It is therefore labelled a *nootropic* drug and seems to influence the bioenergetic metabolism of cells in general, including neurones. It has a number of other actions that affect brain metabolism. Kabes et al (1982) published a double-blind, crossover, placebo-controlled trial of piracetam (4 g single iv dose) in 40 subjects with EPSE, but did not specify how many had akathisia. Piracetam produced a significant effect on akathisia, but the rating scale of akathisia used and the statistical analysis applied can be criticized. A replication of this study is warranted with better methodology.

Electroconvulsive therapy

Hermesh et al (1992) reported a 28-year-old manic patient who developed akathisia and parkinsonism that persisted despite changes in neuroleptics, treatment with anticholinergics on two occasions, benzodiazepines, and a neuroleptic-free period of 5 days. She was treated with right unilateral electroconvulsive therapy (ECT) on five occasions. There was a marked improvement after the first use of ECT and complete remission of all motor symptoms after the fifth. This improvement was sustained for 3 months, after which it recurred, only to respond to a reduction of neuroleptic dosage. The mechanism of action of ECT in this case can only be speculated upon. This report suggests that ECT may have a role in very severe and resistant cases.

I have reviewed a number of studies on akathisia, but the limitations of the research make the final recommendations tentative. The deficiencies of most of the studies have already been highlighted. When encountering akathisia in the clinic, our approach is first to establish the diagnosis, if necessary by repeated assessment and observation of the patient. If the diagnosis is fairly certain, we evaluate the need for the offending drug and the dosage being used. This may mean a reduction of the dosage or complete cessation if it is clinically indicated, or a change in type of neuroleptic to one that is less likely to cause akathisia. Sometimes an effective change in both dosage and type may be necessary. Alternative drugs may be available if a non-neuroleptic is the offending drug. Even when a neuroleptic drug is being used, one may be able to suspend it in some circumstances, eg, in a manic patient for whom lithium may be a suitable alternative, or if the neuroleptic drug is being used to control agitation where a benzodiazepine may be equally effective. It may be possible to reduce or suspend the drug and then reintroduce it by gradually increasing the dosage. As stated earlier in this chapter, the role of iron deficiency should be considered, although the evidence for a significant contribution is conflicting.

Once the diagnosis is established, and the manipulation of the offending drug has not produced significant relief, the introduction of another drug should be considered. We recommend the use of an ACh antagonist as the first-line and a β-antagonist as the second-line drug, but this order may be reversed. If parkinsonian side-effects are present, the ACh antagonist is the obvious choice; the presence of a prominent tremor may suggest the use of a β-antagonist. Vulnerability to side-effects will have to be considered: ACh antagonists are more likely to cause confusion in the elderly, may precipitate urinary retention in elderly men, etc. β-Antagonists have to be used cautiously in patients with bronchial asthma, cardiac disease and diabetes mellitus. If an ACh antagonist is decided on, the actual choice of the drug has not been shown to be of concern. Benztropine and benzhexol are the most commonly used drugs. We initially start with benztropine 2 mg/day, and increase the dosage after 2 days to 4 mg/day. If significant improvement does not occur in 2 days, we increase it to 6 mg/day. Although the response is usually apparent within 2–3 days, an adequate therapeutic trial would be a dosage of 6 mg/day benztropine (or equivalent) for 5 days. The occasional patient is known to respond to a larger dose, and we have used 10 mg/day in a few cases.

If this is unsatisfactory, a β-antagonist trial should be pursued. We recommend propranolol unless a medical condition (eg, bronchial asthma) mandates a β₁-selective drug, in which case metoprolol may be used (a lipophilic drug is necessary). An initial dose of propranolol 10 mg/day tid is appropriate, which can be increased over the succeeding 4–5 days to 90–120 mg/day. An adequate trial would be 120 mg/day (or equivalent) over 5 days, but we have used with benefit dosages as high as 200 mg/day in the occasional patient. We generally taper off the ACh antagonist once the propranolol is introduced unless concomitant EPSE are present. Attention must, however, be drawn to the fact that most research studies of β-antagonists have been conducted in patients already on an ACh antagonist, ie, the combination was being investigated. Combined therapy may, therefore, be indicated if the drugs fail individually.

As a third line, we use benzodiazepines, either lorazepam 1.5–3 mg/day, diazepam 5–15 mg/day or clonazepam 0.5–2 mg/day. Sometimes these are given concomitantly with benztropine or propranolol, especially if the response to these drugs has been partial.

If all these drugs fail, we recommend reassessing the status of the offending drug as described earlier. If significant alteration is not an option, then miscellaneous drugs may be tried. Amantadine or clonidine would be the next obvious choices. In the rare case, if akathisia is very severe and psychosis is difficult to control, the use of ECT may be justified.

The treatment guidelines are presented diagramatically in Fig. 11.1.

Tardive and chronic akathisia

The assessment of the literature on the treatment of TA and CA is problematic for a number of reasons. The most important is, of course, the lack of detailed characterization of the syndrome in many published studies such that cer-

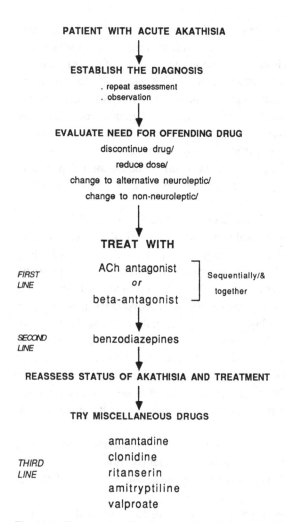

Fig. 11.1. Treatment outline for acute drug-induced akathisia.

tainty of diagnosis cannot be ascertained. The treatment studies reviewed earlier for AA often do not explicitly state the criteria for the diagnosis and may well have included TA or CA in some cases. The publications that explicitly deal with TA are mostly anecdotal and suggest, rather than confirm, the usefulness of particular treatment strategies.

It is important that the pharmacological characteristics of CA with acute or tardive onsets be delineated separately, as they may have distinct, and in some ways opposing, biochemical abnormalities. CA with acute onset may behave like AA, and therefore the same treatment principles will apply. TA and some cases of CA may behave like TD. Alternatively, the pathophysiology of all subsyndromes of CA may have a common basis irrespective of their differences.

The diagnosis of a tardive onset of akathisia is usually based on historical information from the patient or an informant, and is therefore prone to errors due to selective recall of information. In contrast, WA is often directly observed by the physician in the course of its development and yields a more reliable diagnosis.

The variability of TA presents the same problems in investigation as does AA. Furthermore, Remington et al (1993) and Sachdev and Loneragan (1993a,b) highlighted the possibility of a marked placebo response in some patients.

The published literature on the treatment of TA and CA will now be reviewed, with an attempt to characterize the subtype wherever possible.

Modification of the offending drug

Under ideal circumstances, discontinuation of the neuroleptic drug would be the obvious treatment. This is not always practicable, however, considering the continuing psychosis in the patient. As with WA, there may be some worsening of TA if the neuroleptic is suspended, but this is often temporary. Published literature on the long-term outcome of discontinuation of neuroleptics is scanty, but if the TD literature can be taken as a guide, this should lead to the resolution of a proportion of the disorder (American Psychiatric Association, 1992). A few patients who responded to a discontinuation of neuroleptics have been reported (Weiner and Luby, 1983; Shearer et al, 1984). Burke et al (1989) followed up their patients ($n = 48$) over a mean 2.3 (range 0.1–8) years and found that 67% continued to have akathisia. Of the 16 who had no akathisia, only 4 were judged to be in complete remission, and their akathisia had lasted 1.2 ± 0.4 years after discontinuation of the neuroleptic.

It would be premature to make any definitive recommendations since more data are necessary. Until these become available, the recommendations for TD should probably apply to TA. Indeed, the two disorders often co-occur, and even if some pharmacological characteristics of the two are antithetical, the more disabling disorder will take precedence. A reduction in dosage or discontinuation, and the use of alternative drugs, are important considerations. If a modification of neuroleptic dosage is impractical or does not produce the desired result, alternative drugs for the treatment should be considered. The relative risk of the newer antipsychotics (eg, remoxipride and risperidone) for TA is unknown, but preliminary evidence is emerging that clozapine may be an alternative worth considering.

Clozapine

Clozapine has been suggested as a suitable antipsychotic drug for schizophrenic patients with severe and intractable akathisia (Marder and Van Putten, 1988; Lieberman et al, 1989). Some anecdotal support for this was provided by Wirshing et al (1990) and Gardos et al (1987). Levin et al (1992) treated 3 patients suffering from severe and treatment-resistant akathisia with clozapine after the discontinuation of other neuroleptics. Remission of akathisia occurred in all 3 patients within 3 months, and this was maintained over a 2-year follow-up. TD also remitted but more gradually. Safferman et al (1993) examined the impact of clozapine on patients with ($n = 21$) or without ($n = 49$) akathisia at baseline after a 2-week wash-out period. Patients who did not have akathisia at baseline (acute or tardive) did not develop it during the 1 year of treatment with clozapine (mean dosage 565 mg/day). Those with akathisia, which was possibly a mixture of AA and TA and/or agitation, improved considerably in the first 3 weeks and then continued to improve over 3 months even though the dosage of clozapine was increasing. This study, however, suffered from the dual limitations of a 50% drop-out rate over the year (although no patients were withdrawn because of EPSE) and the use of a modified Simpson and Angus (1970) rating scale for the diagnosis of akathisia, which is less than optimal for such purposes.

Preliminary evidence therefore suggests that clozapine may be a suitable alternative in patients with significant TA who have to be continued on an antipsychotic drug. These studies do not help us decide whether the clozapine actually hastened the improvement of akathisia or simply permitted it to remit after the cessation of the offending neuroleptic drug. A placebo-controlled study is necessary to decide this.

ACh antagonists

Case reports of treatment of TA with anticholinergic drugs have appeared with mixed results. The 3 patients reported by Kruse (1960a) did not respond to 'antiparkinsonian drugs', presumably anticholinergics. The 2 patients with WA reported by Braude and Barnes (1983) (1 with procyclidine 5 mg tid) and 1 patient reported by Weiner and Luby (1983) also did not experience any improvement with anticholinergics. Further case reports of no improvement with an anticholinergic were published by Stein and Pohlman (1987) and Yassa et al (1988). Yassa and Bloom (1990) reported a patient who, after having failed a trial of procyclidine 10 mg tid, later responded to a combination of lorazepam 1.5 mg/day and procyclidine 15 mg/day (this patient was followed up for 1 week, and spontaneous fluctuation or improvement cannot be ruled out). Burke et al (1989) treated 10 patients with an anticholinergic drug and reported improvement in 1, worsening in 3 and no change in the rest. Sachdev and Chee (1990) reported an iv challenge of benztropine (2 mg) in a patient with well-established TA and noted a positive response which lasted 2 hours after a single injection. Interestingly, the patient worsened after a challenge of physostigmine (1 mg), an ACh agonist (see Fig. 11.2). The patient had a considerable improvement with oral benztropine, but the dosage had to be increased to 8 mg/day and unacceptable side-effects supervened. It is difficult to draw any conclusions from these reports, except to say that the majority, but not all, were negative, and a few reported worsening. A selective reporting cannot be ruled out, especially because there has been an expectation among investigators that TA will behave like TD in showing either no improvement or worsening with anticholinergics (Jeste and Wyatt, 1982).

That ACh antagonists may be effective in CA (without further specification) is suggested by the emergence of akathisia in studies that examined the effect of withdrawal of these drugs in schizophrenic patients maintained on neuroleptics. While a number of such studies have been published, only a few have examined akathisia with any consistency. Manos et al (1981), in a double-blind study, randomly assigned 98 chronically ill schizophrenic patients who had been treated continuously with antipsychotics for a mean 8.24 years and antiparkinsonian drugs for a mean 4.71 years to either placebo ($n = 75$) or trihexyphenidyl ($n = 23$) over 6 weeks. The mean akathisia ratings (0–4 scale) for objective akathisia increased in the placebo group from 0.28 to 0.79 (vs 0.13 to 0.17 for the drug group, $p < .01$), and the restlessness rating increased from 0.20 to 1.20 (vs 0.04 to 0.13 for the drug group, $p < .001$), thus suggesting that the long-term administration of the anticholinergic drugs was suppressing some akathisia that became manifest upon their withdrawal. Klett and Caffey (1972), in their large study of the withdrawal of anticholinergic drugs in long-term-medicated schizophrenics noted that in many cases the study had to be terminated prematurely because of a poorly definable feeling of restlessness reported by the patients. Some of the worsening was due to a definite akathisia. These studies provide evidence that akathisia responsive to ACh antagonists may persist in long-term-medicated patients, although it is not possible to determine whether this is of acute or tardive onset.

The only controlled investigation (Sachdev and Loneragan, 1993a) was a

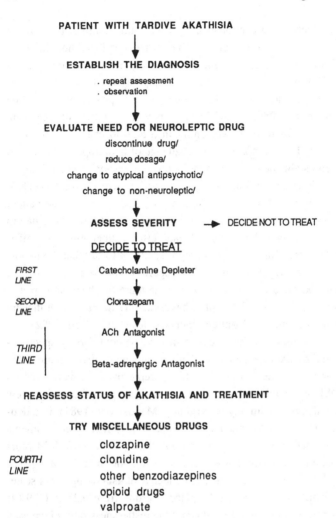

PATIENT WITH TARDIVE AKATHISIA

ESTABLISH THE DIAGNOSIS
. repeat assessment
. observation

EVALUATE NEED FOR NEUROLEPTIC DRUG
discontinue drug/
reduce dosage/
change to atypical antipsychotic/
change to non-neuroleptic/

ASSESS SEVERITY ➔ DECIDE NOT TO TREAT

DECIDE TO TREAT

FIRST LINE   Catecholamine Depleter

SECOND LINE   Clonazepam

                    ACh Antagonist
THIRD LINE
                    Beta-adrenergic Antagonist

REASSESS STATUS OF AKATHISIA AND TREATMENT

TRY MISCELLANEOUS DRUGS
clozapine
FOURTH LINE   clonidine
               other benzodiazepines
               opioid drugs
               valproate

Fig. 11.2. Treatment outline for tardive akathisia.

study of five patients with TA who were challenged with benztropine (2 mg), propranolol (1 mg) and placebo using a random, double-blind, crossover design. Overall, benztropine was judged to be marginally superior in producing improvement ($p = .08$), with the subjective scores showing a significant improvement ($p < .05$). On global ratings, three patients were judged to respond to benztropine, with none showing any worsening. Of these three, two later responded to oral benztropine at dosages up to 10 mg/day. The small number of subjects studied make the findings preliminary, and further studies are needed. Our work suggests that some of the negative results reported may be because of inadequate dosages, and TA may respond to relatively large dosages (greater than the 4–6 mg/day of benztropine usually employed to treat AA). This has some similarity with TDt, which may also respond to large dosages of anticholinergics in some cases (Sachdev, 1993b).

β-Adrenergic antagonist drugs

Reports of the use of propranolol are again mostly anecdotal, and positive reports of cases (eg, Stein and Pohlman, 1987; Yassa et al, 1988) are counterbalanced by the negative ones (eg, Burke et al, 1989). In the Sachdev and Chee (1990) study involving multiple single-drug challenges in one patient, propranolol (40 mg oral) produced a sustained improvement over 4 hours, while metoprolol (100 mg oral; lipohilic, β_1-selective antagonist) produced a mild reduction, noted at 60 minutes and persisting up to 2 hours. With atenolol (a hydrophilic β_1-antagonist), no significant change was noted. Subsequent treatment of the patient with propranolol 80 mg/day was associated with moderate improvement in akathisia in spite of neuroleptics having to be introduced because of a relapse of psychosis.

In the double-blind iv challenge study already cited (Sachdev and Loneragan, 1993a), propranolol led to a significant improvement in both subjective ($p < .01$) and objective features ($p < .05$). Overall, two of the five patients reported improvement. They were subsequently treated with oral propranolol (up to 120 mg/day) with mild improvement in one patient for which it was not significant enough to continue the drug.

In conclusion, the evidence for the usefulness of β-antagonists in TA is weak, but enough to justify a controlled trial.

Other adrenergic drugs

Clonidine was tried in two patients by Burke et al (1989) and in one patient by Sachdev and Chee (1990), with no benefit. Burke et al (1989) also reported having tried phenoxybenzamine without success.

Catecholamine-depleting drugs

This class of drugs, which includes reserpine, tetrabenazine and oxypertine, deplete catecholamines (DA and NE) and, to a smaller extent, indoleamines from the nerve terminals. They are now commonly used in the treatment of TD (Fahn, 1985). Their utility in TA has been documented by Burke et al

(1989) in an open study. Reserpine produced significant improvement in 13 (87%) of 15 patients treated (mean maximum dosage 5.0 mg/day), with complete remission in 3, 1 of whom was weaned off the drug without recurrence of the akathisia. Tetrabenazine helped 7 (58%) of 12 patients, being markedly helpful in 6 of them, but no patient could be weaned off the drug. Of all the drugs used, this class was the most helpful, and about 50% of the patients so treated were still taking the drug on follow-up.

An additional rationale for the use of DA-depleting drugs comes from a study by Sachdev and Loneragan (1993c) in which they challenged 7 patients suffering from TA with low-dosage apomorphine (0.01 mg/kg) by sc injection in a double-blind, placebo-controlled experiment and reported significant reduction in the movement component of the akathisia. One patient was later treated with tetrabenazine, which resulted in marked improvement in both TA and TD; an attempt to reduce the dosage 6 months later resulted in reemergence of the symptoms. The lack of response to oxypertine (60 mg/day) was reported in one case by Kuniyoshi et al (1991).

In conclusion, there is encouraging preliminary evidence that DA depleters may play a significant role in the treatment of TA, and the drugs need to be investigated further. Side-effects should, of course, be kept in mind. Drowsiness, depression and postural hypotension are the most important ones, and the medication should be started at a small dosage and increased gradually. The side-effects may be less with tetrabenazine than reserpine. The drugs should possibly be avoided in depressed patients. It should also be pointed out that DA-depleting drugs can cause AA, and theoretically one could substitute this for TA, although this would be impossible to decide in practice.

GABAergic drugs

Benzodiazepines have been reported to be useful in some cases. Kruse (1960a) reported that two of his three patients with TA experienced considerable relief from a benzodiazepine. Burke et al (1989) treated four patients with lorazepam (mean maximum dosage 7 mg/day) and reported improvement in three (marked in two), in whom the drug was continued over the subsequent few months. Kuniyoshi et al (1991) reported nine patients with TA who had previously failed to respond to anticholinergics (eight cases), flunitrazepam 2 mg (six cases), lorazepam (one case), diazepam 10 mg (one case) and some other drugs and who responded to clonazepam (1–3 mg/day; in 1 case clonazepam 0.5 mg along with diazepam 10 mg). The authors used the criteria applied by Inada et al (1988); ie, in addition to the Burke et al (1989) criteria, the patients showed aggravation of the akathisia with reduction or discontinuation of the neuroleptic and did not respond to antiparkinsonian drugs.

These few case reports make an assessment difficult, especially because sedation may have a nonspecific effect on the manifestations of akathisia. Nevertheless, these are relatively nontoxic drugs, and their role in the treatment of TA should be fully explored.

Opioids

Walters et al (1988b) reported a double-blind trial of opiates (acetaminophen with codeine up to 60 mg qid or propoxyphene up to 100 mg qid) in 5 patients with CA of acute onset and reported significant improvement ($p < .02$), especially in 3 patients. The authors subsequently pointed out that the positive response was in patients with shorter-duration akathisia (mean 2.4 months) rather than in patients with more chronic illness (mean > 1 year) and argued that opiates may be effective in AA rather than TA (Walters and Hening, 1989). Miller and Jankovic (1988) reported a lack of therapeutic response of TA with opiates. Burke et al (1989) tried opiates in 10 patients and obtained a mild improvement in 2, which was short-lived. The available evidence does not, therefore, appear promising.

Other treatments

Viukari and Linnoila (1977) reported a study of fusaric acid, a selective and potent inhibitor of dopamine β-hydroxylase, which decreases brain NE and 5HT levels (and not DA), in 15 patients with TD. Their akathisia ratings were not significantly affected by the drug.

DeKeyser and D'Haenan (1986) reported the amelioration of TA with ECT.

Conclusions

As this review has suggested, the treatment of TA is, in general, unsatisfactory, and the main emphasis should be on its prevention. The principles for its prevention are similar to those for TD, and for a detailed discussion the reader is referred to some excellent texts that have examined this issue (Jeste and Wyatt, 1982; American Psychiatric Association, 1992).

If TA does develop, the first step is to reassess the diagnosis and the need for continued neuroleptic medication at the current dosage. Cessation or modification of the neuroleptic treatment is advisable if it is clinically feasible, along the lines previously discussed. The use of alternative neuroleptics and non-neuroleptic drugs should be considered. Such changes may lead to a temporary worsening of the akathisia, but a longer-term perspective should prevail. The co-occurrence of TD often complicates the management, and sometimes the management of dyskinetic or dystonic movements must take precedence.

The next step should be the assessment of the TA in terms of its severity and impact on the patient. In mild cases, it may be advisable to refrain from treating it, in view of some of the side-effects that the treatment drugs may induce. This is especially true if the objective rather than the distress component of the akathisia is the predominant feature. If a decision to treat TA is made because of the disability it is causing, the choice of the primary drug will depend on the clinical situation in the individual case. We often choose a DA-depleting drug as the first-line drug in a nondepressed patient. Either tetrabenazine or reserpine may be used, but we prefer the former because of its better side-effects profile. We generally initiate the treatment with 25–50 mg/day and build it up gradually to 100–150 mg/day. The highest dosage we have used was 250 mg/day for a short period in a failed trial. Burke et al used a mean maximum dosage of 175 mg/day. With reserpine, we recommend starting with 0.25 mg/day and titrating upwards to about 3–5 mg/day. It is difficult to recommend an adequate duration for a therapeutic trial of a catecholamine depleter, but we minimally treat for 2 weeks at the higher dosage before deciding on a lack of success and gradually withdrawing the drug.

If these drugs fail or produce only incomplete relief, we use clonazepam. Even though the evidence for its benefit is weak, it is relatively nontoxic and has shown more promise than the other benzodiazepines in the preliminary investigations. We start with 0.5 mg/day and titrate the dosage up to 3 mg/day. We often use clonazepam in conjunction with other drugs.

As the next line of management, we try an ACh antagonist or a β-antagonist, in the dosages discussed earlier. With ACh antagonists, the possible exacerbation of a concomitant TD must, of course, be kept in mind. We have not had any clinical experience with opiates, and the reported evidence for their efficacy is not encouraging.

If the preceding treatments fail, and the patient continues to need treatment with antipsychotic medication, we recommend the use of clozapine. Figure 11.2 presents the treatment of TA diagramatically.

Withdrawal akathisia

No definitive guidelines for the management of WA emerge from the published literature, and the following recommendations are based on the small clinical experience with this disorder and the speculation on its theoretical basis.

Since rapid or abrupt cessation of the neuroleptic is the basis for the emergence of this syndrome, a gradual withdrawal is likely to reduce its incidence. If it does occur, a strategy worth considering is to increase the dosage of the neuroleptic to the previous level and to reduce it more gradually. This strategy, unfortunately, is not always practicable and may indeed not work. If increasing the dosage of the neuroleptic does not suppress the akathisia, it is advisable not to persist with the higher dosage as it will possibly delay any spontaneous improvement.

There is an expectation that WA will ameliorate spontaneously with time. While this is awaited, a strategy to reduce its manifestations is worthwhile. The drugs we have utilized are mainly catecholamine depleters (tetrabenazine or reserpine) and benzodiazepines. The dosage schedule is similar to the one discussed for TA. If WA persists beyond 3 months, we change the diagnosis to CA. The management is no different from the one recommended for TA/CA.

Akathisia due to a general medical condition

Little information is available about the management of akathisia secondary to an organic brain disease. In PD, the role of dopaminergic treatment should be considered, and the relationship of the akathisia to the 'on' and 'off' phases delineated. Dopaminergic drugs (eg, bromocriptine and pergolide), benzodiazepines and anticholinergic drugs may be tried. The report by Linazasoro et al (1993) on the use of low-dosage clozapine (mean 26.4 mg/day) in the treatment of 'nocturnal' akathisia in nine patients with PD, with excellent results in all patients, is of interest.

Ethical and legal issues

Because DIA is an iatrogenic disorder which leads to serious distress, may compromise the psychiatric status of the patient, may lead to impulsive actions (aggression or self-harm) and may become chronic and resistant to treatment, it is of much ethical concern and may lead to litigation. A detailed discussion of the ethical and legal issues is beyond the scope of this book. The most common allegations against psychiatrists, in reference to medication side-effects, pertain to two areas: negligence and informed consent (Slawson, 1989).

A negligence or 'tort' action is successful if the plaintiff can establish by a preponderance of evidence (ie, more convincingly than the contrary can be established by the defendant) that the psychiatrist violated his or her duty to care for the patient (by an act of omission or commission), leading to physical or emotional injury to the patient. In the case of akathisia, an appropriate standard of care will involve (i) performing a detailed assessment of the patient to establish the diagnosis that indicates treatment with a neuroleptic or other akathisia-inducing medication; (ii) considering suitable alternatives to the prescription of such medication; (iii) prescribing the drug in the appropriate dosage, and for the proper duration, as is generally considered by the majority of the profession; (iv) recognizing the side-effect early, alerting the patient to it and taking the appropriate measures, which include reviewing the offending medication and monitoring and treating the akathisia when indicated; (v) recognizing the risk of TA and WA, and using generally recommended practices for long-term treatment, while being cognizant of the attendant risks; (vi) consulting with psychiatrist colleagues and, if necessary, experts in the field, in case of doubt.

The obtaining of informed consent has more than medicolegal significance. By involving the patient in the decision-making process, it will also encourage compliance and improve the patient–psychiatrist alliance. The concept of informed consent has been accepted as a legal doctrine in most English-speaking countries in one form or another. The key elements of informed consent are appropriate information dissemination, competence to assess the information and voluntariness of the decision making. Each element has been extensively debated in the literature.

The information imparted to the patient should include the nature of the patient's condition, the proposed treatments and the anticipated benefits and risks, the alternative treatments possible and their anticipated risk and benefits and the consequence of no treatment (Rozovsky, 1990). The extent of the information may vary depending on whether a physician-based or patient-based standard is used. In the case of akathisia, the risk of both AA and TA should be disclosed in routine circumstances. There may be some exceptions to obtaining informed consent for the acute use of neuroleptic drugs: (i) in a psychiatric emergency when treatment is immediately necessary, disclosure is impractical and a delay would be detrimental for the patient; (ii) when the patient is judged to be legally incompetent to make an informed decision (eg, with mental retardation or dementia), in which case a legal guardian may substitute. In some circumstances, the patient may 'waive' his or her right to decide and may ask the physician to decide instead. Or patients may inform the physician that they do not wish to be told.

Obtaining consent from a psychotic patient entails some special considerations. If the patient is judged to be incapable of making a decision, many jurisdictions require that a substitute decision be made by the court or an appropriate authority before the initiation of treatment. Even when the patient is judged to be competent, physicians often fear noncompliance, decompensation or litigation if the full risks of treatment are disclosed (Lidz et al, 1983). Empirical data on these issues are limited (Appelbaum et al, 1987), but a solution offered to these dilemmas is that informed consent be considered a process that occurs over a period of time and not as a single event. This is especially true where long-term treatment is concerned but is also relevant for short-term treatment. The risks and benefits can therefore be gradually discussed. Even when the psychotic patient is judged to be competent to make an informed choice, his or her capacity may be limited by cognitive deficits or the nature of the symptoms, and the full impact of the treatment will become obvious only over a period of time. There are various other ways in which this process of informed consent can be facilitated. The patient should be encouraged to express his or her opinion, so that the psychiatrist can assist in weighing options. The presentation and format of the information should be individualized to the patient. It is useful to involve family members in the decision making, as they may be able to assist in determining the competence of the patient and may be in a better position to assess the risks and benefits of the treatment.

Monitoring for TA, like TD, should occur as long as neuroleptic treatment continues. The psychiatrist prescribing the drug is primarily responsible for this monitoring, but the responsibility may be delegated to a nonphysician on the mental health team, such as a nurse, social worker or a pharmacist (Munetz and Benjamin, 1990). The frequency and method of monitoring will depend on the circumstances and setting of the treatment. It is important that appropriate documentation of the patient's examination, the consenting procedure, any adverse events and the monitoring procedure be maintained. Written consent forms may be used in some circumstances, and they are mandatory for experimental drugs and procedures. They are no substitutes for the clinical process and are not generally recommended for routine use in either the short- or the long-term-care setting.

PART III
Restless legs syndrome

12

Restless legs syndrome: clinical features and pathophysiology

Introduction

The early history of the concept of RLS was discussed in Chapter 1. By the 1960s, the syndrome was well accepted and had found its way into the major textbooks of neurology (Grinker and Sahs, 1966; Brain and Walton, 1969). It was no longer considered a psychogenic or 'psychosomatic' disorder, and its organic basis was generally recognized. However, the descriptions were still sparse, and only a few authors had provided accounts of their clinical experience. The most comprehensive account was, of course, that of a series of 175 personal cases described by Ekbom (1960). Other series published in the 1960s included 22 cases seen by Bornstein (1961), 27 by Gorman et al (1965) and 38 by Morgan (1967).

Subsequent reviews have supported the main features described by these authors, and have also highlighted the diversity of the syndrome, identifying new features and associations. Ekbom (1945) had noted a familial aggregation in some cases. More detailed descriptions of familial RLS have been published (eg, Lugaresi et al, 1965; Coccagna et al, 1966; Boghen and Peyronnard, 1976; Montplaisir et al, 1985; Watson and Hollander, 1987; Walters et al, 1990), and an autosomal inheritance pattern of a proportion of RLS is now recognized. A number of symptomatic cases of RLS have been described in association with neurological, metabolic and vascular disorders (see later).

In 1953, Symonds published the description of intense myoclonic jerks which appeared on falling asleep and persisted throughout sleep. He called this nocturnal myoclonus (NM) and misclassified his cases as 'epilepsy variants'. Four of the five cases described by Symonds had familial RLS. Oswald (1959) questioned the pathological nature of this phenomenon, arguing that it was identical to the physiological 'sleep starts'. One of Oswald's cases also probably had RLS. An association between NM and RLS was therefore suggested. The polysomnographic studies of Lugaresi et al (1965, 1968) estab-

295

lished the association between NM and RLS. Subsequently, NM was described in the absence of RLS. Coleman et al (1980) studied leg movements in relation to sleep disorders and demonstrated that they occurred in normal individuals, especially in the elderly. They proposed the term *periodic leg movements in sleep* (PLMS), which is now most commonly used.

Some other syndromes with restless legs as a predominant feature have been described. These include the painful legs and moving toes syndrome (Spillane et al, 1971), the muscular pain-fasciculation syndrome (Hudson et al, 1978) and the restless red legs syndrome (Metcalfe et al, 1986).

Epidemiology

RLS is recognized to be a common disorder, but there is no consensus on its incidence and prevalence. A major difficulty in establishing its prevalence is the lack of well-accepted diagnostic criteria. Most healthy individuals report minor degrees of uncomfortable leg and bodily sensations at some stage, and the subjective report of RLS patients is variable and 'hard to describe'. The intensity and duration necessary to make a diagnosis have not been established. Epidemiological studies do not generally include polysomnography in their assessments. It is also not certain whether a variant of RLS exists which manifests as PLMS without restless legs, as has been suggested by Walters et al (1990). Furthermore, since many medical 'causes' of RLS have been described, it is not clear whether the term restless legs syndrome should refer only to the idiopathic syndrome or should include the cases in which some cause is apparent.

Ekbom (1945) surveyed 500 healthy individuals in Sweden and reported a prevalence of 5%, which included those with mild symptoms. Between 1945 and 1960, he collected 175 cases, some of them severe, and argued that the severe cases were uncommon but not rare. Strang (1967) surveyed 320 healthy Australians and reported a prevalence of 2.5%. Cirignotta et al (1982) reported a rate of 1.2% in a general population survey in Italy. If a prevalence of 1.2–5% is to be accepted, it is difficult to explain the uncommon presentation of this syndrome in the clinic. Bornstein (1961) and Morgan (1967) noted that the disorder was far more common than the clinical experience would suggest and argued that the symptoms were often mild, regarded as trivial by physicians, dismissed as 'neurotic' or were not displayed by the patients for fear of seeming ridiculous. No incidence figures have been presented.

A few studies have examined rates in special populations. Braude and Barnes (1982) interviewed 54 surgical outpatients in England and found that 8 (15%) complained of unpleasant sensations in the legs associated with an inability to keep them still. A further 7 complained of nonspecific restlessness which was mostly related to anxiety. Feest and Read (1982) disputed these high figures. In their questionnaire survey of 452 patients, only 20 complained of restless legs, and these complaints were determined to be nonspecific on interview. Rates from 24% (Ekbom, 1960) to 42% (Aspenstrom, 1964) have been reported in iron deficiency anaemia. In pregnancy, incidence rates of 11% (Ekbom, 1960) to 27% (Jolivet, unpublished data, 1953) have been reported, with the disorder being more common in late pregnancy. In Ekbom's (1945) report, about half the women had the RLS only while pregnant. Ekbom (1966) reported a rate of 12.6% in patients who had partial gastrectomy. Callaghan (1966) found the symptoms of RLS in 5 (25%) of 20 chronic renal failure patients when directly asked. The author noted that it was uncommon for the complaint to be reported spontaneously. Read et al (1981) reported that about 15–20% of their dialysis patients had symptoms of RLS.

RLS has been reported to result from a number of causes, some of which are listed in Table 12.1. Since these are based mostly on anecdotal evidence, prevalence figures cannot be provided. With regard to PD, the prevalence of RLS is controversial. We have already reviewed the so-called akathisia of PD (Bing–Sicard akathisia) in Chapter 8. Some patients with PD may, however, have a disorder that phenomenologically resembles RLS rather than akathisia. Ekbom (1965) reported RLS in 3 of 28 PD patients, obtained by direct interview. Strang reported RLS in 7% of 600 PD patients but did not state how severe the disorder was.

Clinical features

Age

A wide age range has been described for the onset of the syndrome. In Ekbom's (1960) series, the range was from less than 10 to 82 years, and in his epidemiological survey, it was equally prevalent in all age groups (Ekbom, 1945). Bornstein (1961) and Morgan (1967) described patients as young as 5 and 4 years, respectively. Most patients who consulted Morgan (1967) were middle-aged or elderly, and Coccagna (1990) reported that his patients were around 40–50 years of age but had been ill for a long time. In a family reported by Montagna et al (1983), most affected individuals had an onset in their twenties. The family reported by Walters et al (1990) had affected members as young as 10 and 12 years.

Table 12.1. *Symptomatic restless legs syndrome*

Cause	Reference
Deficiency disorders	
Iron deficiency	Nordlander (1953), Ekbom (1960)
Folate deficiency	Botez and Lambert (1977)
Pregnancy	Jolivet (unpublished data, 1953), Ekbom (1960)
Metabolic and other disorders	
Chronic renal failure	Callaghan (1966), Read et al (1981)
Rheumatoid arthritis	Reynolds et al (1986)
Partial gastrectomy	Ask-Upmark and Meurling (1955), Banerji and Hurwitz (1989)
Cancer	Ekbom (1955)
Acute intermittent porphyria	Stein and Tschudy (1970)
Chronic respiratory insufficiency	Spillane (1970)
Hypothyroidism	Akpinar (1987)
Drug-related	
Caffeine	Ekbom (1966), Missak (1987), Lutz (1978)
Barbiturate withdrawal	Gorman et al (1965)
Antidepressant (eg, mianserin)	Paik et al (1987)
Recovery from spinal anaesthesia	Moorthy and Dierdorf (1990)
β-Antagonist	Morgan (1967)
Phenothiazines[a]	Harriman et al (1970)
Lithium	Heiman and Christie (1986)
Terbutaline	Zelman (1978)
Nifedipine (calcium channel antagonists)	Keidar et al (1982)
Neurological disorders	
Acute poliomyelitis	Luft and Muller (1947)
Neuropathy	Gorman et al (1965)
Diabetes mellitus	Bornstein (1961), Gorman et al (1965)
Alcohol	Gorman et al (1965)
Amyloid neuropathy	Heinze et al (1967), Salvi et al (1990)
Chronic myelopathy	Lugaresi et al (1968)
Parkinson's disease[a]	Ekbom (1965), Strang (1967)
Hyperexplexia (startle disease)	De Groen and Kamphuisen (1978)
Peripheral vascular disorders	
Venous insufficiency	Balmer and Limoni (1980)
Varicose veins	McEwan and McArdle (1971)
Arborizing telangiectasia of lower limbs	Metcalfe et al (1986)
Sleep disorders	
Sleep apnea	Coccagna and Lugaresi (1981), Sieker et al (1960)

[a]Possibly akathisia.

Sex

Ekbom (1960) reported equal prevalence in men and women, as did Bornstein (1961) and Morgan (1967). Jolivet (unpublished data, 1953) and Bonduelle and Jolivet (1953) reported an excess in women, but this may be accounted for by the impact of pregnancy and, to a smaller degree, menopause.

Signs and symptoms

Like akathisia, RLS is characterized by sensory and motor features that are, to some degree, interrelated.

Subjective features

As Ekbom (1960) described it, the main symptom is an unpleasant and uncomfortable sensation frequently localized in the leg ('between the knee and the ankle'). The shin may be more affected than the calf (thus 'anxietas tibiarum'; Morgan, 1967). Typically, the symptoms are bilateral, but they may be asymmetrical, and occasionally they may alternate between the right and left legs but not affect both at the same time. The sensations may affect the thighs or feet, and less often the buttocks and lower back. Sometimes, they may be limited to one region such as the thighs, knees or feet. Some patients localize the sensation to tendons (ie, ankle extensors, hamstrings or the Achilles), and these may be tender. The arms are affected only infrequently, the hands almost never, and even when the arms are affected, the symptoms are usually mild. In Morgan's (1967) series, 5 of 38 patients reported symptoms in the arms on direct enquiry. In 2 of these cases, the arms were as severely affected as the legs.

Patients find the nature of the discomfort difficult to describe and use words like creeping, pulling, stretching, restless sensations, aching and even pain. Less often, they may describe itching, burning, scalding, numb or cold or 'dead' feeling. Ekbom described them typically as creeping sensations felt deeper to the skin in the muscles or bones but not the joints. Some patients are quite graphic in their descriptions (Ekbom, 1960, p. 869; Morgan, 1967, p. 590): 'It feels as if my whole leg was full of worms'; 'As if ants were running up and down in my bones'; 'It feels like an internal itch'; 'As if someone was pulling the sinews out of my legs'; 'It is an indescribable feeling; you have to experience it yourself to know what it is'. Most patients are clear that the sensation does not resemble the 'pins-and-needles' or 'the leg going to sleep' feeling. In many cases, the problem is mild, but it may be severe, unbearable and even 'diabolical' ('I would not wish it on my worst enemy'; 'It is worse than any ordinary illness'). Patients are known to respond to these sensations with frustration, anger, depression and even suicide (Murphy, 1959; Spillane, 1970).

While Morgan emphasized that some of his patients described aching and pain, Ekbom argued that pain as a symptom of RLS was uncommon, although true pain did occur in some cases, usually in association with creeping sensations. Ekbom (1960) considered the cases in which pain, rather than creeping sensation, was predominant as atypical and proposed that these were two subgroups. He subsequently (Ekbom, 1975) argued that pain was characteristic of the syndrome of 'growing pains', which was a distinct syndrome (see later). He did not, however, present detailed clinical material to support this distinction, except for one case, and Wersall (1952) and Morgan (1967) did not support the distinction, stating that pain was an uncommon but integral feature of RLS.

Characteristic features are the effect of posture and time of day on the symptoms. The symptoms appear only when the limbs are at rest. They are relieved by movement and are almost invariably worse in the evening or at night. During the day, the symptoms appear if the patient has to sit still for a period of time, especially in the evening. This may happen in a car, theatre, lecture room or at home while watching television, reading or playing cards. The sensations are worse if the patient is tired. Most patients experience only a mild discomfort during the day, but some may have such severe symptoms that the mere act of sinking into a chair may become intolerable. The symptoms are worst at bedtime, and often the sensation starts 5–30 minutes after the patients get into bed. Depending on the severity of the disorder, these sensations cease after a short while or persist for some hours, in some cases until the early hours of the morning. As stated before, the patient may lie kicking or moving the legs, or massage them, or may get up and move the legs and walk, and in the severe cases, this pattern is repeated many times a night. Eventually, the sensations stop in every case, and the patient usually gets at least 1–2 hours of sleep. Sleep disturbance is therefore an important consequence of the disorder, and this has been objectively confirmed. It is not certain that sleep disturbance in RLS is solely due to the distressing leg sensations and the motor phenomena. Coccagna et al (1966) reported two patients who had episodes of nocturnal insomnia and daytime somnolence irrespective of sensorimotor symptoms. Treatment of the sensorimotor symptoms (eg, with L-dopa; Brodeur et al, 1988a,b), does not necessarily improve sleep.

Other influences on the symptoms are variable in effect. Many patients find heat to have an adverse effect. At night, they tend to remove blankets from the legs and even pour cold water or ice on them. Others find heat comforting and use a hot-water bottle, wear socks or take a hot bath. Some patients have been reported to improve when they are febrile; one of Ekbom's patients obtained relief at the temperature of 39°C or more. Morgan reported a patient who experienced the symptoms in winter and obtained relief in warm weather. Attempts to obtain relief by raising the legs are not helpful.

Psychological factors have been considered important, and the early authors considered RLS to be a psychosomatic disorder. However, the general belief is that psychological factors are peripheral, secondary or incidental. It is often reported that patients are more likely to develop the symptoms if they are sitting through a boring lecture or movie, but this may well be because of a reduced threshold of tolerance in such circumstances. The complaining behaviour of the individuals varies, from some who hide their problem and are acutely embarrassed to discuss it, to those who complain bitterly. To a great extent, this is determined by the premorbid personality of the individual. The problem is exacerbated by the inability of physicians, and even family members, to empathize with the degree of distress that the symptom can entail. Ekbom found most of his patients to be 'well-balanced persons without mental disturbances' (1960, p. 870). Morgan, on the other hand, stated that the majority of his patients were tense or anxious, and reported that their symptoms were exacerbated by anxiety and stress. About half his patients had been treated with antidepressants and a number suffered from 'psychosomatic' problems, eg, migraine, tension headache, asthma, hyperventilation, flatulent dyspepsia. Gorman et al (1965) demonstrated a high frequency of anxiety, tension and depression in their patients, and in many these problems antedated the development of the restless legs. Patients often recognized that stress aggravated their condition.

Psychiatric problems may develop secondarily to the RLS. Involuntary fidgeting and walking may make the individual reclusive or avoidant of other people and may exacerbate their anxiety or make them depressed. They may use alcohol (which does not reportedly improve the symptoms) or smoke excessively at night. Chronic insomnia and daytime drowsiness may also make the individual irritable and tense.

Motor features

Restlessness

Associated with the sensations is an irresistible urge to move the limbs, with some consequent relief in the symptoms. The individual may initially attempt to obtain relief by rubbing the skin, massaging the legs or stretching and kicking. He or she may sit on the edge of the bed and swing the legs or stand and walk. In the more severe cases, walking is the only method to obtain relief. These movements are recognized as being voluntary, with the ostensible purpose of obtaining relief from the sensations. The individual may have to walk for varying periods of time (2–30 minutes according to Morgan) before returning to a sitting or lying position. The sensations may recur, with the need to get up again and walk. One of Ekbom's patients likened the restlessness to that of a caged bear; a middle-aged woman used to dance the Charleston in her bedroom. One of Morgan's patients adopted a yogic headstand for 5 minutes, combined with kicking. Some patients may find the house too small to permit enough walking and may go out, even on winter nights, to walk in the garden. One of Bornstein's patients, a bus driver, had to stop the bus every 2 hours to walk. A woman had to give up the ambition of being a concert pianist and become a music teacher so that she did not have to sit in one place for long periods. Morgan commented that movement of the arms did not usually result in relief of the arm symptoms.

These movements are qualitatively different from those seen in NIA. The two characteristic movements of NIA – marching in place and body rocking – are not prominent in RLS but they do occur. Morgan (1967) described body rocking in a chair and marching in place in some of his patients. Walters et al (1988a) found that 6 out of their 10 patients reported these movements, which were confirmed by videotape analysis in 3.

Involuntary movements

The other characteristic motor feature of RLS is myoclonic jerks. The usual history is of flexion jerks of from one to four extremities in sleep, as noted by the partner or some other observer, and these have been described as NM or PLMS. The jerks may also occur during wakefulness, as was reported in 8 of 10 patients by Walters et al (1988a), and these have been called dyskinesias while awake (DWA), which are probably on a continuum with PLMS. These movements are best documented by simultaneous EMG and videotape.

The usual parameters adopted to perform polysomnography in patients with RLS are described by Coccagna (1990): surface EMG from both tibialis anterior muscles; additional electrodes over the soleus, quadriceps femoris, and biceps femoris muscles and, rarely, if upper limb involvement is suspected, over the brachial biceps and triceps muscles. In a typical recording, EEG, electrooculogram, electrocardiogram and respiration are simultaneously recorded. A TV camera fitted with an infrared device provides information about motor activity.

Motor agitation

The motor restlessness that patients report when they go to bed typically starts a few minutes after they have assumed the recumbent position. Rhythmic alternating EMG activity is seen in the antagonistic muscles in relation to the flexion and extension movements, eg, activity in the tibialis anterior and soleus (Fig. 12.1). The camera shows pedalling movements, or rubbing the calf against the shin, foot against calf, or foot against foot. Upper limb involvement is rare but may manifest as rubbing the forearms, clenching the fists and banging the arms down on the bed (Coccagna, 1990). The patient is awake at this stage of motor agitation. As he or she falls asleep, the phenome-

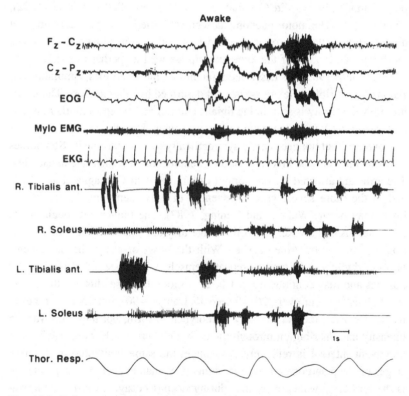

Fig. 12.1. Polysomnographic recording from a patient with restless legs syndrome. The patient was awake; motor agitation (pedalling movements) was displayed by rhythmically alternating contractions of antagonist leg muscles (right tibialis anterior–right soleus). Muscular contractions sometimes resemble myoclonic jerks. Rhythmic discharges of partial myoclonic twitches are present over the different muscles. Reproduced with permission from Coccagna (1990).

non disappears but reappears many times at night on awakening. At times, the patient may be so restless that he or she has to get out of bed, in which case the recording instruments have to be temporarily disconnected. The episodes become less frequent and intense in the early hours of the morning.

Periodic leg movements in sleep or nocturnal myoclonus

RLS is almost invariably associated with PLMS (Lugaresi et al, 1986), although cases of RLS without the myoclonic movements have been described (Ehrenberg, 1992), and, of course, PLMS can occur in healthy individuals and in association with a number of other sleep disorders (see later). Coccagna et al (1990) observed PLMS in all patients examined by polysomnography, as did Coleman et al (1980) and Pelletier et al (1992), among others. The motor phenomena seen are varied. The most common is a dorsiflexion of the big toe and/or the foot and, as the movement becomes more intense, flexion of the knee and hip, as well as perhaps flexion at the elbow. Smith (1985) has described a fanning of the small toes, simulating the Babinski and triple reflex response, not described by other authors. The maximum EMG activity is seen in the tibialis anterior and biceps femoris muscles, with lesser activity in the quadriceps and soleus. Usually, both lower limbs are involved, but not necessarily symmetrically or simultaneously. Sometimes only one limb may be involved, or the phenomenon may alternate in each leg. The arms are affected uncommonly (4 of 11 cases of Coccagna et al, 1966), and in the more severe cases, sequences of movements involving all four limbs may occur (Walters and Hening, 1987). The movements begin while the patient is still awake, and at this stage they are similar to the motor agitation movements described earlier. With the onset of sleep, the movements become rhythmic and tend to repeat themselves in clusters that last several minutes and may continue up to 1 hour or more. In these clusters, the movement tends to occur every 20–40 seconds (range 4–90) with marked regularity. In a cluster, they are usually stereotyped in form, but they may vary in intensity and distribution through the night (Walters and Hening, 1987). The interevent interval is relatively constant in the same individual in different stages of sleep and on consecutive nights (Coleman et al, 1980). The interval is shorter during wakefulness than during sleep (Coccagna, 1990). The movements are most pronounced in stages 1 and 2 of non–rapid eye movement (NREM) sleep and subside considerably, though not necessarily disappear, in stages 3 and 4 and in REM sleep (Coleman et al, 1980; Coccagna and Lugaresi, 1981).

The EMG characteristics of the movements are varied and are usually of longer duration than those of classic myoclonus, typically 1.5–2.5 seconds (range 0.5–5) (Coleman, 1982). There may be an initial myoclonic jerk followed by a tonic contraction, or a polyclonic contraction with or without a tonic component. Less often, the movement may be tonic, rarely followed by a myoclonic contraction. In between the contractions, low-amplitude rhythmic activity may be present, especially in relation to motor agitation.

Lugaresi et al (1972) demonstrated that nocturnal myoclonus is usually associated with an arousal (bursts of K complexes or alpha activity of less than 15 seconds) or an awakening (alpha activity lasting more than 15 seconds). There is also an autonomic arousal manifested by an increase in heart rate and blood pressure, as well as a deepening of breathing. The significance of this will be discussed later.

Dyskinesias while awake

That myoclonic jerks can occur while the RLS patient is awake is generally recognized. Boghen and Peyronnard (1976) reported this in many members of their large RLS family. Lugaresi observed it in about half of his 100 patients investigated with polysomnography (cited in Walters et al, 1988a). Walters et al found it in 8 of their 10 patients in the 1988 study and 9 out of 11 in the 1991 report. In many, these were sufficiently brief to be designated myoclonic jerks (since all were not so brief, the authors preferred the term *dyskinesia*). In others, they were slower and resembled PLMS. DWA occur most commonly when patients are lying in bed at night but can be observed in patients lying or sitting at rest during the day. The movements are stereotypic and repeated in a periodic or aperiodic fashion. They temporarily disappear when the patient makes some voluntary movements, such as shifting the body or walking. Sometimes, a few (four to five) jerks occur rapidly in a cluster. Awareness of these movements can help make a clinical diagnosis.

Montplaisir and colleagues (Montplaisir et al, 1985; Brodeur et al, 1988a) performed a Suggested Immobilization Test (SIT) to quantify RLS. Patients were asked to sit motionless on a bed, legs outstretched and eyes open, for 30 minutes. Every time they experienced a sensation or an urge to move the legs, they pressed a button. EMG was recorded from the tibialis anterior muscle. Four of 6 patients exhibited sensory symptoms and periodic movements during the test. This test provided further evidence for the periodicity of leg movements during wakefulness, which may otherwise be difficult to document because of the presence of voluntary movements. The authors stated that the intermovement interval is shorter during wakefulness and lengthens as the NREM sleep progressively deepens.

Actigraphy

The use of activity monitoring to measure akathisia was discussed in Chapter 10. Actigraphy has been successfully used to quantify the motor symptoms of RLS (Mills et al, 1993), and these measures parallel the questionnaire and polysomnography measures. Since actigraphy measures waking and sleep activity as well as both restlessness and dyskinesias, is simple and relatively inexpensive and can be utilized to measure activity over several days, it may in fact be the preferred method to monitor drug effect in RLS. It can certainly supplement subjective ratings and sleep studies.

The relationship of sensory and motor symptoms in RLS

The following relationships have been proposed: (i) The sensory symptoms are primary, and the motor phenomena are a voluntary response to them. The clinical description of the restlessness seen when the patient is awake is conducive to this interpretation. The myoclonic jerks while awake and the periodic movements in sleep are not. Moreover, the motor phenomena without the sensory ones have been reported in individuals with a prominent family history of RLS (Boghen and Peyronnard, 1976; Walters et al, 1990). (ii) The sensory symptoms result from repetitive muscular contractions, which over time lead to hypersensitivity to the sensations and even pain. The clinical description of sensations in the absence of any movement is against this suggestion, since subclinical contractions are generally unlikely to produce sensory symptoms. (iii) The sensory and motor symptoms are distinct features of the syndrome with perhaps a common neurological basis. The fact that RLS is almost always associated with PLMS (which does not have any appreciable sensory component), and that mild sensory symptoms do not lead to any motor abnormality, suggests that the sensory and motor symptoms may be separate but necessary features.

An empirical study of the association was published by Pelletier et al (1992). They performed all-night polysomnography on 10 well-selected patients with idiopathic RLS and performed the Forced Immobilization Test (FIT) on the evening before the polysomnographic recording. In this test, the patient stayed in bed for 60 minutes in the sitting position, with legs outstretched in a restrictive device to prevent any movement at the knee and considerably limit movements of the ankle and foot. The patients pressed a hand switch as soon as they experienced a disagreeable sensation. In all, 548 movements were recorded during the FIT that met Coleman's (1982) criteria, and only 270 (49%) were associated with sensory detections. On the other hand,

465 sensory events were noted, and 95.7% were associated with leg movements (within 5 seconds before or after the movement). The sensory event occurred after the movement in 76.9% (mean latency 1.4 ± 1.1 seconds), and preceded the movement in 18.8% (mean latency 0.6 ± 0.4 second, range 0.1–2.5). Even accounting for the reaction time between the awareness of the sensation and the pressing of the hand switch, only a proportion of sensations preceded the movement. Some patients identified sensation both before and after the onset of the movement. One patient had several biphasic motor potentials, with sensory events during one or both phases. Although some bias in the reporting of sensations cannot be avoided, the results of the study suggest that the relationship between the two features does not follow any definitive pattern, and it is likely that they represent independent features of the syndrome. The findings of this study need replication.

The sleep disturbance of RLS

RLS leads to significant disruption of sleep – usually difficulty in going to sleep, multiple awakenings at night and daytime somnolence and fatigue – which is often the primary complaint. The difficulty in going to sleep may be explained on the basis of the sensory symptoms, motor restlessness and resting DWA. Increased sleep latency is reported by most investigators (Coccagna and Lugaresi, 1968; Walters et al, 1988a, 1991; Pelletier et al, 1992). Patients also have reduced sleep efficiency (total sleep time/total recording time after sleep onset × 100) and increased number of awakenings at night. The percentage of time spent in deep sleep is reduced. Coccagna and Lugaresi (1968) reported the results of polysomnography on 24 RLS patients. The total sleep duration was 5 hours and 15 minutes, with only 1–2, and rarely 3, sleep cycles per night. Light sleep (stages 1 and 2) was increased (72% vs 48% in controls) and deep sleep decreased (14% vs 18%). The average deep sleep reported by Walters et al (1991) in 11 patients was 9% (range 0–21). REM sleep percentage was also reduced in both studies, significantly so in the Walters et al study (mean 9%, $p < .01$). An increased REM-onset latency was reported by Walters et al. Coccagna (1990) reported that in 1 patient who was sleep-deprived for 40 hours, the sleep time was only slightly lengthened (to 8 hours and 50 minutes), and no increase in deep sleep occurred. However, the sensorimotor symptoms were delayed to the second half of the night. It is uncertain whether PLMS cause the multiple awakenings at night, although the two are associated, and it is recognized that large-amplitude PLMS can cause an awakening. The main abnormalities of sleep in RLS are summarized in Table 12.2.

Table 12.2. *Sleep disturbances in restless legs syndrome*

Symptoms
Difficulty in going to sleep
Multiple awakenings at night
Daytime somnolence
Tiredness

Signs
Periodic leg movements in sleep
Reduced total sleep time
Increased number of awakenings
Reduced sleep efficiency
Increased stage 1 and 2 sleep
Reduced slow-wave sleep
Increased latency to slow-wave sleep
Reduced REM sleep
Increased REM latency (?)

Genetic factors

The fact that a number of patients with RLS have a positive family history of
the disorder has been known since the early writings of Ekbom, who noted it
in one-third of his patients. Ekbom (1960) reported one pair of monozygotic
twins and their mother with RLS. Families with multiple members affected
have been reported by a number of authors (Mussio Fournier and Rawak,
1940; Tuvo, 1949; Bornstein, 1961; Boghen and Peyronnard, 1976; Walters
et al, 1990). An autosomal dominant pattern of inheritance is suggested by
these reports. The first detailed polygraphic study on a family was performed
by Lugaresi et al (1965), who found that the mother and nine children were
definitely affected. A follow-up of this family revealed an onset of RLS in
two members of the next generation (Montagna et al, 1983). Walters et al
(1990) presented a five-generation family with RLS.

The exact proportion of familial vs sporadic cases is not known. A recent
Canadian survey reported that 40–50% of cases were familial (Godbout et al,
1987). It is likely that the diagnosis is often missed in relatives if history only
from the proband is utilized for data collection. RLS is not uncommonly
passed off as a nonspecific sleep complaint, and the onset is often later in life,
at the time when the individual may have lost regular contact with his or her
relatives. Furthermore, the restlessness may be mild in obligate carriers of the
RLS gene, and the diagnosis may only become obvious upon close observation and polygraphy.

It has been suggested that RLS and other familial dysaesthetic syndromes may be genetically linked. Huizinga (1957) described a pedigree of 200 relatives with an autosomal inheritance of restless legs with restless feet that abated with exposure to cold. One family member had recurrent paraesthesiae in her fingers that responded to rubbing her hands. Bornstein (1961) described family members of patients with RLS who had similar sensations in the upper limbs and neck. One family had hereditary RLS and hereditary tremor, usually, but not always, together in the same person. Boghen and Peyronnard (1976) described an association between RLS and PLMT syndrome in two siblings.

Neurological examination and laboratory investigations

In idiopathic RLS, the neurologic examination performed during the day is normal. In severe cases, the abnormal movements may be present during the examination or become obvious if the patient is made to rest for a few minutes. The Suggested Immobilization Test (Brodeur et al, 1988a) will often help provide objective evidence for the presence of the motor abnormality. Routine leg muscle EMG and nerve conduction studies fail to reveal any abnormalities. Harriman et al (1970) did not find any abnormalities of the motor nerve ending in 10 cases of idiopathic RLS.

In symptomatic cases, the appropriate abnormality will be detected, using either a metabolic disorder, neurological illness (usually in association with peripheral neuropathy) or a peripheral vascular disease. The occasional patient with familial RLS has been described who had a peripheral neuropathy associated with a myelopathy (Frankel et al, 1974; Montagna et al, 1983).

Course

The course of idiopathic RLS is quite variable, starting in childhood, adulthood or old age, being progressive or staying the same or even getting better. In the majority, it worsens with age, but as Ekbom reported, in some cases it becomes milder with time. Patients begin showing symptoms in middle or old age, giving a history of many years' duration. In the majority, it is a lifelong disorder. It fluctuates in intensity, with exacerbations and remissions that have no identifiable cause, although in women pregnancy is often an exacerbating factor. Unfortunately, detailed longitudinal studies are lacking. Montagna et al (1983) followed for 20 years a four-generation family with RLS in which the propositus and all his eight siblings were affected. The onset in this family was usually in the second decade, and the course was stationary or very slowly progressive, with wide fluctuations but no definite remission. In one case, it was later complicated with combined degeneration and peripheral neuropathy, but this could have been coincidental.

Diagnosis and differential diagnosis

If the clinician is familiar with the signs and symptoms of the disorder, the diagnosis is relative easy to make. Walters et al (1991) suggested that paraesthesiae, motor restlessness and aggravation of the symptoms by rest and nightfall were necessary for the diagnosis. Other features important but nonmandatory are periodic movements in sleep, dyskinesias while awake, sleep disturbance, a normal neurological examination and a positive family history suggesting an autosomal inheritance.

The first important question to address is that of symptomatic RLS, ie, the features of RLS in a patient with another disorder (local or systemic) known to produce similar symptoms. A tentative list of these causes is presented in Table 12.1, but it is uncertain whether these causes produce RLS de novo or aggravate a mild disorder in a genetically predisposed individual. For a cause to be considered aetiological, a temporal association and sufficient severity are necessary. For example, iron deficiency anaemia is an accepted risk factor for RLS, but is it likely to produce the syndrome only in a predisposed individual, or will it produce it in any individual when sufficiently severe? Do patients with symptomatic RLS have PLMS and DWA in the idiopathic syndrome? The published literature generally lacks such a critical analysis of the symptomatic cases, yet it is important for our understanding of the aetiopathogenesis of RLS. Some attempts have been made. Passouant et al (1970) demonstrated electrophysiologically defined PLMS in patients with renal failure. Bliwise et al (1985) demonstrated a positive relationship between PLMS and urea nitrogen in elderly women. Salvi et al (1990) reported RLS in four siblings in a family with familial amyloid polyneuropathy, and demonstrated PLMS in all four by polysomnography.

There is, therefore, some suggestion that symptomatic RLS may show sleep pathology similar to idiopathic RLS. However, this information is still preliminary, and at this stage a distinction between idiopathic and symptomatic RLS should be maintained, at least in research studies. We propose that RLS be considered idiopathic only if (i) no other disorder known to produce the syndrome is present, or (ii) if such a disorder is present, the symptoms of RLS definitely predate the development of the disorder or persist for months (>3 months) after the disorder has been effectively corrected. A positive history will favour the diagnosis of idiopathic RLS but in itself should not be

Table 12.3. *Diagnostic criteria for restless legs syndrome*

1. Idiopathic RLS (Ekbom's syndrome)[a]
   a. Sensory symptoms, usually in the legs, that are aggravated by rest and are worse at nightfall
   b. Motor restlessness, usually seen in response to the sensory symptoms
   c. Dyskinesia, presenting as myoclonic-like jerks during waking hours or as PLMS
   d. A normal neurological examination
2. Symptomatic RLS
   a. Criteria 1a and 1b
   b. Presence of a systemic or focal (neuropathic or vascular) disorder known to cause RLS and in sufficient severity (Table 12.1)
   c. Onset of RLS subsequent to the disorder considered to be causative
3. RLS not otherwise specified
   a. Criteria 1a and 1b
   b. Other criteria under 1 and 2 not satisfied or uncertain

[a]If first- or second-degree family history is positive, diagnosis is familial; otherwise, sporadic.

considered sufficient for this, since it does not preclude symptomatic RLS. RLS may therefore be categorized as follows:

1. Idiopathic RLS (Ekbom's syndrome)
   a. Familial
   b. Sporadic
2. Symptomatic RLS

Tentative diagnostic criteria for these are presented in Table 12.3. The subcategorization into familial and sporadic is tentative, since the family history is often erroneous or difficult to establish, and no definite clinical differences between familial and sporadic cases have been reported.

An outline for the investigation of a patient with RLS is summarized in Table 12.4. Very often, the diagnosis is obvious, and extensive and expensive investigations are unnecessary. Minimally, disorders like iron deficiency, chronic renal failure, diabetes mellitus and chronic renal failure as well as drug use and pregnancy should be excluded. Polysomnography is not practicable in every case but will aid the difficult diagnosis. The following disorders are important in the differential diagnosis.

PLMS (unrelated to RLS)

PLMS and NM were described earlier as stereotyped, periodic, jerking, nonepileptiform movements of one or both legs, occurring primarily in light

Table 12.4. *Investigation of a patient with restless legs syndrome*

To establish diagnosis
History of illness
Family history and/or examination of relatives
Direct observation of movements
Polysomnography with video recording
To rule out causes of symptomatic RLS
Drug history (including prescription drugs); alcohol history
History of metabolic or neurological disorders
History of pregnancy
Detailed physical (including neurological) examination
Laboratory investigations (if indicated)
Haematological parameters
Serum iron status
Serum folate levels
Urea and creatinine
Fasting blood glucose
ESR and rheumatoid factor
Other biochemical tests if neuropathy suspected
Nerve conduction velocity
EMG
Nerve and muscle biopsy

sleep. Their association with RLS is well established, but PLMS are also seen in a number of other sleep disorders as well as in healthy individuals. The mere presence of PLMS, therefore, is not sufficient to make a diagnosis of RLS, although it has been noted occasionally that members of a family with the RLS gene may manifest PLMS alone.

The polysomnographic characteristics of PLMS have been discussed previously. They are characterized by repetitive movements separated by varying intervals that recur for long periods through the duration of the sleep. The term nocturnal myoclonus, which has a historical legacy, is considered inappropriate because the movements are not exclusively nocturnal, often have a tonic component and are therefore longer than a typical myoclonus. There is a lack of complete consensus on what should be considered a true PLMS episode. The variables to be considered are the duration of each EMG burst, the interval between the bursts and the number of movements necessary to define a myoclonic epoch. The most common interval is 20–40 seconds, but the outer limits vary from author to author, eg, 4–60 seconds (Coleman et al, 1980), 5–120 seconds (Bixler et al, 1982), <120 seconds (Guilleminault et al,

1975). The investigators also vary in the number of jerks they consider necessary to define an epoch: 3 or more (Guilleminault, 1982), 5 or more (Coleman
et al, 1980), 30 or more (Bixler et al, 1982). Another parameter used is that of
movement index (MI), which is the average number of periodic leg movements per hour of sleep. Coleman (1982) considered an MI of 5 or more necessary to establish a diagnosis of PLMS. The Association of Sleep Disorders
Centers (1979) criteria specified three or more series of 30 or more events for
the diagnosis of PLMS.

   PLMS is common in healthy elderly individuals and is reported to increase
with age (Coleman et al, 1983). It is rare in individuals less than 30 years of
age but is present in 5% of 30- to 50-year-old individuals and in 29% of those
over 50 (Bixler et al, 1982). The pathological significance of PLMS has therefore been questioned. The Association of Sleep Disorders Centers (1979)
classifies PLMS under disorders of initiating and maintaining sleep, and disorders of excessive somnolence. Whether PLMS can cause sleep–wake disorders is controversial, with research evidence divided on the issue. Some
authors have reported high rates of PLMS in individuals with chronic insomnia or sleep–wake disorders (9% by Guilleminault et al, 1975; 13% by
Coleman et al, 1978), but these studies lacked healthy control populations,
and a comparable figure (11%) was reported by Bixler et al (1982) in 100
healthy individuals who underwent nocturnal recordings. Whether PLMS is
more common in insomniacs compared with those having daytime hypersom-
nolence is also uncertain (Ohanna et al, 1985; Saskin et al, 1985; Peled and
Lavie, 1987). Zorick et al (1978) presented evidence that people who complain of insomnia may not have abnormal sleep parameters but rather a lower
threshold of arousal with the myoclonias; ie, they wake up easily in response
to stimuli. This arousal threshold decreases with age, possibly explaining the
poorer sleep in the elderly (McDonald et al, 1981). Some drugs (eg, baclofen,
clonazepam) improve sleep in PLMS patients without decreasing the PLMS
episodes (Guilleminault and Flagg, 1984).

   A sleep disorder other than RLS in which PLMS are particularly common
is narcolepsy, although it is again uncertain whether they result in sleep disturbance in this disorder (Wittig et al, 1983). The PLMS in narcolepsy differ
from those in RLS in being evenly distributed throughout the night (Godbout
et al, 1988).

   In summary, PLMS are common in healthy individuals and in association
with a number of sleep disorders (especially RLS and narcolepsy), and their
presence should not lead to a diagnosis of RLS in the absence of other
features.

Sleep starts (massive myoclonic jerks)

These occur in healthy individuals and are sudden involuntary movements of the whole or part of the body that occur when the individual is drowsy (Oswald, 1959).

The axial and proximal limb muscles are those most often involved, and the EMG activity is associated with arousal on EEG and autonomic parameters. They may be associated with hypnogogic hallucinations. They are not repetitive and do not need treatment. The sensory and motor symptoms of RLS are not present.

Painful legs and moving toes syndrome (or dysaesthetic dyskinesia)

This syndrome, originally described by Spillane et al (1971), is characterized by pain in the feet or legs and involuntary movements of the toes, sometimes spreading proximally. The pain is deep aching, pulling, burning or pressure, severe in intensity (ie, can vary from a constant discomfort to 'a torment'), not related to rest or the sleep–wake cycle and not relieved by leg movements or walking. Immersion of the limb in hot or cold water as well as local pressure produce some relief. The movements always involve the toes but may extend proximally to the feet and legs and produce clawing and straightening, fanning and circular movements of the toes. They can be suppressed voluntarily for a few seconds and are difficult to imitate. The movements may be continuous or intermittent, lasting for a few seconds with intervals of some minutes. The problem starts gradually, usually after the age of 40, and may affect one or both limbs. Some patients have associated face, trunk and diaphragm dyskinesias (Schoenen et al, 1984). The disorder has been described in association with radicular or peripheral nerve lesions (Nathan, 1978; Barrett et al, 1981; Schoenen et al, 1984) or following minor trauma to the legs (Schott, 1981) or to the spinal cord and cauda equina (Dressler et al, 1994), but many patients have no identifiable pathology (Spillane et al, 1971; Dressler et al, 1994). EMG patterns of these patients may fall into two subgroups (Schoenen et al, 1984): (i) those with a simple erratic pattern of EMG suggesting a peripheral nerve lesion, for whom local anaesthetics are effective (Nathan, 1978, suggested that the nerve root was involved), and (ii) those with a complex alternating pattern in the EMG suggesting a central origin, for whom there are dyskinesias in other parts and the pain is less severe.

The PMLT syndrome is, therefore, a heterogeneous disorder which can be readily distinguished from RLS if careful attention is paid to its features. The two syndromes may be interrelated. Boghen and Peyronnard (1976) described this in one patient whose sibling suffered from typical RLS. There is no effective treatment.

The muscular pain–fasciculation syndrome

This syndrome, described by Hudson et al (1978), is characterized by fasciculations in the leg and other muscles, and myalgia, cramps, muscular fatigue and paraesthesiae. The pain is described most often in the leg muscles but may also occur in the back, chest, girdle or arm muscles and is usually present in more than one region. The intensity may vary from mild to severe but is usually a constant ache or burning. It usually tends to stay in one region except over long periods, is made worse by physical activity or at the end of the day and is relieved by rest. The symptoms may fluctuate without any obvious reason. Some patients experience painful nocturnal cramps in the calves or feet. The muscular twitches may start with the pain or after a delay of 1–2 years and are usually observed as solitary twitches in the calves and, less commonly, other muscles. The twitching may move from one part of the body to the other and is worse after a period of activity. Patients complain of heaviness or weakness of the affected muscles. Paraesthesiae may occur, but the sensory system is normal on examination. There is no muscle atrophy but ankle jerks may be reduced or absent. The course is variable, with constancy, worsening or improvement all being reported. Electrophysiologic studies suggest axonal degeneration and muscle fibre denervation, most marked in the legs. Mild denervation atrophy of the muscle was demonstrated in one case with light microscopy. The anterior horn cells were not reduced, and the findings therefore suggested a benign polyneuropathy. No satisfactory treatment is available.

Myokymia

Masland (1947) described a syndrome in which irregular muscle twitching and sensory symptoms were reported. There were crawling sensations deep in the calves and thighs and occasionally other parts of the body. Aching and fatigue of the muscles were also present. The symptoms worsened with exercise, nervous tension and cold, and improved with rest. Although Masland did not stress aching, the syndrome may be the same as the muscular pain-fasciculation syndrome just described. The muscle in myokymia displays undulating movements because of rapid motor unit discharges lasting up to several seconds. Myokymia and fasciculation may, however, result from the same cause, the variation merely reflecting the severity of the damage.

Another syndrome of muscular pain and myokymia has been described. These patients have severe cramps, myotonia-like spasms of muscle, profuse sweating and, in some cases, muscular atrophy (Gardner-Medwin and Walton, 1969).

Although superficially resembling RLS, these syndromes can be clearly distinguished when closely examined.

Nocturnal leg cramps

These are sudden, sporadic, painful muscular contractions that occur randomly at night. They usually involve the sural and intrinsic muscles of the foot. Stretching of the muscle relieves the spasm. Electrophysiologically, they are preceded by an arousal on EEG and may occur in any sleep stage. Quinine is known to be effective (Anonymous, 1986). A familial disorder has been described in which intermittent cramps occur in the whole body during sleep, and myoclonic jerks are also present (Jacobsen et al, 1986).

Drug-induced akathisia

The similarities between RLS and DIA are well described in the historical account of the concept of akathisia in Chapter 1. The two syndromes are recognized as distinct, but it is not uncommon for misdiagnosis to occur, since strict criteria are not often applied. RLS secondary to phenothiazines has been reported in the literature (Harriman et al, 1970), but it is uncertain whether this represents an instance of misdiagnosis. Some drugs (eg, lithium and calcium channel antagonists) have been reported to cause both akathisia and RLS. Findings from one syndrome have been applied to the other (eg, the role of iron deficiency in the aetiology, and β-antagonists in the treatment), often with good results. All these data suggest that there are some aspects of the pathophysiology that the two syndromes share, while being distinct in other respects. A detailed comparison of the two syndromes would, therefore, be revealing. The following account summarizes the main similarities and differences (see also Table 12.5).

The subjective symptoms

The characteristic subjective complaints are qualitatively different. In DIA, there is a sense of inner restlessness in the mind or the body, particularly the legs. This is in contrast to RLS, in which the characteristic complaint is of sensory symptoms in the legs. Paraesthesiae can occur in DIA, but they are

Table 12.5. *Contrasting drug-induced akathisia and idiopathic restless legs syndrome*

Features	Akathisia	Restless legs syndrome
Subjective features		
Characteristic symptoms	Inner restlessness	Paraesthesiae/dysaesthesiae in legs
Cognitive symptoms	Present	Lacking
Paradoxical behavioural reactions	Possibly present	Lacking
Motor features		
Characteristic movements	Body rocking, fidgetiness, marching in place, crossing/uncrossing of legs, shifting body position in chair, inability to sit	Rubbing and stretching legs, leg flexion, pacing
Reason for movement	To relieve restlessness	To relieve sensory symptoms
Result of movements	Some relief while movement occurs	Movements ameliorate symptoms temporarily
Exacerbating and relieving factors		
Diurnal variation	No pattern	May appear only, or worsen markedly, at night-time
Effect of posture	Worse when sitting or standing in one place for long	Worse when lying or sitting with legs at rest
Heat or cold	Little effect	May improve or worsen
Involuntary movements		
Dyskinesia while awake	Uncommon; if present, of small amplitude and not prominent	Common, often prominent and of large amplitude
Periodic movements in sleep	Rare	Almost always present
Tremor	Often associated (because of neuroleptics)	No association

Table 12.5. (*cont.*)

Features	Akathisia	Restless legs syndrome
Sleep disturbance		
Complaint	Rare	Usual
Polysomnographic disturbances	Rare	Usual
Neurological examination	Evidence of akathisia and associated EPSE	Usually normal, unless symptomatic RLS
Onset and course		
Onset	Related to drugs (acute or tardive)	Gradual onset
Age	No relation	Worsens with age
Course	AA related to duration of drug use; TA may persist after drug use	Chronic, with relapsing and remitting course; may worsen with age
Family history	Not relevant	Autosomal dominant inheritance in more than one-third of cases
Treatment		
Most effective drugs	ACh and β-A antagonists	Dopaminergic, benzodiazepine and opioid drugs

uncommon. RLS patients may experience paraesthesiae in the arms as well, which would be extremely unusual in DIA. DIA may also be experienced as inner tension, apprehension, irritability, impatience or general unease and may give rise to 'paradoxical behavioural reactions' (exacerbation of psychosis, violence, suicide, sexual torment, etc). This is unusual for RLS, which is recognized as a sensorimotor sleep disorder without a cognitive or affective component, although patients may secondarily develop frustration, anxiety, anger or depression.

Motor manifestations (intentional)

The characteristic intentional movements of DIA are fidgetiness, crossing/uncrossing and pumping up and down of legs, inverting/everting of feet, tapping of toes, shifting body while sitting, rocking, shifting weight from foot to foot while standing, marching in place and pacing. The typical movements of RLS are rubbing of legs, stretching of muscles, leg flexions, deep knee bends, tossing and turning in bed and pacing the floor. The DIA patient moves to relieve the inner restlessness, while the RLS patient moves to relieve the paraesthesiae. Body rocking, marching in place, shifting body position in a chair, and crossing/uncrossing of legs, movements characteristic of DIA, are not commonly seen in RLS, although they do occur intermittently. The movements in RLS are usually successful in relieving the symptoms after a few minutes, but the akathisic patient gets little sustained relief. The classic 'inability to sit', although present in only a proportion of DIA patients, is not typical of RLS, and the pacing of the RLS patient has a quantitatively different basis.

Exacerbating and relieving features

The symptoms of RLS are worst at night-time and when the limbs are at rest. They typically become most distressing when the individual goes to bed, and in mild cases may appear only at this time. The symptoms of DIA do not show a definite diurnal pattern, although they may fluctuate either in relation to neuroleptic administration or for no apparent reason. They are worst when the person maintains a posture, either sitting or standing, for a prolonged period. DIA patients are, in fact, least distressed when they are lying in bed. RLS patients may obtain relief from the application of heat or cold to the legs, which is not the case in DIA.

Involuntary movements

The majority of patients with RLS have myoclonic jerks of the legs during the resting state, especially when the patients are drowsy, and these may be of large amplitude and even violent. Jerks of the legs and feet may be present in DIA, but they are uncommon. PLMS are an important feature in the majority of RLS patients. Their presence in DIA is controversial in the literature, and they certainly are not a prominent feature. Overall, sleep has a marked ameliorating effect on movements in akathisia. Tremor, especially of the hands, may be an associated feature in DIA but is not present in RLS.

Sleep disturbance

While sleep disturbance is the most common complaint in RLS, it is most unusual for it to be prominent in patients with DIA. Sleep is significantly disturbed in RLS, with increased sleep latency, reduced sleep efficiency, multiple awakenings at night and daytime somnolence. Polysomnography reveals increased sleep latency, reduced slow-wave sleep, reduced REM sleep and increased stage 1 and 2 sleep. While sleep disturbance may be seen in DIA, it is relatively mild in comparison. Some increase in sleep latency, with an increased number of awakenings and reduction in sleep efficiency are seen in DIA. It is uncertain whether these disturbances are related to the primary psychiatric disorder, the neuroleptic drugs (irrespective of the akathisia) or to the akathisia itself.

Examination of the patient

Daytime examination of the RLS patient is usually normal except in symptomatic cases. In the more severe cases, the symptoms will appear if the patient is examined after a period of rest. DIA patients will usually manifest the objective features of the disorder during examination. Additionally, they may have parkinsonian side-effects, dyskinesia or dystonia related to neuroleptics.

Onset and course

DIA, in its acute form, begins a short time after the introduction or change in neuroleptic or other drug, reaches a peak soon after and disappears within days of stopping or reducing the dosage of the drug. Tardive akathisia has a more variable onset and ending. Age is not a strong predisposing factor for akathisia. RLS occurs insidiously at any age, has a long-term course with fluctuations, tends to become worse in middle or older age and sometimes remits spontaneously.

Family history

RLS is familial in one-third or more of patients, with evidence of autosomal dominant inheritance. No genetic component is apparent in DIA.

Treatment

The most effective drugs in the management of AA are ACh and βA antagonists, with benzodiazepines, opiates and clonidine producing relief in some cases. Tardive akathisia responds partially to catecholamine depleters and some other drugs. RLS responds best to dopaminergic drugs, benzodiazepines and opiates, with β-antagonists and clonidine being successful sometimes.

Peripheral neuropathy

A discussion of the varied causes and manifestations of peripheral neuropathy are beyond the scope of this book. In general, neuropathy (eg, due to chronic renal failure, diabetes mellitus, amyloid deposition) can produce symptoms resembling RLS. However, an examination of the patient will demonstrate sensory and/or motor deficits, especially in the limbs. EMG and nerve conduction studies will further aid the diagnosis.

Peripheral vascular disorders

RLS-like symptoms can develop with some peripheral vascular disorders. Patients with varicose veins complain of feelings of heaviness in one or both legs, combined with fatigue, that gets progressively worse towards the end of the day. Elevation of the legs produces relief of symptoms, and an examination of the legs makes the diagnosis apparent. The symptoms of acute venous occlusion, being pain, local tenderness and oedema, are difficult to confuse with RLS. Erythromelalgia is a rare disorder in which burning, tingling and often itching of the feet and lower legs appear as the ambient temperature rises above a critical level (range 31.7–36.1°C), and these body parts become bright red.

Metcalfe et al (1986) reported 2 patients with arborizing telangiectasia of the lower limbs in whom disabling sensory symptoms similar to RLS were observed (restless red legs). The first patient developed intermittent tingling in both feet and the left leg, followed by an aching discomfort, which made her get up and pace the floor in search of relief. The second patient complained of severe aching of the legs and feet and a feeling of being gripped with an ice-cold band. The discomfort was worse in bed at night, and moving the legs produced relief. In a previous report of 13 cases of essential telangiectasia (McGrae and Winkelmann, 1963), 5 patients had numbness, tingling and burning in the dependent limbs. Even though the skin lesion in these cases suggests a vascular abnormality, a 'neuropathic' aetiology cannot be ruled out.

Growing pains

The report of aching pain in the legs, which is often unilateral, and can be intense and intolerable, is not unusual in children 3–6 years of age. The literature on this symptom is scanty, and a review was provided by Oster (1972). It is different from RLS in that aching is the prominent symptom, the symptoms are variable and, even though they appear in the first few hours of the night, do not occur every night. It is unusual to find the symptom in adults. The aetiology of 'growing pains' is unknown, but they may involve oedema of the muscle bodies within tight fascial sheaths following vigorous exercise during the day. Ekbom considered it to be distinct from RLS and described an adult with both growing pains and RLS. Unlike RLS, the pain responds to analgesic medication such as acetylsalicylic acid. The application of local heat and massage may help, and if severe, quinine sulphate may be administered at bedtime.

Aetiopathogenesis

The pathogenesis of RLS is poorly understood, and a number of hypotheses have been proposed. These hypotheses stem from the following general facts regarding RLS.

1. Some drugs, in particular dopaminergic drugs, opiates and benzodiazepines, are effective in the treatment of RLS. These have implicated dopaminergic, opiate and GABAergic mechanisms. In addition, noradrenergic and serotonergic mechanisms have been discussed. These findings suggest, as will be discussed later, that disturbances in certain neurotransmitters play a role in the pathogenesis of RLS. Whether these disturbances are primary or secondary to some other disturbance is unclear.
2. RLS is associated with certain neurological and metabolic or other disorders. The association with neuropathy has led to speculation that RLS is a consequence of subclinical neuropathy. Evidence does not support this, since patients with idiopathic RLS have normal leg muscle EMG and nerve conduction. Furthermore, while peripheral vascular disorders can cause symptoms resembling those of RLS, patients with RLS do not have any evidence of such abnormality. Any hypothesis of the pathogenesis of RLS must account for the fact that the syndrome worsens with iron deficiency, chronic renal failure and pregnancy. Unfortunately, a parsimonious hypothesis that accounts for all this has not been proposed. It is possible

that RLS is a heterogeneous syndrome with multiple causes and pathome-chanisms. Alternatively, it is possible that an underlying vulnerability is necessary, and the manifestations of the disorder depend on the presence of an additional factor.

3. RLS has an autosomal inheritance in a number of cases. However, until the responsible gene is discovered, this fact does not provide any new patho-genetic hypotheses.

4. The association of RLS and PLMS is strong and a common pathophysio-logical mechanism for the two is likely. This is in spite of the fact that one can occur without the other. The evidence that PLMS without RLS can occur in families with the RLS gene provides a further argument that the pathophysiology of the two are linked. Both peripheral and central mecha-nisms have been suggested, but some evidence points to the presence of a central, subcortical disturbance, probably based in the reticular formulation.

The evidence that dopaminergic mechanisms may be involved in the patho-physiology comes from many sources but is largely indirect. L-Dopa and bromocriptine have been shown to be effective in treating RLS and PLMS, suggesting reduced dopaminergic activity as a pathomechanism. PLMS asso-ciated with PD improves with treatment using L-dopa or anticholinergic drugs. The similarities between RLS and NIA also implicate DA. Do-paminergic mechanisms are consistent with the relationship of RLS with iron deficiency (see Chapter 9 for a discussion of DA–iron interactions), hypothy-roidism and fever (Akpinar, 1987). There is evidence for a decreased turnover of homovanillic acid, a DA metabolite, and a loss of DA receptor sites in aging, suggesting reduced function (Severson et al, 1982; Stahl et al, 1985). PLMS is associated with narcolepsy in which a decreased bioavailability of DA is likely (Faull et al, 1983). Montplaisir et al (1986) reported a family with RLS in which the propositus exhibited an increase of free DA and homovanillic acid in the CSF but not in the serum. On the basis of this, they suggested reduced sensitivity of DA receptors as being responsible for RLS. Disturbances in dopaminergic transmission may, however, be secondary to disturbance in other transmitters.

The involvement of endogenous opiates is suggested by the dramatic improvement in some patients with opiate drugs. In two cases of familial RLS, iv naloxone reactivated the myoclonus while patients were on opiates (Hening et al, 1983). The endogenous opioid system has been shown to play a regulatory role in the control of sleep (Sandyk, 1985a). Since the opiate pep-tides are rich in the striatum and have a close functional relationship with DA, they may produce their effects through dopaminergic mechanisms (Diamond and Borison, 1978; Stefano, 1982).

The evidence for the role of GABAergic (based on the efficacy of benzodi-azepines, valproate and baclofen, in some cases, though baclofen actually increased the number of leg movements), serotonergic (involvement of 5HT activity in myoclonus in animals; Magnussen and Braengaard, 1982) and noradrenergic (based on the occurrence of RLS secondary to antidepressants like mianserin and the doubtful efficacy of clonidine) mechanisms is also indirect and more tentative. Sandyk (1989) suggested a role for the melanocyte-stimulating hormone (MSH), basing it primarily on an anecdotal observation by Kastin et al (1968) that the administration of MSH to amenor-rhoeic women produced motor restlessness and MSH-like symptoms.

Some attempts have been made to understand the neurophysiological basis of PLMS and, by corollary, RLS. Both central and peripheral mechanisms have been suggested, although the weight of the evidence suggests a central mechanism. Askenasy et al (1987) argued that a 2–6 per minute pacemaker in the striatopallidal loop was responsible for PLMS in PD, which improved upon treatment with antiparkinsonian drugs. This explained why PLMS is fre-quent in stage 2 of sleep and decreased in deep sleep. Two studies (Wechsler et al, 1986; Martinelli et al, 1987) have documented that PLMS are associated with hyperexcitability in the blink reflexes, somatosensory evoked responses, long latency motor responses and H reflexes, ie, mono- and polysynaptic reflexes of both the brain stem and the spinal cord. This suggests that the descending influences are abnormal with PLMS and places the abnormality at the pontine level or rostral to it. Some authors have still argued, however, for an abnormality at the spinal level, and the controversy is not totally resolved. Alpha- and gamma-motoneurone dissociation has been suggested by some authors (Bergonzi et al, 1981; Mano et al, 1982), but the evidence for this with PLMS and RLS is not strong. Moorthy and Dierdorf (1990) reported a patient who developed RLS during recovery from spinal anaesthesia. They suggested that this was due to different rates of recovery of sensory and motor nerve fibres, with disruption of the normal proprioceptive feedback system leading to the restlessness. The demonstration of DA (Lindvall et al, 1983) and opiate (Levin et al, 1982) neurones in the spinal cord has been argued to support the role of spinal mechanisms.

Mosko and Nudleman (1986) demonstrated normal lower- and upper-extremity somatosensory-evoked responses, as well as normal brainstem auditory-evoked responses, in 10 patients with PLMS, providing evidence that a primary sensory disturbance was lacking. Backaveraging the EEG in relation to the muscle jerks with PLMS does not reveal a cortical onset (Lugaresi et al, 1986). The periodicity of the movements suggests a subcorti-cal pacemaker. In addition, PLMS are associated with arousal and autonomic phenomena. The brain stem reticular system is one candidate as the site for the pacemaker. It does not mean, however, that the pathology is localized at this level, as cortical and subcortical influences impinge on this area to modify its activity. Another suggestion that has been put forward (Coleman et al, 1980) is that disturbance in the 24-hour circadian rhythm may underlie the disturbance with PLMS. Altered function of the circadian rhythm pacemaker in the suprachiasmatic nucleus (SCN) has also been suggested, leading to nocturnal encroachment of daytime-like CNS activity (leg movements or alpha activity in EEG; Ehrenberg, 1992). The SCN is rich in GABA receptors, possibly explaining the efficacy of benzodiazepines, valproate and baclofen in RLS. The circadian rhythm is closely associated with the daily temperature cycle, which may explain the intriguing finding of Ekbom that fever could ameliorate RLS. Spinal influences are still likely as modifying factors. Spinal inhibitory medication has been reported to reduce the amplitude (but not the number) of PLMS (Guilleminault and Flagg, 1984). Shifts in body position cause a decline in PLMS, again suggesting spinal influences (Dzvonik et al, 1986).

As is apparent from this discussion, the pathophysiology of RLS and PLMS is poorly understood and further research is clearly necessary.

Conclusion

RLS is a common but underrecognized disorder that produces great distress in individuals and families. It is a chronic disorder which may start at any age and last a lifetime, with fluctuations in its severity and variable periods of remission. Fortunately, it is mild in most cases, so that many patients do not consult a physician. A number of causes of symptomatic RLS are recognized, but comparisons of idiopathic and symptomatic cases are not available. Many patients with an idiopathic but mild disorder may first become distressed during pregnancy or medical illness. There has been recent interest in sleep disorders and movement disorders associated with RLS, in particular PLMS and DWA. The diagnosis is usually clinically apparent, and extensive investigations are rarely necessary. The more severe cases may need drug therapy, and the details for this are discussed in Chapter 13. Given its importance at the primary health care level as well as in specialist centres, its relative neglect by researchers is surprising.

13

Treatment of restless legs syndrome

An interesting array of drugs and other therapies has been used in the treatment of RLS. An early aetiological hypothesis that guided much treatment was that the symptoms were due to the accumulation of metabolites caused by reduced blood flow at rest. Ekbom (1960) recommended the use of peripheral vasodilators like tolazoline and carbachol, suggesting that they ameliorated symptoms in two-thirds of patients. Other drugs reported to have good results included *meso*-inositol hexanicotinate and nitroglycerine (Allison, 1943). These drugs are no longer used in the treatment of RLS, and one questions the earlier results as possibly placebo effects. Other substances recommended in the literature include ascorbic acid (Swedberg, 1952), aldehydes (Brenning, 1957), dextran (Nordlander, 1953), heparin and quinine (Bornstein, 1961). Nonspecific methods like massage or the use of vibration and the administration of sedative-hypnotics and analgesics were recommended by Ekbom (1960). Unilateral lumbar sympathectomy was unsuccessful in one case (Ekbom, 1960).

In patients with iron deficiency anaemia, Ekbom (1960) reported good results with iron injections. Iron therapy was also recommended for those without anaemia or other evidence of iron deficiency (Nordlander, 1953), but no empirical evidence was presented to support this. Roger et al (1991) studied the effect of epoetin (Exprex, Janssen-Cilag), used for the correction of anaemia in uraemic patients on chronic renal dialysis. They gave 40 units/kg iv three times a week titrated to maintain haemoglobin between 90 and 100 g/l. The haemoglobin concentration was a mean 66 g/l at baseline and rose to 99 and 96 g/l at 6 and 12 months, respectively. Seventeen patients had RLS at baseline. Their mean ratings (on a scale of 1–7) dropped from 4.1 to 2.3 and 1.9 at 6 and 12 months respectively ($p < .01$). The 10 patients without RLS at baseline did not develop the symptoms in the 1 year of treatment. Even though iron was supplemented if ferritin concentration was less than 100 µg/l, there was no relation between the presence of RLS and initial ferritin concentration or the subsequent need for iron supplementation. Folate supplementation was recommended, especially in pregnant women with RLS (Botez and Lambert, 1977).

A number of drugs have recently been investigated for the treatment of RLS with good results, and the studies will be briefly summarized here. It is important to recognize that the symptoms of RLS fluctuate in intensity spontaneously, and treatment cannot, therefore, be based on case reports. Further, placebo response tends to be strong, requiring that a double-blind placebo-controlled design be used in drug studies. Because of the possibility of the development of tolerance, studies should be long term (Coccagna, 1990). Polysomnography should be performed on at least some patients to assess the effect on PLMS.

Dopaminergic drugs

L-Dopa

The greatest number of published treatment studies concern the use of L-dopa. Akpinar (1982) treated 5 subjects with L-dopa (and benserazide) in a single bedtime dose (200/50 mg in 4 subjects, 500–750 mg in 1) and reported complete relief of symptoms, with recurrence upon cessation of the drug. Akpinar (1987) later published a double-blind, placebo-controlled, crossover study (2 weeks each) in 13 patients (mean age 50.8 years, range 29–75) using a single dose of L-dopa (200/50 mg) 1 hour before bedtime. The subjective evaluation of the sleep improved in all cases, being rated very good in 10 and good in 3. The total number of nocturnal awakenings and time spent awake decreased significantly (effect size = −10.23, adjusted effect size = −9.52). Patients were subsequently maintained on L-dopa for various periods (0.5–5 years) and showed fluctuations in their symptoms, with periods of spontaneous improvement. Two subjects could not tolerate L-dopa because of hypothyroidism.

Von Scheele (1986) reported a double-blind, placebo-controlled study on 20 patients (mean age 58.2 years, range 10–83), who were given L-dopa and placebo on alternate days until the patient stated a preference for one of the treatments or was unable to distinguish the two. Seventeen preferred L-dopa and 3 were unable to discriminate, with none preferring placebo. The dose of L-dopa was individually titrated in a pretrial period of 14 days; 14 of the 17 were given 100 mg at bedtime (range 50–200 mg). All 17 responders obtained complete relief. The same author (von Scheele and Kempi, 1990) published his experience of the long-term use of L-dopa. Of 36 patients, 30 responded (who had RLS for a median 27 years) to L-dopa with benserazide

(50–250 mg, median 100) and were followed up for two years. Two had a loss of effect after 1 month but were satisfactorily treated with bromocriptine. One improved spontaneously, and 1 developed paraplegia (from a traffic accident). The remaining 26 were maintained on L-dopa for the 2 years; 8 on the same dosage, 9 on an increased dosage (100–600 mg, median 250) and 9 on a reduced dosage. At 2 years, 22 reported improved sleep (additional 1–5 hours, median 2), and 17 reported a reduced number of awakenings. There were no significant side-effects except for transient nausea in 2 patients.

Some studies have been published by Montplaisir and colleagues, who included polysomnography in their investigations. In their 1986 open study, they reported the effect of L-dopa on seven patients (mean age 40.7 years, SD 12.5) over 4 weeks using 100–200 mg drug (with benserazide) as a single dose 1 hour before bedtime. All reported improvement in the RLS and sleep, with two showing complete recovery. On a severity scale of 0–3, the mean RLS ratings dropped from 2.8 (SD 0.1) to 0.8 (SD 0.4), and the movements in sleep dropped from 2.4 (SD 0.3) to 1.2 (SD 0.3). The total number of PLMS per night, and the PLMS index, did not decrease, but the PLMS decreased in the first third of the night and increased in the last third, often leading to a patient's report of recurrence of movements in the early morning. The subjective report of sleep depth and the refreshing value of sleep showed improvement (tending to significance), and the patients ranked L-dopa superior to clonazepam or baclofen. The same group (Bedard et al, 1987) reported the efficacy of L-dopa in narcolepsy-related PLMS in one patient. In 1988, they (Brodeur et al, 1988a) reported a double-blind, placebo-controlled, crossover study in six patients (mean age 51.3 years, SD 12.4) over 7 weeks (2 weeks baseline, each treatment 2 weeks and wash-out between treatments 1 week). Two doses of L-dopa (100/25 mg with benserazide) were given, 1 hour before and 3 hours after bedtime, with the second dose intended to suppress the early morning rebound in PLMS. Patients underwent polysomnography at baseline and at the end of each treatment, as well as completing morning and evening questionnaires about movements and sleep. Patients reported significantly greater improvement in paraesthesiae of the arms and legs and reduced sleep latency with L-dopa. The number of PLMS improved considerably in both halves of the night. Patients reported an improved quality of life.

In an open study, Sandyk et al (1987) treated eight patients (58–70 years) suffering from RLS associated with chronic renal failure with L-dopa/carbidopa (up to 100/25 mg to 250/25 mg twice daily) for 1–3 months. All showed some improvement, with satisfactory relief in six. Symptoms relapsed within 48 hours of discontinuation of the drug.

An interesting report of medium- to long-term L-dopa use was published by

Guilleminault et al (1993). They treated 20 patients (mean age 64 years, SD 9) with Sinemet CR (25/100 mg) sustained release at bedtime. All subjects were monitored at 3–7 weeks and both subjective and objective indicators suggested complete elimination of the RLS in all subjects. The subjects were followed up for 8–20 months (mean 11). Thirteen reported continued efficacy of the drug. Seven (mean age 62 years, SD 10) reported reappearance of the symptoms in the morning between 8 AM and 11 AM, with monitoring suggesting a rebound. Withdrawal of Sinemet in 4 of these 7 resulted in the disappearance of worsening in the morning and reappearance of nocturnal disruption within 2–6 days. These 7 patients were given a twice daily dose (bedtime and morning) with complete improvement. One patient subsequently developed symptoms in the afternoon requiring a 24-hour prescription, effective over the 4.5 months of follow-up.

In conclusion, the use of L-dopa in the treatment of RLS is convincing, with a number of open studies and three double-blind, placebo-controlled studies attesting to its efficacy. The effect on the subjective symptoms and sleep is impressive, but that on the associated PLMS is less so. A single bedtime dose (Sinemet 100/25 mg to 250/25 mg) is usually sufficient, but a sustained release preparation may be necessary to avoid an early morning rebound. The drug is effective over at least some years, but dosage adjustments may be necessary, and the occasional patient may show tolerance. Some patients may need an additional early morning dose to treat the rebound increase in movements, and rarely a 24-hour schedule may be necessary. Patients show spontaneous exacerbations and remissions and this should be taken into account in the management.

Bromocriptine

Akpinar (1987) reported two patients with RLS and hypothyroidism who could not tolerate L-dopa and were treated with 2.5 mg bromocriptine given 1 hour before bedtime with good results, which were maintained in the 1-year follow-up period. In the von Scheele and Kempi (1990) report, two patients did not continue their improvement with L-dopa but improved with bromocriptine. The only double-blind, placebo-controlled, crossover study of bromocriptine was published by Walters et al (1988b), who used 7.5 mg bromocriptine or placebo in 30-day phases, with a 2-week wash-out between phases. Six patients (mean age 61 years, range 40–68) with idiopathic RLS were studied. Five reported improvement in restlessness and paraesthesiae with the drug compared to placebo, and expressed a desire to continue the medication. There was a reduction in the PLMS per hour of sleep (43% from baseline and 57% from placebo). Sleep parameters were modestly improved with bromocriptine, but not to a statistically significant degree. One patient experienced transient nasal stuffiness and light-headedness.

In short, bromocriptine (2.5–7.5 mg 1–3 hours before bedtime in 1–2 doses) is effective in treating RLS, but the improvement may not be as marked as that with L-dopa. However, some patients may respond preferentially to this drug, and it may therefore be utilized as a second-line drug. The published literature is not extensive but suggests its good tolerability.

Piribedil

Akpinar (1987) used piribedil, another DA agonist, with one patient at a dosage of 40 mg at bedtime, with good improvement that was maintained over a year.

The use of dopaminergic drugs in treating RLS is summarized in Table 13.1.

Benzodiazepines

The use of benzodiazepines in the treatment of RLS has a long history. Ekbom (1965) reported treating 15 patients with 2–10 mg diazepam with very good results in 12. He found diazepam to be superior to chlordiazepoxide. Some of Ekbom's patients had previously not responded to narcotics. Morgan (1967) used 5–10 mg diazepam at bedtime with 19 patients; 15 showed complete improvement and another 12 were much improved. The improvement usually occurred within 1–3 days, almost always within a week. After 1–2 weeks of improvement, the drug could be given intermittently in some cases (on two successive nights every 1–2 weeks, or on every second or third night).

Most recent investigations of benzodiazepines have used clonazepam. A number of anecdotal reports have been published that attest to its efficacy (Matthews, 1979; Handwerker and Palmer, 1985; Montplaisir et al, 1985; Egawa, 1987; Salvi et al, 1990). More detailed reports using clonazepam have also been published.

Read et al (1981) studied the effect of clonazepam in 15 patients (18–66 years) on maintenance haemodialysis who had RLS with no overt evidence of peripheral neuropathy. The patients had previously been treated ineffectively with various sedative-hypnotic drugs (temazepam, diazepam, nitrazepam, chlordiazepoxide and lorazepam). A split-evening or a twice-daily dose of clonazepam was used, starting with 0.5 mg twice a day and increasing if necessary. Six patients responded immediately, 8 others after an increase in dosage. Only 1 patient responded partially (at >2 mg/day). Two patients had a

Table 13.1. Treatment of restless legs syndrome with dopaminergic drugs

Drug	N	Mean age, years (range)	Dosage (mg)	Duration	Percent change	Effect size[a]	Adjusted effect size[a]	Study type[b]	Comments	Reference
L-Dopa	5	43.5 (33–54)	200/50[c]	6–18 months	100	—	—	Open	Subjective report used	Akpinar (1982)
	13	50.8 (29–75)	200/50[c]	2 weeks	—	−10.23	−9.52	DB, placebo crossover	Number of awakenings	Akpinar (1987)
	20	58.2 (10–83)	50–200	1 week	85	—	—	DB, placebo	Subjective preference for drug	von Scheele (1986)
	7	40.7 ± 12.5	100–200	4 weeks	71	—	—	Open	Scale, 0–3	Montplaisir et al (1986)
	6	51.3 ± 12.4	200/50[c]	1–3 months	25	−2.05	−1.89	DB, placebo crossover	Symptoms, PLMS, quality of life, improved	Brodeur et al (1988a)
	8	64 (58–70)	100/25–250/25[d]	1–3 months	25	—	—	Open	Clinical assessment	Sandyk et al (1987)
	28	52.5	50–600	2 years	50	—	—	Open	Improved sleep	von Scheele and Kempi (1990)

Table 13.1. (cont.)

Drug	N	Mean age, years (range)	Dosage (mg)	Duration	Percent change	Effect size[a]	Adjusted effect size[a]	Study type[b]	Comments	Reference
L-Dopa	20	64 ± 9	100/25[d]	3-7 weeks	83	—	—	Open	Long-term follow-up	Guilleminault et al (1993)
Bromo-criptine	2	—	2.5	1 year	100	—	—	Open	Could not tolerate L-dopa	Akpinar (1987)
	6	61 (40–68)	7.5	30 days	—	-1.85	-1.71	DB, placebo, crossover	5/6 improved	Walters et al (1988b)
	2	—	—	—	100	—	—	Open	Tolerance to L-dopa	von Scheele and Kempi (1990)
Piribedil	1	—	40	1 year	100	—	—	Open	—	Akpinar (1987)

[a]For an explanation of effect size and adjusted effect size, see Table 11.1.
[b]DB denotes double-blind study.
[c]L-Dopa with benserazide.
[d]L-Dopa with carbidopa.

recurrence of their symptoms when they stopped the drug, and relief when they restarted it. Of particular note in this open study was the differential efficacy of clonazepam in comparison with other benzodiazepines.

Montagna et al (1984) published the first double-blind, placebo-controlled, crossover trial of clonazepam. Six patients (44–64 years) with idiopathic RLS who had been refractory to treatment with iron and benzodiazepines (flurazepam and lorazepam) were treated with 1 week each of clonazepam 1 mg, placebo and vibratory stimulation of the sural muscles, with 3-day intervals between treatments. Clonazepam produced significantly greater improvement in the subjective quality of sleep and leg dysaesthesiae. Five of six patients favoured clonazepam. Vibration produced some subjective improvement but it was not statistically significant.

Boghen et al (1986) studied the effect of clonazepam in six patients (31–61 years) using a double-blind, placebo-controlled, crossover design. The drug (0.5–2 mg) and placebo were each given for 4 weeks, and there was a baseline drug-free period of 1 week. A 5-point scale was used to assess the degree of daily discomfort. Clonazepam resulted in a 34.5% reduction, whereas placebo produced a 15.3% reduction (not significant). Three patients were judged to have improved with the drug and two with placebo.

Horiguchi et al (1992) reported the results of open clonazepam (0.5–1.5 mg) treatment of 15 RLS patients (age range 62–88 years), who also underwent all-night polysomnography before and after the treatment. All patients reported subjective improvement of restlessness and dysaesthesiae within 3 days. Clonazepam also reduced the total and per hour PLMS, but did not affect the mean intermovement interval.

A number of researchers have examined the efficacy of clonazepam in nocturnal myoclonus, with or without RLS. Oshtory and Vijayan (1980) noted that clonazepam (1 mg at bedtime) significantly reduced nocturnal myoclonic jerks and improved sleep in two patients. Ohanna et al (1985) studied 20 patients who met the Coleman et al (1980) criteria for PLMS (8 had insomnia and 12 hypersomnia; 1 had RLS) and were treated with clonazepam 0.5–2 mg at bedtime. There was subjective improvement and decrease in the number of leg movements without affecting the intermovement interval or movement duration. The percentage of movements associated with arousal did not change. The findings of Mitler et al (1986) were somewhat different. They treated 10 patients suffering from nocturnal myoclonus with clonazepam (1 mg hs) and temazepam (30 mg hs) for 1 week each, with a 2-week wash-out. Both drugs improved sleep efficiency, sleep duration, wake time and stage-2 sleep, as is typical of benzodiazepines. They did not reduce the total number of leg movements, although movements per hour were reduced. The number of jerks with EEG arousal and awakening were reduced. Subjects preferred both drugs to baseline conditions. Peled and Lavie (1987) studied 20 patients suffering from PLMS associated with daytime sleepiness in 11 and insomnia in 9 (3 had RLS), using a double-blind, parallel group design. Clonazepam (0.5–2 mg) was effective, with 7 patients reporting marked improvement. Sleep latency, sleep efficacy, total sleep time, movement index and arousal index all improved significantly with the drug but not with placebo. Moldofsky et al (1986) followed up 13 patients with PLMS for a mean 6 months on treatment with nitrazepam (2.5–10 mg) and found it useful in suppressing PLMS and improving sleep physiology and daytime symptoms.

In conclusion, there is good evidence that benzodiazepines are useful in the treatment of patients with RLS, and those with PLMS and disturbed sleep but no RLS. Clonazepam seems to be the most promising drug, but the reasons for this are uncertain. These drugs are safe, although tolerance and dependence is an issue the clinician has to remember when using them for a chronic problem such as RLS. A summary of the studies of benzodiazepines in the treatment of RLS is presented in Table 13.2.

Opioid drugs

The use of opioid drugs in the treatment of RLS was suggested by Willis (1685), who tried opium with success in one case. Ekbom (1960) found codeine, hydrocodeine and opium useful, but he recommended their use in only the most severe cases because of the risk of dependence.

A number of papers published in the past decade support the use of opioid drugs in RLS, but no double-blind study has been published. Trzepacz et al (1984) reported three patients, one treated with methadone (20 mg) and two with oxycodone (2.5 mg), with complete improvement in one and partial in two. Lang (1987) treated a 67-year-old man with 15 mg/day codeine, with complete recovery of his RLS. Egawa (1987) reported marked amelioration in one patient with a single 25-mg dose of codeine. Kavey et al (1987) reported improvement with propoxyphene (130–195 mg) in four out of five patients with RLS. Improvement is generally reported in the dysaesthesia and restlessness, as well as in sleep. The drugs most commonly used include methadone (5–20 mg), codeine sulphate (15–120 mg), oxycodone (2.5–4.5 mg) and propoxyphene (65–290 mg), usually given 1–2 hours before bedtime. Hening and Walters (1989) reported that the beneficial effects are long term. In their opinion, based on their 7-year experience (Walters et al, 1991), tolerance or addiction is not usually a problem.

A number of case reports revealed that opioids significantly reduce daytime

Table 13.2. *Treatment of restless legs syndrome with benzodiazepines*

Drug	N	Mean age, years (range)	Dosage (mg)	Duration	Percent change	Effect size[a]	Adjusted effect size[a]	Study type[b]	Comments	Reference
Diazepam	15	—	2–10	—	80	—	—	Open	Clinical impression	Ekbom (1965)
	19	—	5–10	Long	89	—	—	Open	Clinical impression	Morgan (1967)
Clonazepam	2	42 and 65	1	—	85	—	—	Open	Clinical impression	Matthews (1979)
	15	42 (18–66)	1–2	—	58	—	—	Open	Clinical impression	Read et al (1981)
	6	59.3 (44–64)	1	1 week	—	−0.71	−0.66	DB, placebo crossover	5/6 favoured clonazepam	Montagna et al (1984)
	1	36	4	2 days	100	—	—	Open		Montplaisir et al (1985)
	6	46 (31–61)	0.5–2	4 weeks	34.5	−0.34	−0.32	DB, placebo, crossover	3 drug and 2 placebo improved	Boghen et al (1986)
	2	—	0.5–2.5	1 day	—	—	—	Open		Egawa (1987)
	4	(54–71)	1	—	75	—	—	Open		Salvi et al (1990)
	15	69 (62–88)	0.1–1.5	—	—	−0.67	−0.65	Open	All improved	Horiguchi et al (1992)

Note: Other authors have examined clonazepam with PLMS (Oshtory and Vijayan, 1980; Ohanna et al, 1985; Peled and Lavie, 1987; Mitler et al, 1986; Moldofsky et al, 1986).
[a]For an explanation of effect size and adjusted effect size, see Table 11.1.
[b]DB denotes double-blind study.

and nocturnal myoclonic jerks (DWA and PLMS) in some patients, but only modestly in some others (Hening et al, 1986; Walters et al, 1986; Kavey et al, 1987; Montplaisir et al, 1991). Sleep and PLMS may improve in some patients in the absence of RLS (Kavey et al, 1988). In one study (Walters et al, 1986), two opioid-treated patients experienced a recurrence of myoclonic jerks when challenged with naloxone but not with placebo.

In conclusion, the anecdotal evidence for the efficacy of opioid drugs is impressive, but controlled studies are recommended. For this reason, and because of the small but significant risk of dependence, they cannot be recommended as first-line treatment. They may, however, be used if dopaminergic drugs and benzodiazepines fail. Codeine, propoxyphene or oxycodone may be used, and some patients may require two or three tablets (given 2 hours and 1 hour before bedtime), and even another tablet in the middle of the night if sleep is interrupted. A summary of the studies of opioids in the treatment of RLS is presented in Table 13.3.

Adrenergic drugs

Clonidine

Clonidine is an α_2-agonist that reduces the activity of the adrenergic system. There have been some anecdotal reports of its success and one placebo-controlled study, but the evidence is still far from definitive.

Handwerker and Palmer (1985) reported 3 patients who responded well to clonidine (0.1–0.3 mg), but the duration of the treatment was not stated. Steiner (1987) reported 15 patients in an open study who had a good response. These patients were independently reviewed by Walters et al (1991), who were convinced of the efficacy of clonidine in some patients, although their own experience with the drug was largely negative. Neither group of authors employed polysomnography in the evaluation.

Ausserwinkler and Schmidt (1989) performed a double-blind study comparing clonidine ($n = 10$) with placebo ($n = 10$) in 20 uraemic patients with RLS, 9 of whom were on chronic renal dialysis. Clonidine (0.075 mg twice daily over 3 days) produced complete relief of symptoms in 8, marked improved in 1, and no change in 1. In the placebo group, only a mild improvement was noted in 1 patient.

While more empirical evidence is necessary, clonidine may be a worthwhile drug to try in cases where other drugs have failed. It is well tolerated in the low dosages (0.1–0.3 mg at bedtime or, if necessary, in a twice-a-day schedule) used.

Table 13.3. *Treatment of restless legs syndrome with opioid drugs*

Drug	N	Daily dosage (mg)	Duration	Improvement	Comments	Reference
Opium	1	—	—	Good	Clinical impression	Willis (1685)
Codeine, hydrocodeine, opium	Many	—	—	Good	Risk of dependence highlighted	Ekbom (1960)
Methadone	1	20	Few days	Complete	—	Trzepacz et al (1984)
Oxycodone	2	2.5	Few days	Partial		
Methadone/codeine	2	5–20	4 weeks	Good	Polysomnography	Hening et al (1986)
Propoxyphene	3	130–260				
Methadone	1	20	1 day	Very good	Polysomnography	Walters et al (1986)
Propoxyphene		195–260	—			
Codeine	1	25	1 day	Complete	—	Egawa (1987)
Propoxyphene	5	130–195	—	(Effect size –1.48)	—	Kavey et al (1987)
Codeine	1	15	1 week	Complete	—	Lang (1987)
Codeine	1	120	1 day	Very good	Polysomnography	Montplaisir et al (1991)

Note: No double-blind studies have been published.

Propranolol

Propranolol is curiously documented to be both a cause (Morgan, 1967) and a treatment of RLS. Ginsberg (1986) reported a patient who responded to 40 mg tid of propranolol. It was, in fact, the report by Strang that prompted the use of propranolol in NIA, in which it has been found to be more useful. More evidence is necessary before propranolol can be recommended for RLS.

Carbamazepine

Two double-blind studies examining carbamazepine have been published, although neither used polysomnography. In a large Norwegian multicentre general practice study (N = 174), Telstad et al (1984) compared carbamazepine (n = 84) with placebo (n = 90) using random assignment and a double-blind design. The median dosage of carbamazepine used was 236 mg/day (serum concentration 1–27 mmol/l, median 12), and patients were assessed at baseline and at 3 and 5 weeks using a visual analogue scale and a record of the number of attacks of restless legs per week. Carbamazepine was significantly more effective than placebo at both 3 and 5 weeks ($p < .01$), and the mean number of attacks was reduced from 4.95 in the first to 1.85 in the fifth week with the drug (cf 5.26 to 2.87 with placebo). The authors emphasized the pronounced placebo effect in the disorder.

Lundvall et al (1983) compared carbamazepine (600 mg/day) with placebo in a double-blind, crossover study of six patients (age range 37–71 years) over 4 weeks for each phase. A daily global rating on a scale of 0–3 was used, and the patient and physician gave their preference to continue or not at the end of the trial. Carbamazepine performed better overall, and three patients preferred to continue the drug (none preferred placebo). The authors suggest that the drug may be worthwhile in some patients. They also recommend increasing the dosage to 1,000 mg day or more for the occasional patient.

Zucconi et al (1989) treated nine patients (six with familial RLS) with carbamazepine, administered as a single oral dose (3–7 mg/kg), 1–2 hours before bedtime, for 30 days. Seven of the nine reported marked improvement in RLS (self-rating dropped from a mean 4.4 to 2.4 on a scale of 1–5, $p < .01$), with four showing complete recovery. Subjective evaluation of sleep improved in eight out of nine, with sleep latency and sleep efficiency showing improvement. The authors performed polysomnography before and after treatment and found that periodic movements were not significantly modified.

These studies suggest that carbamazepine may be a useful drug, although it is likely to produce improvement only in some patients and will possibly not improve the associated PLMS.

Other drugs

The following drugs have also been examined, as summarized in Table 13.4.

Baclofen

Baclofen is a derivative of the inhibitory neurotransmitter GABA and has been used mainly for the treatment of muscle spasticity. Guilleminault and Flagg (1984) assessed its efficacy in PLMS in five patients (mean age 59.6 years) in a double-blind polysomnographic study, at a dosage of 20–160 mg/day. Baclofen reduced the number of awakenings and improved sleep, but it actually increased the number of PLMS, although their amplitude was decreased during NREM sleep. There were fewer alpha EEG arousals and K complexes, suggesting decreased sleep fragmentation. The sleep of one patient with RLS improved. Dosages of 20–40 mg at bedtime were the most effective.

Amitriptyline

Sandyk et al (1988) treated a 63-year-old man suffering from RLS with 25 mg amitriptyline at bedtime, with complete remission of the symptoms.

L-Tryptophan

Because of the reported involvement of serotonergic mechanisms in myoclonus, Sandyk (1986) treated two patients having RLS (one with chronic renal failure) with 2 g L-tryptophan over 3–4 days, noting complete improvement in their symptoms.

Recommendations

On the basis of this review, we make the following recommendations in the management of RLS:

1. The patient should be investigated for various local and systemic disorders that may produce or exacerbate RLS. A list is provided in Table 12.1. The clinician should be guided by the history and physical examination in an individual case. It is important to correct the disorder wherever possible.
2. The role of iron is much disputed, but it would be reasonable clinical practice to investigate for iron deficiency anaemia and correct it, if present. Folate deficiency should also be corrected.

Table 13.4. *Treatment of restless legs syndrome with other drugs*

Drug	N	Dosage (mg/day)	Duration	Improvement	Study type	Comment	Reference
Clonidine	3	0.1–0.3	—	100%	Open	Scale, 0–3	Handwerken and Palmer (1985)
	7	0.1–0.3	—	No benefit	Open	Subjective response	Bamford and Sandyk (1987)
	15	0.1–0.3	—	—	Open	Subjective response	Steiner (1987)
	10	0.15	3 days	9/10 drug 1/10 placebo	DB, placebo	Uraemic patient	Ausserwinkler and Schmidt (1989)
Propranolol	1	120	—	100%	Open	Single case study	Ginsberg (1986)
Carbamazepine	6	600	4 weeks	$g = -.075$	DB, placebo	3 preferred carbamazepine	Lundvall et al (1983)
	174	236	5 weeks	$g = -0.40$ $d = -0.4$ ($p < .01$)	DB, placebo	General practice study	Telstad et al (1984)
Baclofen	9	3–7/kg	30 days	77.8%[a]	Open	PLMS not improved	Zucconi et al (1989)
	5	20–160	10 days	70%[a]	DB, placebo	PLMS studied	Guilleminault and Flagg (1984)
Amitriptyline	1	25	15–30 minutes	100%	Open	Single case study	Sandyk et al (1988)
L-Tryptophan	2	28	3–4 days	100%	Open	Uraemic patient	Sandyk (1986)

Note: g is effect size; d, adjusted effect size; DB, double-blind study.
[a]Improvement on sleep disturbance index.

3. The severity of the RLS must be judged so that a decision whether to use drug therapy can be made. Many mild cases do not need any treatment.
4. Strategies should be used to improve sleep hygiene (Becker and Jamieson, 1992). In particular, avoiding caffeine and nasal decongestants in the evenings and refraining from excess use of alcohol are important. Patients should abstain from exercise in the 3 hours before bedtime.
5. If a decision is made to use drugs, the choice of the initial drug will to some extent be guided by the side-effects profile and the personal experience of the clinician. No comparative studies have been conducted.

We recommend a trial of clonazepam first. Although evidence for the efficacy of L-dopa is the most convincing, problems with the long-term use of this drug make clonazepam a better first drug. One can begin with 0.5 mg 1 hour before bedtime, and the dose may be increased with another 0.5 mg 2 hours before bedtime. Some patients may need 2 mg/day, and occasionally daytime medication may also be necessary. The effect is apparent within a few days, and a trial of 1 week at the higher dosage is usually sufficient.

If clonazepam is unsuccessful, a dopaminergic drug may be used, in most cases L-dopa. A single bedtime dose (usually L-dopa/carbidopa 100/25 to 250/25 mg) is usually sufficient, but a sustained-release preparation may be necessary to avoid an early morning rebound. Some patients may need an additional early morning dose to treat the rebound increase in movements, and rarely a 24-hour schedule may be necessary.

If L-dopa is not tolerated, bromocriptine may be used, and there is some evidence that the latter may even be useful in patients who do not respond to L-dopa or develop tolerance to it.

The next group of drugs to be tried is the opioids, and codeine, oxycodone or propoxyphene may be used. Strict monitoring of the dosage is important. In the resistant case, any of the other drugs may be tried, in particular carbamazepine.

Long-term studies are few, with the suggestion that L-dopa, benzodiazepines and the opioids may be effective for many years, but dosage adjustments may be necessary, and the occasional patient may show tolerance. Patients sometimes show spontaneous exacerbations and remissions and this should be taken into account in the management.

Part IV
Conclusions

14

Summary and recommendations for future research

Life is the art of drawing conclusions from insufficient premises.

Samuel Butler, *Notebooks* (1912)

Why do some neuropsychiatric patients develop mental and motoric restlessness? What are the determinants of its intensity and duration? What is its pathophysiology? Why do some drugs, used ostensibly to tranquillize behaviourally and emotionally disturbed patients, paradoxically produce restlessness? Why are some drugs that 'seize the neurone' disliked by the patients who take them to treat their illnesses? Why are some patients, and families, unable to go to bed for fear of distressing feelings in the legs? How do we help these restless individuals suffer their illnesses in tranquillity? These and many similar questions have been addressed in this book.

The major limitation, repeatedly emphasized, has been the lack of sufficient data. In many ways, the syndromes that we have discussed are too complex and poorly delineated to lend themselves to 'tight' research. Many of the phenomena vary from normal behaviours only in degree. Their significantly subjective nature sets up the possibility of trivialization by an unempathic medical and research community. The occurrence of some of the disorders in psychiatrically ill patients further compromises their distinctive nature and associated disability. These are some of the reasons that only a few research groups have attempted to investigate this field. As an example, the contrast between the magnitude of research effort on TD and akathisia in the past 30 years is a testimony to the neglect of 'restlessness'. This is despite the fact that akathisia is apparent soon after prescription of the drug, is extremely distressing and significantly affects the short-term management of serious mental disorder. This book is an attempt at a synthesis of diverse information and sets the stage for further research into the syndromes of restlessness, akathisia, restless legs, and related disorders. Some directions became appar-

345

ent as the individual syndromes were discussed. In the next few paragraphs, I will try to summarize what I consider to be important avenues for research in each of the major areas.

Restlessness

Restlessness is a diffuse and varied concept, and the research literature lacks strict operational definitions. I have attempted one such definition, acknowledging that there will be other attempts in the future. The relative emphasis on the subjective and objective aspects of restlessness presents the same problems as does akathisia – the specific case of restlessness addressed by this book. It is true that motor or mental features are emphasized in different contexts, but the presence of both is necessary, although the subjective aspects may have to be presumed in the absence of testimony from the patient. In addition to its usage in the clinical setting, restlessness has a lay meaning which has been insufficiently explored. In Chapter 2, I described a number of syndromes in which restlessness is a major feature. A composite description of restlessness will result only when it has been pedantically described in each of the syndromes. With a few exceptions, the published literature is largely anecdotal on this issue. For example, while depressed patients are recognized to be commonly agitated or retarded, detailed descriptions of their restlessness have been generally lacking until recently. Such descriptions will aid easy recognition of restlessness in different contexts – an important initial step. The recent interest in restlessness can partly be attributed to the problem of managing increasing number of patients with dementia. Some prevalence studies have, therefore, been attempted, but large epidemiological studies using randomly selected populations are still lacking.

The final purpose of clinical description and epidemiological research is, of course, to help us understand the pathophysiology of the syndrome so that rational treatment or prevention may ensue. This understanding will be aided by functional imaging studies and the development of animal models, as discussed in Chapter 10, where I proposed a neuroanatomical model of restlessness that purports to account for the varied aetiology. This and similar models may bring cohesiveness to a splintered syndrome and suggest avenues for management. Most current interventions are empirically derived, and yet lack rigorous evaluation of their usefulness. More treatment studies are, therefore, necessary, and they should be based on an understanding of the underlying mechanisms.

Neuroleptic-induced dysphoria

The dislike of therapeutic drugs is a common phenomenon, but the unpleasantness produced by neuroleptics stands out as sufficiently extreme and distinctive to warrant separate study. Any clinician will attest to the various ways in which patients express their dislike of antipsychotic drugs, but the overall literature on this problem is scanty. The manifestations of this syndrome were categorized in Chapter 5. Some of the more valuable descriptions have been provided by healthy volunteers and Tourette's syndrome patients, who, unlike psychiatric patients, can more easily distinguish drug-induced states from symptoms of the underlying illness. An attempt has been made in my descriptions to distinguish NID from akathisia, while accepting that dysphoria is an important feature of the latter syndrome. This decision highlights the fact that there are a number of causes of NID and that akathisia is a more complex disorder that deserves distinctive recognition. In spite of the influential papers by Van Putten and colleagues, NID is still underrecognized, resulting in much unnecessary suffering. We also do not understand the determinants of this response, nor do we have enough information on its longitudinal course. Examination of animal models will help us to understand its pathophysiology, and I have reviewed some animal models in Chapters 5 and 10. The subjective responses of the patients to the newer antipsychotic drugs should also be evaluated.

The definition of drug-induced akathisia

One of the major reasons for the dearth of research studies on akathisia is the difficulty in defining the syndrome precisely. In Chapter 4, I examined the various published definitions and proposed a set of operational criteria. I invite challenges to these criteria, from both a conceptual viewpoint and empirical examination, so that tested and valid definitions may emerge. Different aspects of the definition do lend themselves to empirical testing. For example, the decision to regard definitive akathisia as being characterized by both subjective and objective features can be tested by the longitudinal follow-up of patients who have either the subjective or the objective features but not both, to determine whether they do develop the complete syndrome. Pharmacological strategies, such as varying the dosages of antipsychotic drugs, may be used to support the diagnosis. The proposed definition draws largely upon the literature on AA, and its suitability for akathisia of tardive or withdrawal onset remains to be examined. Furthermore, its suitability for akathisia not related to drugs is unknown. While the proposed criteria may seem too strict, they are intended for research into akathisia, especially that involving pharmacological intervention. A less strict set of criteria may be suitable for clinical use or epidemiological studies. While examining and criticizing the proposed criteria, investigators of akathisia will have to make decisions regarding inclusion criteria and definitions so that their studies may proceed. These investigations should include enough diagnostic data so that different sets of criteria can be applied, post hoc if necessary. Investigators should be cognizant of the possible subtypes of akathisia even if these do not form the basis of the investigation. The existence of subtypes should be considered in any calculation of sample size so that the data collected in these studies can be used to examine the definitional schema. One of the reasons for a poor understanding of akathisia is the lack of an appreciation of its subtypes in the past. The application of strict criteria which take into account the temporal relationship between drug treatment and the development of akathisia, as well as its duration, will remedy this deficiency.

Epidemiology

The limitations of the epidemiological data on akathisia were highlighted in Chapter 5. The major lessons from a review of the published literature that can be applied to any future investigations are that (i) strict operational criteria for diagnosis are necessary, (ii) the various subtypes of akathisia have to be taken into consideration, (iii) the studies have to be longitudinal in order to understand the relationship between drug use and side-effects, as well as to examine the development of the syndrome over time, and (iv) detailed psychiatric evaluation of the subjects is necessary to distinguish akathisia from anxiety, agitation, etc. With the recent introduction of many antipsychotic drugs that differ from the conventional ones in their pharmacological profiles, the examination of the incidence and prevalence of akathisia has received a renewed emphasis. An example is the discrepant findings on the incidence of akathisia in response to clozapine (see Chapter 5), which calls for not only a fresh examination but also an adequate explanation for the previous results. The published literature on akathisia provides a mix of incidence and prevalence data which are difficult to interpret, especially because the natural history of akathisia is poorly understood. Future studies should redress this deficiency.

Epidemiology is, of course, concerned not only with the distribution of akathisia in various populations, but also in examining the factors that influence that distribution. The first steps to achieve the latter have been taken for AA, but the literature is extremely deficient for the other subtypes. The examination of akathisia in special populations, and in response to non-neuroleptic drugs, will further assist the understanding of its pathophysiology and the factors that predispose its development. At the risk of repetition, I would like to emphasize the importance of conducting prospective studies when epidemiological factors of akathisia are being examined.

Acute akathisia

This is the syndrome of akathisia that has been best investigated, and we now recognize its clinical features and some of the factors that predispose its development. Atypical manifestations of akathisia have been described by a few authors, and the veracity of these descriptions should receive greater scrutiny in future studies. The relationship of akathisia with suicidal behaviour and violence, which has aroused some emotive debate, is based on anecdotes that have to be placed in the proper perspective. Some authors have suggested that predisposing factors (eg, age, psychiatric diagnosis, drug potency) should receive focused attention. It is unlikely that any single factor, other than drug dosage and type, will be found to contribute overwhelmingly to the development of AA. It is therefore important that studies are large in sample size and use a broad approach, so that the relative contributions of the various predisposing factors can be examined using regression models. The issue of iron deficiency as a risk factor highlights this point, since the conflicting findings of different studies may be explained by the suggestion that this is a minor risk factor that reaches statistical significance in some studies owing to sample size, special subject characteristics or methodological factors. The diagnosis of AA will continue to be plagued by the overlap of its manifestations with a number of other syndromes commonly encountered in acutely psychotic individuals. It is unlikely that tests that use pharmacological strategies or quantitative measures will emerge, and clinicians will still need to rely on their clinical judgements to make a diagnosis. A high index of suspicion and being sensitive to patients' reports are the two main factors likely to increase early and accurate diagnosis. The clearest message from the study of akathisia is 'Listen to the patient, even when he or she is acutely psychotic'.

Tardive and chronic akathisia

Tardive akathisia has not been universally accepted as a distinct syndrome, and I have discussed some of the reasons for this in Chapter 7. While the arguments presented in the literature are convincing enough for most investigators, a sceptical researcher is likely to demand direct evidence that a prospective long-term study of patients assessed at baseline and followed up while being maintained on neuroleptics can provide. Strictly speaking, such a study should have a control group of patients treated with placebo and be double-blind, but this would be impossible because of ethical and practical objections. The ongoing longitudinal studies of schizophrenia could adequately address the issue of the tardive emergence of akathisia for most purposes. A number of such studies are currently in progress for TD and can easily be adapted to study TA as well. The clinical characteristics of TA have been investigated, but since these studies have been cross-sectional, the possibility remains that what is been described is a mix of AA, CA and TA. TA is further plagued by the overlap with TD, making it difficult to attribute confidently a particular abnormal movement in a patient to one or the other syndrome. For example, irregular respiratory movements have been variously attributed to TD and TA. Some behavioral symptoms have been considered to be analogues of either TD or TA by different investigators. The features that distinguish TA from TD are not well established. The description of TA is often modelled on AA, and that of TD is overly influenced by the OBLF syndrome, thus limiting the range of abnormalities that can be seen in these syndromes. The definition of TA with regard to the relative emphasis on subjective or objective features presents the same difficulties as with AA. This is further confounded by the somewhat ambiguous concept of pseudoakathisia, which I believe to be of little clinical or research use.

Considering that the concept of TA is still struggling for widespread recognition, it is not surprising that its predisposing factors and pharmacological characteristics are poorly understood. Longitudinal studies are again necessary to examine the factors that predispose an individual to develop TA, and such studies are difficult and expensive. One issue that has received much recent attention is the relationship of the tardive syndromes, including TA, with the negative symptoms and cognitive dysfunction seen in schizophrenia. Our work suggests that TA is an appropriate syndrome to investigate this association. Pharmacological challenge studies may yield clues to effective treatment, as well as validate the distinctiveness of the syndrome in relation to other tardive disorders. Investigation of the pathophysiology using functional imaging and, if possible, animal models may yield important insights. The latter are, however, even more difficult to establish for TA than for AA.

Akathisia due to general medical condition, or 'organic' akathisia

In the past few decades, the term *akathisia* has become synonymous with DIA, but the fact that the term predates the introduction of neuroleptic medication argues for its additional application to an organically based syndrome. Indeed, epidemic encephalitis has been suggested as a model for many drug-induced states including akathisia. The study of akathisia associated with neurological disorders presents an opportunity to examine some hypotheses relating to the pathophysiology of akathisia. Its recognition is also of clinical importance, with reports that in disorders like PD, akathisia may significantly affect the patient's welfare. The concept of 'organic' akathisia will, however, remain tentative until more extensive and detailed studies have been performed and the manifestations of 'organic' akathisia are compared with the drug-induced syndrome.

Assessment and measurement of akathisia

The complexity of the phenomena seen in akathisia, the subjective nature of some of the features, the lack of a well-accepted definition and the variability of the disorder over time make its assessment extremely difficult. The various methods used to quantify akathisia were discussed in Chapter 9. All methods have limitations, but multi-item rating scales have been the most popular. Many rating scales are available, and their relative merits must be examined. Videotape measures are currently underutilized but hold the potential for providing excellent records. No instrumental method of measurement has been proved to be completely successful, but a combination of strain-gauge measures and actigraphy may provide an accurate measure of the motor component of akathisia. Any instrumental methods developed in the future must be validated against the more conventional measures before they are accepted for clinical or research use. It is likely that rating scales will continue to dominate the research literature, but the use of instrumental techniques as adjunctive measures will increase in popularity as their validity becomes established.

Pathophysiology

Understanding the pathophysiology of akathisia is important if effective preventative and treatment strategies are to emerge. In Chapter 10, I have discussed the putative risk factors for AA and TA, all of which need further study to delineate their contributions to the development of the syndromes. The appropriate strategies to investigate this are discussed in the relevant sections, and I will not repeat them here. What is needed is one or more models that integrate the findings. A pathogenetic model of akathisia must account for the diversity of the clinical manifestations (including both subjective and objective features), the various aetiological agents and the risk factors. The models discussed in the past account for some but not all features of akathisia. Such partial models have heuristic importance and are more readily testable, but they should be compatible with each other so that a cohesive model may finally emerge. In other words, the dopaminergic, noradrenergic, serotonergic and other models probably all contribute to an overall understanding of the syndrome, but none of these accounts for all its features. There are important questions that need addressing: Why is it that both DA and 5HT antagonists can produce similar symptoms? Why do antiadrenergic drugs sometimes alleviate these symptoms? Why do akathisic symptoms worsen when a posture is maintained? Why is there a particular reference to the legs? The integration of the information will depend on the progress in our understanding of brain–behavior relationships in general, and the investigation of akathisia will contribute to such an understanding. The study of in vivo brain metabolism and receptor function by newer imaging techniques, such as PET, may be one way to achieve this. More suitable animal models may be another.

Treatment of akathisia

Given the level of our understanding of akathisia, it is not surprising that the available strategies for its treatment or prevention are generally poor. The most effective measure is a modification of the offending agent, but the reality of the clinical situation may preclude such an intervention. It is encouraging that newer antipsychotic drugs are less likely to cause akathisia, but there is still no drug available that is completely free of this side-effect. This ideal may be unattainable since the neurochemical changes necessary to ameliorate the psychotic symptoms may not have such a high degree of specificity. Treatment studies must take into account the vagaries of the akathisia diagnosis and the fact that subtypes may have different pharmacological profiles. Acute akathisia is the most troublesome type of akathisia and is, fortunately, the easiest to define for a research study. The fact that it occurs in acutely ill patients, who are often unwilling or unavailable for research, makes its investigation difficult in practice. Published studies reflect this difficulty in that they recruit small numbers of subjects and are unable to control for important confounding variables, such as drug dose, type of drug, rate of dosage increment, dosing schedule and use of other psychotropic drugs such as benzodiazepines. Because of a lack of effective treatment, there is also a danger that new treatments will be accepted without rigorous investigation. My review of the literature on βA antagonists in akathisia highlights this point. The recent spate of studies on these drugs may conceal the fact that double-blind-controlled investigations are few, and there is a need to replicate them by independent groups before they become well accepted.

Restless legs syndrome

Akathisia and RLS are distinct, and yet they have an overlapping history and share many clinical features. They are both extremely distressing to the sufferer but are underrecognized and undertreated. The primary focus of this book has been akathisia, and my own research has exclusively been on the drug-induced syndrome. The two syndromes have, however, been partners in many developments. The iron deficiency hypothesis of akathisia had its origin in the observations that RLS was common in patients with iron deficiency anaemia. The use of dopaminergic drugs in RLS was a logical corollary to the fact that similar symptoms were produced by DA antagonists. The two syndromes are treated by different medical disciplines, with akathisia being largely a psychiatric disorder, by virtue of its occurrence in psychiatric patients, and RLS being neurological because of the possibility of a neuropathic or other aetiology. Both disciplines will benefit from comparing notes on their understanding of the syndromes. Some recent publications (eg, those examining the polysomnographic characteristics of akathisia) are therefore encouraging.

Much of what has been said for the clinical, aetiological and treatment aspects for akathisia can probably be repeated for RLS. The most important message, in my opinion, is that RLS should not be treated as a trivial disorder, and its relative neglect should be addressed. Its epidemiology and genetics need to be better understood, and more rigorous treatment studies are necessary. The latter must be long term, since RLS is a chronic disorder and its natural history is not completely known.

This is the first book-length review of akathisia and related syndromes. Experience with other neuropsychiatric disorders suggests that there is usually a 3- to 5-year delay before another treatise is published, and the growth is exponential thereafter. The syndrome is poised for an explosion of information, and we may not have to wait for very long.

Appendix A: Haskovec's *Akathisie*

Translated by Alexandra Walker and Perminder Sachdev

[First case]

In 1897, I had the occasion to examine a man aged 40, employed, who complained of the following symptoms:

For three weeks, he had trembling in his whole body, and he could not remain standing. In the standing position he was dizzy, weak and his legs shook, and he thought that he would fall over. He could walk well.

Seated, he rose up and down as though he were astride a horse.

Fifteen days ago he suddenly developed pins and needles in his fingers, and at the same time his mouth was twisted, but that was of short duration. He needed to urinate frequently, which disturbed his sleep. If he held back from urinating, the above symptoms worsened.

Compressions of cold water on the area of his heart calmed him. His pulse was sometimes irregular.

[Medical history]

When he was 30 years old, he had fainted on hearing that his mother was suffering from smallpox. As a student, he had a soft chancre from which he was cured. In 1891, he had influenza. In 1894, he lost his voice some time after having a cold and that then happened after each cold. He did not suffer from headaches and his memory was good.

His father died of tuberculosis and his mother died after a cardiovascular attack.

[Examination]

The patient was of average height, bone structure and build. The organs of the chest and abdomen were normal.

The points typically painful to pressure were infraclavicular, around the nipples and in the region of the heart. His skin sensitivity was slightly increased, as was the vasomotor excitability of the skin. The tendon reflexes were quick. The mechanical excitement of the muscles was increased. His visual fields were restricted on both sides. Pressure on the spinal column was very painful.

The patient was slightly tense and timid.

The strength of all his muscles were normal. All his movements, passive and active, of the head, the trunk and the extremities were made without pain and totally correctly.

His gait was quite normal and flowing.

From time to time, the patient had clonic seizures of the diaphragm and spasms of the larynx. He could partially stop these phenomena when one told him to keep still, to speak slowly and to breathe calmly.

But over and above his inability to remain standing as described, what particularly interested me about this patient was the following phenomenon, which was seen objectively.

When he was required to stay seated, he rose up and down quickly and involuntarily, sitting down again and repeating this behaviour. These movements impressed one as being automatic, involuntary and compulsive, and the patient also considered them this way.

These compulsive movements made him repeatedly rise up and sit down again so frequently that sitting was almost impossible for him. They were made with the complete awareness of the patient and against his will. There was no other symptom during these movements. I therefore chose to talk to the patient while he was walking, because then he was quite calm with no irregularities in the innervation of his muscles.

[Diagnosis]

I then considered that this was a case of hysteria and that the above phenomenon was a class of the varied and peculiar movements that one describes under the name *rhythmic chorea*, although I acknowledge that this name does not fit well with phenomena of a hysterical type because they have nothing to do with the chorea itself. One could also consider the above phenomenon an analogue of the saltatory spasm reflex.

I did not see the patient again and thought no more of the case. A year later I had the occasion to examine another case.

[Second case]

JB, aged 54 years, unmarried, whose father died of marasmus and mother of pneumonia. Of four brothers and sisters, three were alive and healthy. One brother had died of tuberculosis.

There was no family history of nervous or mental illness.

The patient had always enjoyed good health. He was agile and hard working.

In 1890, while walking, he had suddenly felt hot throughout his body and had a sense of sadness, and he fell without losing consciousness. Since this time, he had been overcome from time to time by trembling and a feeling of agitation in his whole body. He always recovered during summer in the countryside. The doctors told him that he was suffering from neurasthenia. In addition, he suffered from fleeting pains in the legs and the area of the sacrum. He sensed a pressure and a trembling in the stomach, the latter particularly after meals.

Sometimes he was constipated and he suffered dyspepsia.

At times he could not walk. He had the feeling of being drawn towards the ground, of having atrophy of his muscles and as if his legs did not have a solid foundation and could not function.

Since the end of the past year he found that he could not remain seated. When he was seated, he rose up and down compulsively and violently; this could happen at home or in any public place, so that he could not stay seated for a fixed time. He needed to hold on to the table to stop himself from rising up involuntarily. Sometimes when seated, he would have an uncertain feeling that he would jump up.

From time to time he felt well; at other times he had a feeling of agitation in his whole body, especially in his back.

Apart from that, he worked well. He did not have headaches. The senses functioned well, appetite was normal, as was sphincter function.

No excesses in alcohol use and sexuality.

[Examination]

The patient was of average height and bone structure; his build was frail and his skin was yellowish in colour. The organs of the chest, temperature and pulse were normal. Slight arteriosclerosis. The muscles were developed, normal, symmetrical and their electrical excitability was also normal. The electrical excitability of the motor nerves was normal. All his movements, active and passive, were normal. Skin sensitivity was normal.

Apart from a slight increase in the vasomotor excitability of the skin and the mechanical excitement of the muscles, and quick tendon reflexes, the somatic examination was negative.

I saw the patient again in 1900. He told he that the compulsive and involuntary movements up and down when seated had stopped, and he felt better except for his stomach. He had lost a little weight and his colour was more yellowish. On local examination I could not establish symptoms of cancer of the stomach or liver. The patient died some time later with symptoms of acute enteritis.

[Summary]

In this case of neuroasthenia we see that the patient experiences a feeling which makes him move from a seated to an upright position, a feeling which can be so intense that he has to hold onto the table. Moreover, he displays the same phenomenon that we saw in the preceding case; he was forced to quickly rise up and sit down again, against his will and with perfect awareness. (I have tried to find another similar case but unfortunately I have not succeeded. However, I draw attention to this type of compulsive movement which interferes with the normal seated position.)

Perhaps one could better study this phenomenon with more cases.

I think that what we have here is an analogue of the astasia-abasia of the French school or of the atremia [inability to walk, stand or sit] of Neftel (*Virchow's Archiv,* 1883).

Just as the harmony of the innervation involving normal walking or standing still can be impaired by a number of causes, the same harmony of innervation involved in remaining seated can perhaps be impaired by the same causes.

We have seen it in hysteria and neurasthenia. We can accept as a hypothesis only that this concerns the excitability of the subcortical centres and that this concerns transitory lesions and is certainly functional in nature.

It is fairly probable that in our second case, some visceral sensations could be the agent provocateur of this sudden discharge from the subcortical centres.

If one finds the phenomenon described more often and if one can place it in the nosological framework next to astasia-abasia, one could well give it the name 'akathisie'.

It is clear that this akathisia has nothing to do with the restless, voluntary, sudden and almost convulsive jumps of the anxious neurasthenic, the hypochondriacs and the melancholics.

Likewise this akathisia is not the same as the akathisias that one sees in the different psychoses under the influence of delirious ideas, fixed ideas and hallucinations. Children attacked by helminthiasis often exhibit phenomena resembling akathisia, but these phenomena are not related to the akathisia that we have described.

The prognosis and the therapy of the syndrome described are those of a primary illness.

Appendix B: Prince Henry Hospital Akathisia Scale

(This scale was developed by Sachdev, 1994c, based on the Braude et al, 1983, questionnaire.)

Instructions

Perform objective before subjective ratings.

Objective ratings (by observer)

Patient should be seated in a comfortable chair with full body visible to examiner, preferably with arms and legs unclothed. Engage in neutral conversation for the first 5 minutes, observing the patient's movements. Perform two 'distracting' procedures (counting from 30 backwards, and tapping fingers of right and left hand for 15 seconds each) to see effect on movements. Play a recording of a passage for 2 minutes on which patient has to concentrate (optional: observe patient while he or she is watching a 2-minute video cartoon clip). Make the patient stand in one spot and engage in neutral conversation for 2 minutes, with the examiner standing as well. Repeat distracting procedures while standing. Encircle the rating that applies to each item. Rate sitting and standing separately. If in doubt, rate conservatively.

Subjective ratings

Elicit from patient by direct questioning the best responses to the items listed below. Offer choices in case of indecision. Rate patient's experience currently (for the duration of this assessment only).

Key

0 = Absent
1 = Mild and present some of the time
2 = Mild and present most of the time or severe and present some of the time
3 = Severe and present all of the time

Note: There is a categorical shift between 0 and 1, with a rating of 1 representing a definite presence of the feature.

Global rating

Take overall observations and report into consideration to make a global judgement on the movements and the subjective symptoms.

| Project | Date of assessment: __/__/__ | Rater ID _____ |
| ID no. _____ | Time begin: | end: | Initials _____ |

Objective ratings
I. Sitting
1. Semipurposeful/purposeless leg/foot movements   0 <u>1 2 3</u>
2. Semipurposeful/purposeless hand/arm movements   0 <u>1 2 3</u>
3. Shifting body position in chair   0 <u>1 2 3</u>
4. Inability to remain seated   0 <u>1 2 3</u>

II. Standing
1. Purposeless/semipurposeless leg/foot movements   0 <u>1 2 3</u>
2. Shifting weight from foot to foot and/or walking in one spot   0 <u>1 2 3</u>
3. Inability to remain standing in one spot (walking or pacing)   0 <u>1 2 3</u>

Sum score _____

Subjective ratings
1. Feelings of restlessness, especially in the legs   0 <u>1 2 3</u>
2. Inability to keep legs still   0 <u>1 2 3</u>
3. Inability to remain still, standing or sitting   0 <u>1 2 3</u>

Sum score _____
Total score _____

Global rating (by rater)

Absent	Mild	Moderate	Severe
0	1	2	3

Appendix C: Barnes (1989) Akathisia Rating Scale

Patients should be observed while they are seated and then standing while engaged in neutral conversation (for a minimum of 2 minutes in each position). Symptoms observed in other situations, eg, while the patient is engaged in activity on the ward, may also be rated. Subsequently, the subjective phenomena should be elicited by direct questioning.

Objective

0 = Normal, occasional fidgety movements of the limbs

1 = Presence of characteristic restless movements; shuffling or tramping movements of the legs/feet, or swinging of one leg, while sitting, and/or rocking from foot to foot or 'walking on the spot' when standing, but movements present for less than half the time observed

2 = Observed phenomena, as described in 1, which are present for at least half the time observed

3 = Patient constantly engaged in characteristic restless movements and/or unable to remain seated or standing without walking or pacing, during the time observed

Subjective

Awareness of restlessness

0 = Absence of inner restlessness

1 = Nonspecific sense of inner restlessness

2 = Awareness of an inability to keep the legs still, or a desire to move the legs, and/or a complaint of inner restlessness aggravated specifically by being required to stand still

3 = Awareness of an intense compulsion to move most of the time and/or report of a strong desire to walk or pace most of the time

Distress related to restlessness

0 = No distress
1 = Mild
2 = Moderate
3 = Severe

Global clinical assessment of akathisia

0 = Absent

No evidence of awareness of restlessness. Observation of characteristic movements of akathisia in the absence of a subjective report of inner restlessness or compulsive desire to move the legs should be classified as pseudoakathisia.

1 = Questionable

Nonspecific inner tension and fidgety movements.

2 = Mild akathisia

Awareness of restlessness in the legs and/or inner restlessness worse when required to stand still. Fidgety movements present, but characteristic restless movements of akathisia not necessarily observed. Condition causes little or no distress.

3 = Moderate akathisia

Awareness of restlessness as described for mild akathisia, combined with characteristic restless movements such as rocking from foot to foot when standing. Patient finds the condition distressing.

4 = Marked akathisia

Subjective experience of restlessness includes a compulsive desire to walk or pace. However, patient is able to remain seated for at least 5 minutes. Condition is obviously distressing.

5 = Severe akathisia

Patient reports a strong compulsion to pace up and down most of the time and is unable to sit or lie down for more than a few minutes. Patient experiences constant restlessness, which is associated with intense distress and insomnia.

Appendix D: Hillside Akathisia Scale (version 4)

(This scale was developed by Fleischhacker et al, 1989.)

Subjective subscale (items 1 and 2)

0 = Absent
1 = Questionable
2 = Present and easily controlled
3 = Present and barely controlled
4 = Present and not controllable

Objective subscale (items 3, 4 and 5)

0 = No akathisia
1 = Questionable
2 = Small-amplitude movements part of the time
3 = Small-amplitude movements all of the time or large-amplitude movements part of the time
4 = Large-amplitude movements all of the time

Subjective items

	Sitting	Standing	Lying	Total
1. Patient has sensation of inner restlessness	___	___	___	___
2. Patient has the urge to move	___	___	___	___

Objective items

	Sitting	Standing	Lying	Total
3. Akathisia present in the head and trunk	_____	_____	_____	_____
4. Akathisia present in the hands and arms	_____	_____	_____	_____
5. Akathisia present in the feet and legs	_____	_____	_____	_____

Other neuropsychiatric phenomena present

	Yes	No
Akathisia	_____	_____
Parkinsonism	_____	_____
Choreoathetosis	_____	_____
Anxiety	_____	_____
Agitation	_____	_____
Sleep disturbance	_____	_____

Clinical global impression

Severity of akathisia   Score _____

Considering your total clinical experience with this particular population, how akathisic is the patient at this time?

0 = Not assessed
1 = Normal, not akathisic
2 = Borderline akathisic
3 = Mildly akathisic
4 = Moderately akathisic
5 = Markedly akathisic
6 = Severely akathisic
7 = Among the most akathisic of patients

Global improvement   Score _____

Rate of total improvement whether or not, in your judgement, it is entirely due to drug treatment. Compared with his or her condition at admission to the study, how much has he or she changed?

0 = Not assessed
1 = Very much improved
2 = Much improved
3 = Minimally improved
4 = No change
5 = Minimally worse
6 = Much worse
7 = Very much worse

References

Achenbach TM, Edelbrook CS (1983) *Manual for the Child Behavior Checklist and Revised Child Behavior Profile.* New York: Queen City Printers.

Adler L, Angrist B, Peselow E, et al (1985) Efficacy of propranolol in neuroleptic-induced akathisia. *J Clin Psychopharmacol* 5:164–166.

Adler L, Angrist B, Peselow E, et al (1986) A controlled assessment of propranolol in the treatment of neuroleptic-induced akathisia. *Br J Psychiatry* 149:42–45.

Adler L, Duncan E, Angrist B, et al (1989a) Effects of a specific beta 2-receptor blocker in neuroleptic-induced akathisia. *Psychiatry Res* 27:1–4.

Adler LA, Angrist B, Peselow E, et al (1987a) Clonidine in neuroleptic-induced akathisia. *Am J Psychiatry* 144:235–236.

Adler LA, Angrist B, Reiter S, et al (1989b) Neuroleptic-induced akathisia: a review. *Psychopharmacology* (Berl) 97:1–11.

Adler LA, Peselow E, Rosenthal M, et al (1993) A controlled comparison of the effects of propranolol, benztropine, and placebo on akathisia: an interim analysis. *Psychopharmacol Bull* 29:283–286.

Adler LA, Reiter S, Angrist B, et al (1987b) Pindolol and propranolol in neuroleptic-induced akathisia. *Am J Psychiatry* 144:1241–1242.

Adler LA, Reiter S, Corwin J, et al (1987c) Differential effects of propranolol and benztropine in patients with neuroleptic-induced akathisia. *Psychopharmacol Bull* 23:519–521.

Adler LA, Reiter S, Corwin J, et al (1988) Neuroleptic-induced akathisia: propranolol versus benztropine. *Biol Psychiatry* 23:211–213.

Akpinar S (1982) Treatment of restless legs syndrome with levodopa plus benserazide. *Arch Neurol* 39:739.

Akpinar S (1987) Restless legs syndrome treatment with dopaminergic drugs. *Clin Neuropharmacol* 10:69–79.

Albin RL, Young AB, Penney JB (1989) The functional anatomy of basal ganglia disorders. *Trends Neurosci* 12:366–375.

Allain PP, Lechat P (1970) Action of psychotropic drugs on emotional defecation in mice. *Therapie* 25:655–662.

Allen JC, Gralla R, Reilly L, et al (1985) Metoclopramide: dose-related toxicity and preliminary antiemetic studies in children receiving cancer chemotherapy. *J Clin Oncol* 3:1136–1141.

Allison FG (1943) Obscure pains in the chest, back and limbs. *Can Med Assoc J* 48:36.

American Psychiatric Association (1987) *Diagnostic and Statistical Manual of Mental Disorders* (DSM-III-R). 3rd ed, revised. Washington, DC: American Psychiatric Association Press.

American Psychiatric Association (1994) Diagnostic and Statistical Manual of Mental Disorders (DSM-IV). 4th ed., revised. Washington, DC: American Psychiatric Association Press.

American Psychiatric Association (1992) *Tardive Dyskinesia: A Task Force Report of the American Psychiatric Association* (Chairman: JM Kane). Washington, DC: American Psychiatric Association.

Ancill RJ, Carlyle WW, Liang RA, et al (1991) Agitation in the demented elderly, a role for benzodiazepines? *Int Clin Psychopharmacol* 6(3):141–146.

Ancill RJ, Holliday SG (1988) The assessment and management of dysfunctional behaviour in the cognitively impaired elderly. *Psychiatry* April:20–24.

Andersen J, Korner A, Ostergaard P, et al (1990) A double blind comparative multicentre study of remoxipride and haloperidol in schizophrenia. *Acta Psychiatr Scand* (Suppl) 358:104–107.

Anderson BG, Reker D, Cooper TB (1981) Prolonged adverse effects from haloperidol in normal subjects. *N Engl J Med* 305:643–644.

Anonymous (1986) Treatments for restless legs syndrome. *West J Med* 145:522–523.

Appelbaum PS, Lidz CW, Meisel A (1987) *Informed Consent: Legal Theory and Clinical Practice*. New York: Oxford University Press.

Appleton DB, Eadie MJ, Sutherland JM (1970) Amantadine hydrochloride in the treatment of parkinsonism: a controlled trial. *Med J Aust* 2:626–629.

Arnt J, Hyttel J, Bach-Lauritsen T (1986) Further studies of the mechanism behind scopolamine-induced reversal of antistereotypic and cataleptogenic effects of neuroleptics in rats. *Acta Pharmacol Toxicol* 59:319–324.

Ashkenazi R, Ben-Shachar D, Youdim MBH (1982) Nutritional iron and dopamine binding sites in the rat brain. *Pharmacol Biochem Behav* 17(suppl):43–47.

Ask-Upmark E (1959) Contribution to the pathogenesis of the syndrome of restless legs. *Acta Med Scand* 164:231.

Ask-Upmark E, Meurling S (1955) On the presence of a deficiency factor in the pathogenesis of amyotrophic lateral sclerosis. *Acta Med Scand* 152:217.

Askenasy JJ, Weitzman ED, Yahr MD (1987) Are periodic movements in sleep a basal ganglia dysfunction? *J Neural Transm* 70:337–347.

Asnis GM, Leopold MA, Duvoisin RC, et al (1977) A survey of tardive dyskinesia in psychiatric outpatients. *Am J Psychiatry* 134:1367–1370.

Aspenstrom G (1964) Pica och restless legs vid jardbist. *Svenska Lakartidn* 61: 1174–1177.

Association of Sleep Disorders Centers (1979) Diagnostic classification of sleep and arousal disorders. 1st ed. Prepared by the Sleep Disorders Classification Committee. (Chairman: HP Roffwang). *Sleep* 2:1–137.

Atakan Z, Cooper JE (1989) Behavioural Observation Schedule (BOS), PIRS, 2nd ed. *Br J Psychiatry* 155(suppl 7):78–80.

Ausserwinkler M, Schmidt P (1989) [Successful clonidine treatment of restless leg syndrome in chronic kidney insufficiency] Erfolgreiche Behandlung des "restless legs"-Syndroms bei chronischer Niereninsuffizienz mit Clonidin. *Schweiz Med Wochenschr* 119:184–186.

Axelsson R, Nilsson A, Christensson E, et al (1991) Effects of amperizode in schizophrenia: An open study of a potent 5-HT2 receptor antagonist. *Psychopharmacology* 104(3):287–292.

Ayd FJ (1961) A survey of drug-induced extrapyramidal reactions. *JAMA* 175: 1054–1060.

Ayd FJ Jr (1965) Psychopharmacology in Europe. Presented at the annual meeting of the American College of Neuropharmacology; December 13–15; San Juan, Puerto Rico.

Ayd FJ Jr (1974) Side effects of depot fluphenazines. *Compr Psychiatry* 15(4): 277–284.

Ayd FJ Jr (1988) Akathisia and suicide: fact or myth. *International Drug Therapy Newsletter* 23(9):37–39.

Azima H, Ogle W (1954) Effects of largactil in mental syndromes. *Can Med Assoc J* 71:116–121.

Bain PG, Findley LJ, Atchison P, et al (1993) Assessing tremor severity. *J Neurol Neurosurg Psychiatry* 56:868–873.

Baldessarini RJ, Cohen BM, Teicher MH (1988) Significance of neuroleptic dose and plasma level in the pharmacological treatment of psychoses. *Arch Gen Psychiatry* 45:79–91.

Baldessarini RJ, Marsh E (1990) Fluoxetine and side effects [letter]. *Arch Gen Psychiatry* 47:191–192.

Balfour DJK (1982) The effects of nicotine on brain neurotransmitter systems. *Pharmacol Ther* 16:269–282.

Balldin J, Alling C, Gottfries CG, et al (1985) Changes in dopamine receptor sensitivity in humans after heavy alcohol intake. *Psychopharmacology (Berl)* 86:142–146.

Ballinger BR (1970) The prevalence of nail-biting in normal and abnormal populations. *Br J Psychiatry* 117:445–446.

Balmer A, Limoni C (1980) Clinical, placebo-controlled double-blind study of venoruton in the treatment of chronic venous insufficiency [in German]. *Vasa – Journal of Vascular Diseases* 9:76–82.

Balsara JJ, Jadhav JH, Chandorkar AG (1979) Effect of drugs influencing central serotonergic mechanisms on haloperidol-induced catalepsy. *Psychopharmacology* 62:67–69.

Bamford CR, Sandyk R (1987) Failure of clonidine to ameliorate the symptoms of restless legs syndrome [letter]. *Sleep* 10(4):398–399.

Banerji NK, Hurwitz LJ (1989) Restless legs syndrome, with particular reference to its occurrence after gastric surgery. *Br Med J* 4:774–775.

Bannon MJ, Roth RH (1983) Pharmacology of mesocortical dopamine neurons. *Pharmacol Rev* 35:53–68.

Bard P, Macht MB (1958) The behaviour of chronically decerbrate cats. In: Wolstenholme GEW, O'Connor CM, eds. *Neurological Basis of Behaviour.* Ciba Foundation Symposium. London: I. and A. Churchill. pp. 55–75.

Barnes TR (1989) A rating scale for drug-induced akathisia. *Br J Psychiatry* 154:672–676.

Barnes TR, Braude WM (1984) Persistent akathisia associated with early tardive dyskinesia. *Postgrad Med J* 60:359–361.

Barnes TR, Braude WM (1985) Akathisia variants and tardive dyskinesia. *Arch Gen Psychiatry* 42:874–878.

Barnes TR, Kidger T, Gore SM (1983) Tardive dyskinesia: a 3-year follow-up study. *Psychol Med* 13:71–81.

Barnes TRE, Halstead SM (1988) A scale for rating drug-induced akathisia (abstract: Biennial Winter Workshop on Schizophrenia, Badgastein, Austria, January). *Schizophr Res* 1:249.

Barnes TRE, Halstead SM, Little P (1990) Akathisia variants: prevalence and iron status in an inpatient population with chronic schizophrenia. *Schizophr Res* 3:79. (Abstract).

Barnes TRE, Trauer T (1982) Reliability and validity of a tardive dyskinesia videotape rating scale. *Br J Psychiatry* 140:508–515.

Barrett RE, Singh N, Fahn S (1981) The syndrome of painful legs and moving toes. *Neurology* 31(suppl 1):79.

Barsa JA, Kline MS (1956) Use of reserpine in disturbed psychiatric patients. *Am J Psychiatry* 13:155–162.

Bartels J, Gaertner HJ, Golfinopoulos G (1981) Akathisia syndrome: involvement of noradrenergic mechanisms. *J Neural Transm* 52:33–39.

Bartels M, Heide K, Mann K, et al (1987) Treatment of akathisia with lorazepam: an open clinical trial. *Pharmacopsychiatry* 20:51–53.

Bartholini G, Stadler H, Godes Ciria M, et al (1976) The use of push-pull cannula to estimate the dynamics of acetylcholines within various brain areas. *Neuropharmacology* 15:515–519.

Barton A, Bowie J, Ebmeier K (1990) Low plasma iron status and akathisia. *J Neurol Neurosurg Psychiatry* 53:671–674.

Barton JL (1982) Amoxapine-induced agitation among bipolar depressed patients [letter]. *Am J Psychiatry* 139:87.

Barton R, Hurst L (1966) Unnecessary use of tranquilizers in elderly patients. *Br J Psychiatry* 989:990.

Bartzokis G, Wirshing WC, Hill MA, et al (1989) Comparison of electromechanical measures and observer ratings of tardive dyskinesia. *Psychiatry Res* 27: 193–198.

Bathien N, Kentlidis RM, Rondot P (1984) EMG patterns in abnormal involuntary movements induced by neuroleptics. *J Neurol Neurosurg Psychiatry* 47: 1002–1008.

Baxter LR Jr, Schwartz JM, Phelps ME, et al (1989) Reduction of prefrontal cortex glucose metabolism common to three types of depression. *Arch Gen Psychiatry* 46:243–250.

Beani L, Bianchi C (1973) Effect of amantadine on cerebral acetylcholine release and content on the guinea pig. *Neuropharmacology* 12:283–289.

Beard GM (1880) *A Practical Treatise on Nervous Exhaustion.* 2nd ed. New York: William Wood. pp. 41–42.

Beasley CM, Mascia DN, Potvin JH (1992) Fluoxetine: a review of receptor and functional effects and their clinical applications. *Psychopharmacology* 107: 1–10.

Beasley CM Jr, Masica DN, Heiligenstein JH, et al (1993) Possible monoamine oxidase inhibitor – serotonin uptake inhibitor interaction: fluoxetine clinical data and preclinical findings. *J Clin Psychopharmacol* 13(5):312–320.

Becker PM, Jamieson AO (1992) Common sleep disorders in the elderly: diagnosis and treatment. *Geriatrics* 47(3):41–52.

Bedard MA, Montplaisir J, Godbout R (1987) Effect of L-dopa on periodic movements in sleep in narcolepsy. *Eur Neurol* 27:35–38.

Belmaker RH, Wald D (1977) Haloperidol in normals. *Br J Psychiatry* 131:222–223.

Berger B, Gaspar P, Verney C (1991) Dopaminergic innervation of the cerebral cortex: unexpected differences between rodents and primates. *Trends Neurosci* 14(1):21–27.

Berger BD (1972) Conditioning of food aversions by injections of psychoactive drugs. *J Comp Physiol Psychol* 81:21–26.

Bergonzi P, Gigli GL, Laudisio A, et al (1981) The problem of the spinal myoclonus. *J Neurosurg Sci* 25(3–4):163–167.

Bernick C (1988) Methysergide-induced akathisia. *Clin Neuropharmacol* 11:87–89.

Bersani G, Grispini A, Marini S, et al (1986) Neuroleptic-induced extrapyramidal side effects: clinical perspectives with ritanserin (R 55667), a new selective 5-HT2 receptor blocking agent. *Curr Ther Res* 40:492–499.

Bignami G (1991) Neuroleptic dysphoria in animals [letter]. *Biol Psychiatry* 30: 844–848.

Binder RL, Kazamatsuri H, Nishimura T, et al (1987) Smoking and tardive dyskinesia. *Biol Psychiatry* 22:1280–1282.

Bing R (1923) Über einige bemerkenswerte beglieterscheinungen der 'extrapyramidalen rigidat' (On some outstanding side effects of extrapyramidal rigidity) (Akathisie–Mikrographie–Kinesia Paradoxa). *Schweiz Med Wochenschr* 4:167–171.

Bing R (1939) *Textbook of Nervous Diseases*. 5th ed. London: Henry Kimpton. pp. 758–759.

Bischoff S, Vassout A, Delina-Stula A, et al (1986) Interactions of cipazoxapine, citatepine, eresepine, and maroxepine with central dopamine (DA) receptors: effects of in vivo (3H)spiperone binding, DA metabolism, and behavioral parameters. *Pharmacopsychiatry* 19:306–307.

Bishop MP, Gallant DM, Sykes TF (1965) Extrapyramidal side effects and therapeutic response. *Arch Gen Psychiatry* 13:155–162.

Bixler EO, Kales A, Vela-Bueno A, et al (1982) Nocturnal myoclonus and nocturnal myoclonic activity in a normal population. *Res Commun Chem Pathol Pharmacol* 36:129–140.

Bjorklund A, Skagerberg G (1979) Evidence for a major spinal cord projection from the diencephalic A11 dopamine cell group in the rat using transmitter-specific fluorescent retrograde tracing. *Brain Res* 177:170–175.

Blandina P, Goldfarb J, Green JP (1988) Activation of a 5-HT3 receptor releases dopamine from rat striatal slice. *Eur J Pharmacol* 155:349–350.

Blass JP, Plum F (1983) Metabolic encephalopathies in older adults. In: Katzman R, Terry RD, eds. *The Neurology of Aging*. Philadelphia: Davis. pp. 189–220.

Blessed G, Tomlinson B, Roth M (1968) The association between quantitative measures of dementia and senile change in the cerebral grey matter of elderly subjects. *Br J Psychiatry* 114:797–811.

Bleuler E (1911) *Dementia Praecox, or the Group of Schizophrenias*. An English translation by J Zinkin. Monograph Series on Schizophrenia, No 1. New York: International Universities Press.

Bliss J (1980) Sensory experiences of Gilles de la Tourette syndrome. *Arch Gen Psychiatry* 37:1343–1347.

Bliwise D, Petta D, Seidel W, et al (1985) Periodic leg movements during sleep in the elderly. *Arch Gerontol Geriatr* 4:273–281.

Boghen D, Lamothe L, Elie R, et al (1986) The treatment of the restless legs syndrome with clonazepam: a prospective controlled study. *Can J Neurol Sci* 13:245–247.

Boghen D, Peyronnard JM (1976) Myoclonus in familial restless legs syndrome. *Arch Neurol* 33:368–370.

Bonduelle M, Jolivet B (1953) Les impatiences. *Bull Med* (Paris) 67:316–318.

Borenstein P, Bles G (1965) Effects clinques et electroencephalographiques du metoclopramide en psychiatrie. *Therapie* 29:975–995.

Borison RL, Diamond BI, Sinha D, et al (1988) Clozapine withdrawal rebound psychosis. *Psychopharmacol Bull* 24:260–263.

Borland BL, Heckman HK (1976) Hyperactive boys and their brothers: a 25-year follow-up study. *Arch Gen Psychiatry* 33:669–675.

Bornstein B (1961) Restless legs. *Psychiatr Neurol* (Basel) 141:165–201.

Botez MI, Lambert B (1977) Folate deficiency and restless-legs syndrome in pregnancy. *N Engl J Med* 297:670.

374   *References*

Bozzola FG, Gorelick PB, Frels S (1992) Personality changes in Alzheimer's disease. *Arch Neurol* 49:297–300.
Brain Lord, Walton JN (1969) *Brain's Diseases of the Nervous System*. 7th ed. London: Oxford University Press.
Branchey MH, Branchey LB, Bark NM, et al (1979) Lecithin in the treatment of tardive dyskinesia. *Commun Psychopharmacol* 3:303–307.
Braude W, Barnes T (1982) Clonazepam: effective treatment for restless legs syndrome in uraemia. *Br Med J (Clin Res Ed)* 284:510.
Braude WM, Barnes TR (1983) Late-onset akathisia – an indicant of covert dyskinesia: two case reports. *Am J Psychiatry* 140:611–612.
Braude WM, Barnes TR, Gore SM (1983) Clinical characteristics of akathisia: a systematic investigation of acute psychiatric inpatient admissions. *Br J Psychiatry* 143:139–150.
Braude WM, Charles IP, Barnes TR (1984) Coarse, jerky foot tremor: tremographic investigation of an objective sign of acute akathisia. *Psychopharmacology (Berl)* 82:95–101.
Breggin PR (1993) Parallels between neuroleptic effects and lethargic encephalitis: the production of dyskinesias and cognitive disorders. *Brain Cogn* 23:8–27.
Brenning R (1957) Restless legs. *Svenska Lakartidn* 54:2293.
Broadhurst PL (1957) Determinants of emotionality in the rat. I. Situational factors. *Br J Psychol* 48:7–12.
Brodeur C, Montplaisir J, Godbout R, et al (1988a) Treatment of restless legs syndrome and periodic movements during sleep with L-dopa: a double-blind, controlled study. *Neurology* 38:1845–1848.
Brodeur C, Montplaisir J, Godbout R, et al (1988b) Polygraphic features of L-dopa in restless legs syndrome (RLS) and periodic movements during sleep (PMS): a double-blind controlled study. *Sleep Res* 17:149.
Brooke MM, Questad KA, Patterson DR, et al (1992) Agitation and restlessness after closed head injury. *Arch Phys Med Rehabil* 73:320–323.
Brown KW, Glen SE, White T (1987) Low serum iron status and akathisia. *Lancet* 1:1234–1236.
Brown KW, White T (1991a) Pseudoakathisia and schizophrenic negative symptoms. *Acta Psychiatr Scand* 84:107–109.
Brown KW, White T (1991b) The psychological consequences of tardive dyskinesia: the effect of drug-induced parkinsonism and the topography of the dyskinetic movements. *Br J Psychiatry* 159:399–403.
Brown KW, White T (1992) The influence of topography on the cognitive and psychopathological effects of tardive dyskinesia. *Am J Psychiatry* 149:1385–1389.
Brune GG, Morpurgo C, Bielkus A, et al (1962) Relevance of drug-induced extrapyramidal reactions to behavioral changes during neuroleptic treatment. I. Treatment with trifluoperazine singly and in combination with trihexyphenidyl. *Compr Psychiatry* 3(4):227–234.
Bruun R (1982) Dysphoria phenomena associated with haloperidol treatment of Tourette syndrome. In: Friedhoff AJ, Chase TN, eds. *Gilles de la Tourette Syndrome*. New York: Raven Press. pp. 433–436.
Bruun RD (1988) Subtle and underrecognized side effects of neuroleptic treatment in children with Tourette's disorder. *Am J Psychiatry* 145:621–624.
Bucci L (1969) Acute psychotic episodes in patients treated with fluphenazine enanthate [letter]. *Br J Psychiatry* 115:1346.
Bucy PC (1979) Jean Athanse Sicard. In: Haymaker W, Schiller F, eds. *The Founders of Neurology*. Springfield, IL: Thomas. pp. 517–579.

Bui NB, Marit G, Albin H, et al (1982) High dose metoclopramide during cancer chemotherapy: phase II study in 80 consecutive patients. *Bull Cancer* 69: 330–335.

Burke AL, Diamond PL, Hulbert J, et al (1991) Terminal restlessness: its management and the role of midazolam. *Med J Aust* 155:485–487.

Burke RE (1992) Neuroleptic-induced tardive dyskinesia variants. In: Lang AE, Weiner WJ, eds. *Drug-Induced Movement Disorders.* Mt. Kisco, NY: Futura. pp. 167–198.

Burke RE, Kang UJ (1988) Recognizing akathisia as a movement disorder. *Curr Opin Neurol Neurosurg* 1:316–318.

Burke RE, Kang UJ, Fahn S (1987) Tardive akathisia: motor phenomena and treatment. *Neurology* 37(suppl 1):124–125.

Burke RE, Kang UJ, Jankovic J, et al (1989) Tardive akathisia: an analysis of clinical features and response to open therapeutic trials. *Mov Disord* 4:157–175.

Burns A, Jacoby R, Levy R (1990) Psychiatric phenomena in Alzheimer's disease. IV. Disorders of behaviour. *Br J Psychiatry* 157:86–94.

Butler B, Bech P (1987) Neuroleptic profile of cipazoxapine (Savoxepine), a new tetracyclic dopamine antagonist: clinical validation of the hippocampus versus striatum ratio model of dopamine receptors in animals. *Psychopharmacopsychiatry* 20:122–126.

Caine ED, Margolin DI, Brown GL, et al (1978) Gilles de la Tourette's syndrome, tardive dyskinesia and psychosis in an adolescent. *Am J Psychiatry* 135: 241–243.

Caine ED, Polinsky RJ (1979) Haloperidol-induced dysphoria in patients with Tourette Syndrome. *Am J Psychiatry* 136:1216–1217.

Caliguiri MP, Lohr JB, Bracha MS, Jeste DV (1991) Clinical and instrumental assessment of neuroleptic-induced parkinsonism in patients with tardive dyskinesia. *Biol Psychiatry* 29:139–148.

Callahan N (1966) Restless legs syndrome in uremic neuropathy. *Neurology* 16:359–361.

Calmels JP, Sorbette F, Montastruc JL, et al (1982) Iatrogenic hyperkinetic syndrome caused by an antihistaminic (letter). *Nouv Presse Med* 11(30):2296–2297.

Calne DB (1992) Involuntary movements: an overview. In: Joseph AB, Young RR, eds. *Movement Disorders in Neurology and Psychiatry.* Boston: Blackwell Scientific. pp. 1–4.

Carlsson A (1978) Antipsychotic drugs, neurotransmitters, and schizophrenia. *Am J Psychiatry* 135(2):165–173.

Carlsson M, Carlsson A (1989) The NMDA antagonist MK-801 causes marked locomotor stimulation in monoamine-depleted mice. *J Neural Transm* 75:221–226.

Carlsson M, Carlsson A (1990) Interactions between glutamatergic and monoaminergic systems within the basal ganglia: implications for schizophrenia and Parkinson's disease. *Trends Neurosci* 13:272–276.

Carney MWP, Roth M, Garside RF (1965) The diagnosis of depressive syndromes and the prediction of ECT response. *Br J Psychiatry* 3:659–674.

Carp JS, Anderson RJ (1982) Dopamine receptor mediated depression of spinal monosynaptic transmission. *Brain Res* 242:247–254.

Carrazana E, Rossitch E Jr, Martinez J (1989) Unilateral "akathisia" in a patient with AIDS and a toxoplasmosis subthalamic abscess. *Neurology* 39:449–450.

Carrazana EJ, Rossitch E Jr (1989) Unilateral akathisia: reply. *Neurology* 39:1648.

Casey DE (1989) Clozapine: neuroleptic-induced EPS and tardive dyskinesia. *Psychopharmacology (Berl)* 99(suppl):S47–S53.

Casey DE (1993) Serotonergic and dopaminergic aspects of neuroleptic-induced extrapyramidal syndromes in nonhuman primates. *Psychopharmacology* 112: S55–S59.

Casey DE, Denney D (1977) Pharmacological characterization of tardive dyskinesia. *Psychopharmacology* 54:1–8.

Casey DE, Rabins T (1978) Tardive dyskinesia as a life-threatening illness. *Am J Psychiatry* 135(4):486–488.

Chaffin DS (1964) Phenothiazine-induced acute psychotic reaction: the "psychotoxicity" of a drug. *Am J Psychiatry* 121:26–32.

Channabasavanna SM, Goswami U (1984) Akathisia during lithium prophylaxis. *Br J Psychiatry* 144:555–556.

Chen JC, Hardy PA, Clauberg M, et al (1989) T2 values in the human brain: comparison with quantitative assays of iron and ferritin. *Radiology* 173:521–526.

Chevalier G, Deniau JM (1990) Disinhibition as a basic process in the expression of striatal functions. *Trends Neurosci* 13:277–280.

Chien C-P, DiMascio A (1967) Drug-induced extrapyramidal symptoms and their relations to clinical efficacy. *Am J Psychiatry* 123:1490–1498.

Chien CP, DiMascio A, Cole JO (1974) Antiparkinson agents and depot phenothiazine. *Am J Psychiatry* 131:86–90.

Chiles JA (1978) Extrapyramidal reactions in adolescents treated with high-potency antipsychotics. *Am J Psychiatry* 135:239–240.

Chouinard G (1982) Neuroleptic-induced supersensitivity psychosis. In: De Veaugh-Geiss J, ed. *Tardive Dyskinesia and Related Involuntary Movement Disorders*. Bristol, UK: John Wright. pp. 109–115.

Chouinard G, Annable L, Ross-Chouinard A (1986) Supersensitivity psychosis and tardive dyskinesia: a survey of schizophrenic outpatients. *Psychopharmacol Bull* 22:891–896.

Chouinard G, Annable L, Ross-Chouinard A, et al (1979) Factors related to tardive dyskinesia. *Am J Psychiatry* 136:79–82.

Chouinard G, Creese I, Boisvert D, et al (1982) High neuroleptic plasma levels in patients manifesting supersensitivity psychoses. *Biol Psychiatry* 17:707–711.

Chouinard G, Jones B (1980) Neuroleptic-induced supersensitivity psychosis: clinical and pharmacologic characteristics. *Am J Psychiatry* 137:16–21.

Chouinard G, Jones BD, Annable L (1978) Neuroleptic-induced supersensitivity psychosis. *Am J Psychiatry* 135:1409–1410.

Chouinard G, Ross-Chouinard A, Annable L, et al (1980) Extrapyramidal rating scale. *Can J Neurol Sci* 1:233.

Chouza C, Scaramelli A, Caamano JL, et al (1986) Parkinsonism, tardive dyskinesia, akathisia, and depression induced by flunarizine. *Lancet* 1:1303–1304.

Cirignotta F, Zucconi M, Mondini S, et al (1982) Epidemiological data on sleep disorders. *Sleep* 211. Abstract.

Claghorn J, Honigfeld G, Abuzzahab FS, et al (1987) The risks and benefits of clozapine versus chlorpromazine. *J Clin Psychopharmacol* 7:377–384.

Clarke J, Gannon M, Hughes I, et al (1977) Adjunctive behavior in humans in a group gambling situation. *Physiol Behav* 18:159–161.

Clouet DH (1986) *Phencyclidine: An Update*. NPIDA Research Monograph 64. Rockville, MD: US Department of Health and Human Sciences.

Coccagna G (1990) Restless legs syndrome: periodic leg movements in sleep. In: Thorpy MJ, ed. *Handbook of Sleep Disorders*. New York: Dekker. pp. 457–478.

Coccagna G, Lugaresi E (1968) Insomnia in the restless legs syndrome. In: Gastaut H, Lugaresi E, Berti Ceroni G, et al, eds. *The Abnormalities of Sleep in Man*. Bologna: Gaggi. pp. 139–144.

Coccagna G, Lugaresi E (1981) Restless legs syndrome and nocturnal myoclonus. *Int J Neurol* 15:77–87.

Coccagna G, Lugaresi E, Tassarini CA, et al (1966) La sindrome delle gambe senza riposo (restless legs). *Onnia Med Ther* (new series) 44:619–684.

Cohen BM, Keck PE, Satlin A, et al (1991) Prevalence and severity of akathisia in patients on clozapine. *Biol Psychiatry* 29:1215–1219.

Cohen BM, Tsuneizumi T, Baldessarini RJ, et al (1992) Differences between antipsychotic drugs in persistence of brain levels and behavioral effects. *Psychopharmacology* 108:338–344.

Cohen S, Leonard CV, Farberow NL, et al (1964) Tranquilisers and suicide in the schizophrenic patient. *Arch Gen Psychiatry* 11:312–321.

Cohen-Mansfield J (1986) Agitated behaviors in the elderly. II. Preliminary results in the cognitively deteriorated. *J Am Geriatr Soc* 34:722–727.

Cohen-Mansfield J, Billig N (1986) Agitated behaviours in the elderly. I. A conceptual review. *J Am Geriatr Soc* 34:711–721.

Cohen-Mansfield J, Marx MS, Rosenthal AS (1989) A description of agitation in a nursing home. *J Gerontol* 44:M77–84.

Cole J, Gardos G, Gelernter J (1984) Supersensitivity psychosis. *McLean Hosp J* 9:46–72.

Cole JO, Clyde DJ (1961) Extrapyramidal side effects and clinical response to phenothiazines. *Rev Can Biol* 20:565–574.

Coleman RM (1982) Periodic movements in sleep (nocturnal myoclonus) and restless legs syndrome. In: Guilleminault C, ed. *Sleeping and Waking Disorders: Indications and Techniques.* Menlo Park, CA: Addison-Wesley. pp. 265–295.

Coleman RM, Bilwise DL, Sajben N, et al (1983) Epidemiology of periodic movements during sleep. In: Guilleminault C, Lugaresi E, eds. *Sleep/Wake Disorders: Natural History, Epidemiology, and Long-Term Evolution.* New York: Raven. pp. 217–229.

Coleman RM, Pollack CP, Weitzman ED (1978) Periodic nocturnal myoclonus in a wide variety of sleep-wake disorders. *Trans Am Neurol Assoc* 103:230–235.

Coleman RM, Pollak CP, Weitzman ED (1980) Periodic movements in sleep (nocturnal myoclonus): relation to sleep disorders. *Ann Neurol* 8:416–421.

Concise Oxford Dictionary of Current English. (1994) Oxford University Press.

Connolly ME, Kersting F, Dollery CT (1976) The clinical pharmacology of beta-adrenergic blocking agents. *Prog Cardiovasc Dis* 19:203.

Cookson JC, Natorf B, Hunt N, et al (1989) Efficacy, safety and tolerability of raclopride, a specific D2 receptor blocker, in acute schizophrenia: an open trial. *Int Clin Psychopharmacol* 4:61–70.

Cooper JR, Bloom FE, Roth RH (1991) *The Biochemical Basis of Neuropharmacology.* 6th ed. New York: Oxford University Press.

Corrigan JD, Mysiw WJ (1988) Agitation following traumatic head injury: equivocal evidence of a discrete stage of cognitive recovery. *Arch Phys Med Rehabil* 69:487–492.

Cortes R, Palacios JM(1986) Muscarinic cholinergic receptor subtypes in the rat brain: quantitative autoradiographic studies. *Brain Res* 362:227–238.

Cortes R, Probst A, Tobler HJ (1986) Muscarinic cholinergic receptor subtypes in human brain: quantitative autoradiographic studies. *Brain Res* 362:239–253.

Costall B, Naylor RJ (1975) The behavioural effects of dopamine applied intracerebrally to areas of the mesolimbic system. *Eur J Pharmacol* 32:87–92.

Crane GE (1972) Pseudoparkisonism and tardive dyskinesia. *Arch Neurol* 27:426–430.

Crane GE (1973) Persistent dyskinesia. *Br J Psychiatry* 122:395–405.

Crane GE, Naranjo EK, Chase C (1971) Motor disorders induced by neuroleptics: a proposed new classification. *Arch Gen Psychiatry* 24:179–184.

Creese I, Burt DR, Snyder SH (1976) Dopamine receptor binding predicts clinical and pharmacological potencies of antischizophrenic drugs. *Science* 192:481–483.

Creese I, Burt DR, Snyder SH (1977) Dopamine receptor binding predicts clinical and pharmacological potencies of antischizophrenic drugs. *Science* 197:596–598.

Critchley M (1955) The pre-dormitum. *Rev Neurol* 93:101.

Csernansky J, Hollister L (1982) Probable case of supersensitivity psychosis. *Hosp Formulary* 17:395–399.

Csernansky JG, Solman CA, Bonnett KA, et al (1983) Dopaminergic supersensitivity at distant sites following induced epileptic foci. *Life Sci* 32:385–390.

Culver CM, Gert B (1982) *Philosophy in Medicine*. London: Oxford University Press.

Cunningham SL, Richardson GS, Dorsey CM (1991) Polysomnographic features of akathisia syndrome in two patients. *Sleep Res* 20:62.

Curson DA, Barnes TR, Bamber RW, et al (1985) Long-term depot maintenance of chronic schizophrenic out-patients: the seven year follow-up of the Medical Research Council fluphenazine/placebo trial. II. The incidence of compliance problems, side-effects, neurotic symptoms and depression. *Br J Psychiatry* 146:469–474.

Dahl SG (1986) Plasma level monitoring of antipsychotic drugs. *Clin Pharmacokinet* 11:36–61.

Dahlstrom A, Fuxe K (1965) Existence of monoamine-containing neurons in the central nervous system. I. Demonstration of monoamines in the cell bodies of brain stem neurons. *Acta Physiol Scand* 232(suppl):22.

Dallman PR, Siimes MA, Manies EC (1975) Brain iron: persistent deficiency following short-term iron deprivation in the young rat. *Br J Haematol* 31:209–215.

Danel T, Servant D, Goudemand M (1988) Amitriptyline in the treatment of neuroleptic-induced akathisia. *Biol Psychiatry* 23:186–188.

Davis JM (1976) Comparative doses and costs of antipsychotic medication. *Arch Gen Psychiatry* 33:858–861.

Davis K, Rosenberg G (1979) Is there a limbic equivalent of tardive dyskinesia? *Biol Psychiatry* 14:699–703.

Davis RJ, Cummings JL (1988) Clinical variants of tardive dyskinesia. *Neuropsychiat Neuropsychol Behav Neurol* 1(1):31–38.

De Alarcon R, Carney MWP (1969) Severe depressive mood changes following slow-release intra-muscular fluphenazine injection. *Br Med J* 3:564–567.

Deardoff PA, Finch AJ, Royall LR (1974) Manifest anxiety and nail-biting. *J Clin Psychol* 30:378.

Decina P, Mukherjee S, Caracci G, et al (1992) Painful sensory symptoms in neuroleptic-induced extrapyramidal syndromes. *Am J Psychiatry* 149:1075–1080.

De Groen JH, Kamphuisen HA (1978) Periodic nocturnal myoclonus in a patient with hyperplexia (startle disease). *J Neurol Sci* 38:207–213.

De Keyser J, D'Haenen H (1986) Disappearance of akathisia following electroconvulsive treatment. *Clin Neuropharmacol* 9:563–565.

Delay J, Deniker P (1952) 38 cas de psychoses traites par la cure prolongee et continue de 4560 RP. *Rapports et Comptes Rendus: Congrès des Médicins*

Alienistes et Neurologistes de France et des Pays de Langues Françaises 50:503–513.

Delay J, Deniker P (1961) Apport de la clinique a la connaisance de l'action des neuroleptiques. In: Bordeleau J, ed. *Extrapyramidal System and Neuroleptics.* Montreal: Editions Psychiatriques. pp. 301–327.

DeLong MR (1990) Primate models of movement disorders of basal ganglia origin. *Trends Neurosci* 13(7):281–285.

Demars JPCA (1966) Neuromuscular effects of long-term phenothiazine medication, electroconvulsive therapy and leucotomy. *J Nerv Ment Dis* 143:73–79.

Denham P, Carrick DJEL (1961) Therapeutic value of thioproperazine and the importance of the associated neurological disturbances. *J Ment Sci* 107:326–345.

Deniker P (1960) Experimental neurological syndromes and the new drug therapies in psychiatry. *Compr Psychiatry* 1:92–102.

Denny-Brown D (1945) Disability arising from closed head injury. *JAMA* 127: 429–436.

Derom E, Elinck W, Buylaert W, et al (1984) Which beta-blocker for the restless leg? *Lancet* 1:857.

Detre TP, Jarecki HG (1971) *Modern Psychiatric Treatment.* Philadelphia: Lippincott.

DeVeaugh-Geiss J (1982) Prediction and prevention of tardive dyskinesia. In: DeVeaugh-Geiss J, ed. *Tardive Dyskinesia and Related Involuntary Movement Disorders.* Bristol, UK: John Wright, pp. 161–178.

DeVries DJ, Beart PM (1985) Competitive inhibition of [3H]spiroperidol binding to D-2 dopamine receptors in strial homogenates by organic clacium channel antagonists and polyvalent cations. *Eur J Pharmacol* 106:133–139.

Diamond IB, Borison LR (1978) Enkefalins and nigrostriatal function. *Neurology* 28:1085–1088.

Dilsaver SC (1990) Heterocyclic antidepressant, monoamine oxidase inhibitor and neuroleptic withdrawal phenomena. *Prog Neuropsychopharmacol Biol Psychiat* 14:137–161.

Dilsaver SC, Greden JF (1984) Antidepressant withdrawal-induced activation (hypomania and mania): mechanism and theoretical significance [review]. *Brain Res* 319(1):29–48.

DiMascio A, Bernardo DL, Greenblatt DJ, et al (1976) A controlled trial of amantadine in drug-induced extrapyramidal disorders. *Arch Gen Psychiatry* 33:599–602.

DiMascio A, Demirgian E (1970) Antiparkinson drug overuse. *Psychosomatics* 11:596–600.

Director KL, Muniz CE (1982) Diazepam in the treatment of extrapyramidal symptoms: a case report. *J Clin Psychiatry* 43:160–161.

Divry P, Bobon J, Colland J, et al (1960) Psychopharmologie d'un troisieme neuroleptique de la serie des butyrophenones: le R-2498 ou triperidol. *Acta Neurol Beg* 60:465–480.

Donlon PT (1973) The therapeutic use of diazepam for akathisia. *Psychosomatics* 14:222–225.

Donlon PT (1981) Amoxapine: a newly marketed tricyclic antidepressant. *Psychiatric Annals* 11:379–383.

Dorland WAN (1951) *American Illustrated Medical Dictionary.* 22nd ed. Philadelphia: Saunders.

Drake RE, Ehrlich J (1985) Suicide attempts associated with akathisia. *Am J Psychiatry* 142:499–501.

Drayer B, Burger P, Darwin R, et al (1986) Magnetic resonance imaging of brain iron. *AJNR* 7:373–380.

Dressler D, Thompson PD, Gledhill RF, et al (1994) The syndrome of painful legs and moving toes. *Mov Disord* 9(1):13–21.

Dubin WR (1988) Rapid tranquilization: antipsychotics or benzodiazepines. *J Clin Psychiatry* 49(12, suppl):5–11.

Dufresne RL, Wagner RL (1988) Antipsychotic-withdrawal akathisia vesus antipsychotic-induced akathisia: further evidence for the existence of tardive akathisia. *J Clin Psychiatry* 49:435–438.

Dumon JP, Catteau J, Lanvin F, et al (1992) Randomized, double-blind, crossover, placebo-controlled comparison of propranolol and betaxolol in the treatment of neuroleptic-induced akathisia. *Am J Psychiatry* 149:647–650.

Dupuis B, Catteau J, Dumon JP, et al (1987) Comparison of propranolol, sotalol, and betaxolol in the treatment of neuroleptic-induced akathisia. *Am J Psychiatry* 144:802–805.

Dustan R, Jackson DM (1976) The demonstration of a change in adrenergic receptor sensitivity in the central nervous system of mice after withdrawal from long-term treatment with haloperidol. *Psychopharmacology* 48:105–114.

Dzvonik ML, Kripke DF, Klauber M, et al (1986) Body position changes and periodic movements in sleep. *Sleep* 9(4):484–491.

Editorial (1986) Akathisia and antipsychotic drugs. *Lancet* 2:1131–1132.

Egawa I (1987) A polysomnographic study of restless legs syndrome in patients under haemodialysis treatment. *Sleep Res* 16:330.

Egger M, Smith GD, Teuscher AU, et al (1991) Influence of human insulin on symptoms and awareness of hypoglycaemia: a randomised double blind crossover trial. *Br Med J* 303:622–626.

Ehlert FJ, Roeske WR, Itoga E, et al (1982) The binding of [3H]nitrendipine to receptors for calcium antagonists in the heart, cerebral cortex and ileum of rats. *Life Sci* 30:2191–2202.

Ehrenberg BL (1992) Sleep pathologies associated with nocturnal movements. In: Joseph AB, Young RR, eds. *Movement Disorders in Neurology and Neuropsychiatry.* Boston: Blackwell Scientific. pp. 634–648.

Ehyai A, Kilroy AW, Fenichel GM (1978) Dyskinesia and akathisia induced by ethosuximide. *Am J Dis Child* 132:527–528.

Ekblom B, Eriksson K, Lindstrom L (1984) Supersensitivity psychosis in schizophrenic patients after sudden clozapine withdrawal. *Psychopharmacology* 83:293–294.

Ekbom KA (1944) Asthenia crurum parasthetica (irritable legs). *Acta Med Scand* 118:197–198.

Ekbom KA (1945) Restless legs: a clinical study. *Acta Med Scand Suppl* 158:1–6.

Ekbom KA (1946a) Restless legs. *JAMA* 131:481–486.

Ekbom KA (1946b) Parastesier. *Nord Med* 31:1651.

Ekbom KA (1950) Restless legs: a report of 70 new cases. *Acta Med Scand Suppl* 246:64.

Ekbom KA (1955) Restless legs som tidisymtom vid cancer. *Svenska Lakartidn* 52:1875–1878.

Ekbom KA (1960) Restless legs syndrome. *Neurology* 10:868–873.

Ekbom KA (1965) Restless legs. *Swed Med J* 62:2376–2378.

Ekbom KA (1966) Restless legs syndrome after partial gastrectomy. *Acta Neurol Scand* 42:79–84.

Ekbom KA (1975) Growing pains and restless legs. *Acta Paediatr Scand* 64:264–266.

Eli Lilly Pty Ltd (1993) *Fluoxetine: Product Information.* Eli Lilly Pty Ltd.

Emery VOB, Oxman TE (1992) Update on the dementia spectrum of depression. *Am J Psychiatry* 149:305–317.

Engel J, Berggren U (1980) Effects of lithium on behavior and central monoamines. *Acta Psychiatr Scand* 61(suppl 280):133–142.

Evans JH (1965) Persistent oral dyskinesia in treatment with phenothiazine derivatives. *Lancet* 1:458–460.

Evans LK (1987) Sundown syndrome in institutionalized elderly. *J Am Geriatr Soc* 35:101–108.

Eysenck HJ, Eysenck SBG (1964) *Manual of the Eysenck Personality Inventory.* Sevenoaks, Kent: Hodder & Stoughton.

Fabre L, Slotnick V, Jones V, et al (1990) ICI 204.636, a novel atypical antipsychotic: early indications for safety and efficacy in man. In: *Abstracts of the 17th Congress of CINP.* Kyoto, Japan. p. 223.

Fahn S (1985) A therapeutic approach to tardive dyskinesia. *J Clin Psychiatry* 46:19–24.

Fahn S, Marsden D, Van Woert MH (1986) Definition and classification of myoclonus. *Adv Neurol* 43:1–5.

Fallon JH, Allen JD, Butler JA (1979) Assessment of adjunctive behaviors in humans using a stringent control procedure. *Physiol Behav* 22:1089–1092.

Fann WE, Lake CR (1974) On the coexistence of parkinsonism and tardive dyskinesia. *Dis Nerv Syst* 35:324–326.

Fann WE, Lake CR, Gerber CJ, et al (1974) Cholinergic suppression of tardive dyskinesia. *Psychopharmacology (Berlin)* 37:101–107.

Fann WE, Stafford JE, Malone RL, et al (1977) Clinical research techniques in tardive dyskinesia. *Am J Psychiatry* 134:759–762.

Farde L, Grind M, Nilsson MI, et al (1988) Remoxipride – a new potential antipsychotic drug: pharmacological effects and pharmacokinetics following repeated oral administration in male volunteers. *Psychopharmacology (Berlin)* 95:157–161.

Farde L, Nordstrom A, Weisel F, et al (1992) Positron emisson tomographic analysis of central D1 and D2 dopamine receptor occupancy in patients treated with classical neuroleptics and clozapine. *Arch Gen Psychiatry* 49:539–544.

Faull KF, Guilleminault C, Berger PA, et al (1983) Cerebrospinal fluid monoamine metabolites in narcolepsy and hypersomnia. *Ann Neurol* 13:258–263.

Feest T, Read D (1982) Response to Braude & Barnes. *Br Med J* 284:510.

Feinberg M, Carroll BJ (1982) Separation of subtypes of depression using discriminant analyses. *Br J Psychiatry* 140:384–391.

Feindel W (1970) Thomas Willis. In: Haymaker W, Schiller F, eds. *The Founders of Neurology.* Springfield, IL: Thomas. pp. 91–98.

Findley L, Gresty M, Halmagyi G (1981) Tremor, the cogwheel phenomenon and clonus in Parkinson's disease. *J Neurol Neurosurg Psychiatry* 44:534–546.

Fleischhacker WW, Bergmann KJ, Perovich R, et al (1989) The Hillside Akathisia Scale: a new rating instrument for neuroleptic-induced akathisia. *Psychopharmacol Bull* 25:222–226.

Fleischhacker WW, Miller CH, Barnes C, et al (1993) The effect of activation procedures on neuroleptic-induced akathisia. *Br J Psychiatry* 163:781–784.

Fleischhacker WW, Miller CH, Schett P, et al (1991) The Hillside Akathisia Scale: a reliability comparison of the English and German versions. *Psychopharmacology (Berlin)* 105:141–144.

Fleischhacker WW, Roth SD, Kane JM (1990) The pharmacologic treatment of neuroleptic-induced akathisia [see comments]. *J Clin Psychopharmacol* 10:12–21.

Fleischhauer J (1978) [Dose-effect relations. Double-blind study on two different doses of pimozide (author's transl.)] Beziehungen zwischen Dosishohe und Behandlungsergebnis. Doppelbinduntersuchung mit Pimozid in zwei Dosierungen. *Arzneimittelforschung* 28:1491–1492.

Fornazzari L, Remington G, Jeffries J (1991) Akathisia, porphyria and low iron. *Can J Psychiatry* 36:548.

Forrest DV, Fahn S (1979) Tardive dysphrenia and subjective akathisia. *J Clin Psychol* 40:206.

Fowler HW (1983) *A Dictionary of English Usage.* Oxford: Oxford University Press, 1983.

Frankel BL, Patten BM, Gillin JC (1974) Restless legs syndrome: sleep-electroencephalographic and neurologic findings. *JAMA* 230:1302–1303.

Freedman DX, De Jong J (1961) Factors that determine drug-induced akathisia. *Dis Nerv Syst* 22(suppl):69–76.

Freyhan FA (1957) Psychomotility and parkinsonism in treatment with neuroleptic drugs. *Arch Neurol Psychiatry* 78:465–472.

Freyhan FA (1958) *Extrapyramidal Symptoms and Other Side Effects in Trifluoperazine: Clinical and Pharmacological Aspects.* Philadelphia: Lea & Febiger.

Freyhan FA (1959) Therapeutic implications of differential effects of new phenothiazine compounds. *Am J Psychiatry* 115:577–585.

Freyhan FA (1961) The relationship of drug-induced neurological phenomena and therapeutic outcome. *Rev Can Biol* 20:579–582.

Friedman E, Gershon S (1973) Effects of lithium on brain dopamine. *Nature* 243:520–521.

Friedman JH (1992) Drug-induced parkinsonism. In: Lang AE, Weiner WJ, eds. *Drug-induced Movement Disorders.* New York: Futura. pp. 41–83.

Friis T, Christensen TR, Gerlach J (1983) Sodium valproate and biperiden in neuroleptic-induced akathisia, parkinsonism and hyperkinesia: a double-blind cross-over study with placebo. *Acta Psychiatr Scand* 67:178–187.

Fuxe K, Bolme P, Agnati L, et al (1976) The effect of DL- and D-propranolol on central monoamine neurones. I. Studies on dopamine mechanisms. *Neurosci Lett* 3:45–52.

Gagrat D, Hamilton J, Belmaker RH (1978) Intravenous diazepam in the treatment of neuroleptic-induced acute dystonia and akathisia. *Am J Psychiatry* 135:1232–1233.

Galan P, Hercberg S, Touitou Y (1984) The activity of tissue enzymes in iron-deficient rat and man: an overview. *Comp Biochem Physiol* 77B:647–653.

Galdi J (1983) The causality of depression in schizophrenia. *Br J Psychiatry* 142:621–625.

Galdi J, Bonato RR (1988) Relationship of adverse drug reactions to length of hospital-stay in genetically subgrouped schizophrenics. *Can J Psychiatry* 33:816–818.

Galdi J, Reider RO, Silber D, et al (1981) Genetic factors in the response to neuroleptics in schizophrenia: a psychopharmacogenetic study. *Psychol Med* 11:713–728.

Galey D, Simon H, Le Moal M (1977) Behavioural effects of lesions in the A10 dopaminergic area of the rat. *Brain Res* 124:83–97.

Gallagher-Thompson D, Brooks JO III, Bliwise D, et al (1992) The relations along caregiver stress, "sundowning" symptoms, and cognitive decline in Alzheimer's disease. *J Am Geriatr Soc* 40:807–810.

Ganesh S, Murti Rao J, Cowie VA (1989) Akathisia in neuroleptic mediated mentally handicapped subjects. *J Ment Defic Res* 33:323–329.

Ganzini L, Heintz R, Hoffman WF, et al (1991) Acute extrapyramidal syndromes in neuroleptic-treated elders: a pilot study. *J Geriatr Psychiatry Neurol* 4:222–225.

Gardner-Medwin D, Walton JN (1969) Myokymia with impaired muscular relaxation. *Lancet* 1(601):943–944.

Gardos G, Cole JO (1980) Problems in the assessment of tardive dyskinesia. In: Fann WE, Smith RC, Davis JM, eds. *Tardive Dyskinesia, Research and Treatment.* New York: Spectrum. pp. 201–214.

Gardos G, Cole JO, La Brie R (1977) The assessment of tardive dyskinesia. *Arch Gen Psychiatry* 34:1206–1212.

Gardos G, Cole JO, Salomon M, et al (1987) Clinical forms of severe tardive dyskinesia. *Am J Psychiatry* 144:895–902.

Gardos G, Cole JO, Sniffin C (1976) An evaluation of papaverine in tardive dyskinesia. *J Clin Pharmacol* 16:304–310.

Gardos G, Cole JO, Tarsy D (1978) Withdrawal syndromes associated with antipsychotic drugs. *Am J Psychiatry* 135:1321–1324.

Gardos G, Teicher MH, Lipinski JF Jr, et al (1992) Quantitative assessment of psychomotor activity in patients with neuroleptic-induced akathisia. *Prog Neuropsychopharmacol Biol Psychiatry* 16:27–37.

Gattaz WF, Riederer P, Reynolds GP, et al (1983) Dopamine and noradrenaline in the cerebrospinal fluid of schizophrenic patients. *Psychiatry Res* 8:243–50.

Gawin FH, Ellinwood EH Jr (1988) Cocaine and other stimulants: actions, abuse and treatment. *N Engl J Med* 318:1173–1182.

Gelenberg AJ (1978) Amantadine in the treatment of benztropine refractory extrapyramidal disorders induced by antipsychotic drugs. *Curr Ther Res* 22:375–380.

Gerber MR, Connor JR (1989) Do oligodendrocytes mediate iron regulation in the human brain? *Ann Neurol* 26:95–98.

Gerlach J (1991) New antipsychotics: classification, efficacy, and adverse effects. *Schizophr Bull* 17:97–118.

Gerlach J, Korsgaard S (1983) Classification of abnormal involuntary movements in psychiatric patients. *Neuropsychiat Clin* 2:201–208.

Gerlach J, Korsgaard S, Clemmesen P, et al (1993) The St. Hans Rating Scale for extrapyramidal syndromes: reliability and validity. *Acta Psychiatr Scand* 87:244–252.

Giannini AJ, Houser WL, Lorselle RH, et al (1984) Antimanic effects of verapamil. *Am J Psychiatry* 141:1602–1603.

Giardini V (1985) Conditioned taste aversion to chlorpromazine, but not to haloperidol. *Psychopharmacology* 86:81–83.

Gibb WR, Lees AJ (1986a) The clinical phenomenon of akathisia. *J Neurol Neurosurg Psychiatry* 49:861–866.

Gibb WR, Lees AJ (1986b) The restless legs syndrome. *Postgrad Med J* 62:329–333.

Gilbert GJ (1975) Response of hemiballismus to haloperidol. *JAMA* 233:535–536.

Gimenez-Roldan S, Mateo D (1991) Cinnarizine-induced parkinsonism: susceptibility related to aging and essential tremor. *Clin Neuropharmacol* 14:156–164.

Gingrich JA, Caron MG (1993) Recent advances in the molecular biology of dopamine receptors. *Annu Rev Neurosci* 16:299–321.

Ginsberg HN (1986) Propranolol in the treatment of restless legs syndrome induced by imipramine withdrawal. *Am J Psychiatry* 143:938.

Glazer WM, Morgenstern H, Niedzwiecki D, et al (1988) Heterogeneity of tardive
    dyskinesia: a multivariate analysis. *Br J Psychiatry* 124:253–259.
Godbout R, Montplaisir J, Poirier G (1987) Epidemiological data in familial rest-
    less legs syndrome. *Sleep Res* 16:338.
Godbout R, Montplaisir J, Poirier G, et al (1988) Distinctive electrographic mani-
    festations of periodic leg movements during sleep in narcoleptic vs insomnic
    patients. *Sleep Res* 17:182.
Godwin-Austen RB, Lee PN, Marmot MG, et al (1982) Smoking and Parkinson's
    disease. *J Neurol Neurosurg Psychiatry* 45:577–581.
Goetz CG, Tanner C, Levy M, et al (1986) Pain in Parkinson's disease. *Mov
    Disord* 1:45–49.
Goff DC, Midha KK, Brotman AW, et al (1991) An open trial of buspirone added
    to neuroleptics in schizophrenic patients. *J Clin Psychopharmacol* 11:193–197.
Goldberg E (1985) Akinesia, tardive dysmentia and frontal lobe disorder in schizo-
    phrenia. *Schizophr Bull* 11:255–263.
Goldman D (1958) The results of treatment of psychotic states with newer phe-
    nothiazine compounds effective in small doses. *Am J Med Sci* 235:67–77.
Goldman D (1961) Parkinsonian and related phenomena from administration of
    drugs: their production and control under clinical conditions and possible rela-
    tion to therapeutic effect. *Rev Can Biol* 20:549–560.
Goldstein JA (1984) Calcium and neurotransmission. *Biol Psychiatry* 19:465–466.
Gorman CA, Dyck PJ, Pearson JS (1965) Symptom of restless legs. *Arch Intern
    Med* 115:155–160.
Goswami U, Channabasavanna SM (1984) Is akathisia a forerunner of tardive
    dyskinesia? A clinical report with brief review of literature. *Clin Neurol
    Neurosurg* 86:107–110.
Graham-Pole J, Weare J, Engel S, et al (1986) Antiemetics in children receiving
    cancer chemotherapy: a double-blind prospective randomized study comparing
    metoclopramide with chlorpromazine. *J Clin Oncol* 4:1110–1113.
Grahame-Smith DG (1971) Studies in vivo on the relationship between brain tryp-
    tophan, brain 5-HT synthesis and hyperactivity in rats treated with a mono-
    amine oxidase inhibitor and L-tryptophan. *J Neurochem* 18(6):1053–1066.
Grandy DK, Civelli O (1992) G-Protein-coupled receptors: the new dopamine re-
    ceptor subtypes. *Curr Opin Neurobiol* 2:275–281.
Graybiel AM (1990) Neurotransmitters and neuromodulators in the basal ganglia.
    Trends Neurosci 13:244–254.
Green AR, Grahame-Smith DG (1974) The role of brain dopamine in the hyperac-
    tivity syndrome produced by increased 5-hydroxytryptamine synthesis in rats.
    Neuropharmacology 13:949–959.
Greendyke RM, Kanter DR (1986) Therapeutic effects of pindolol on behavioral
    disturbances associated with organic brain disease: a double-blind study. *J
    Clin Psychiatry* 47:423–426.
Greendyke RM, Kanter DR (1987) Plasma propranolol levels and their effect on
    thioridazine and haloperidol concentrations. *J Clin Psychopharmacol* 7:178–
    182.
Grillner S (1973) Locomotion in the spinal cat. In: Stein RB, Pearson KG, Smith RS,
    et al, eds. *Control of Posture and Locomotion.* New York: Plenum. pp. 515–
    535.
Grinker RR, Sahs AL (1966) *Neurology.* 6th ed. Springfield, IL: Thomas.
Gualtieri C, Quade D, Hicks R, et al (1984) Tardive dyskinesia and other clinical
    consequences of neuroleptic treatment in children and adolescents. *Am J
    Psychiatry* 141:20–23.

Gualtieri CT (1993) The problem of tardive akathisia. *Brain Cogn* 23:102–109.

Gualtieri CT, Barnhill J, McGinsey J, et al (1980) Tardive dyskinesia and other movement disorders in children treated with psychotropic drugs. *J Am Acad Child Psychiatry* 19:491–510.

Gualtieri CT, Schroeder SR, Hicks RE, et al (1986) Tardive dyskinesia in young mentally retarded individuals. *Arch Gen Psychiatry* 43:335–340.

Guilleminault C (1982) *Sleeping and Waking Disorders.* Menlo Park, CA: Addison-Wesley.

Guilleminault C, Cetel M, Philip P (1993) Dopaminergic treatment of restless legs and rebound phenomenon. *Neurology* 43:445.

Guilleminault C, Flagg W (1984) Effect of baclofen on sleep-related periodic leg movements. *Ann Neurol* 15:234–239.

Guilleminault C, Raynal D, Weitzman ED, et al (1975) Sleep related periodic my-oclonus in patients complaining of insomnia. *Trans Am Neurol Assoc* 100: 19–21.

Gunne L-M, Haggstrom J-E, Sjoquist B (1984) Association with persistent neu-roleptic-induced dyskinesia of regional changes in brain GABA synthesis. *Nature* 309:347–349.

Haase HJ (1959) The role of drug-induced extrapyramidal syndromes. In: Kline N, ed. *Psychopharmacology Frontiers.* Boston: Little, Brown. pp. 197–208.

Haase HJ (1961) Extrapyramidal modification of fine movements: a 'condition sine qua non' of fundamental therapeutic action of neuroleptic drugs. *Rev Can Biol* 20:425–449.

Hagan RM, Butler A, Hill JM, et al (1987) Effect of the 5-HT3 receptor antago-nist, GR38032F, on responses to injection of a neurokinin agonist into the ventral tegmental area of rat brain. *Eur J Pharmacol* 138:303–305.

Haines J, Sainsbury P (1972) Ultrasound system for measuring patients' activity and movement disorder. *Lancet* 2:802–803.

Hall CS (1934) Emotional behavior in the rat. I. Defecation and urination as mea-sures of individual differences in emotionality. *J Comp Psychol* 18:385–483.

Hallberg L, Bengtsson B, Garby L, et al (1979) An analysis of factors leading to a reduction in iron deficiency in Swedish women. *Bull W H O* 57:947–954.

Hallgren B, Sourander P (1958) The effect of age on the non-hemin iron in the hu-man brain. *J Neurochem* 3:41–51.

Hamel M, Gold DP, Andres D, et al (1990) Predictors and consequences of aggres-sive behavior by community-based dementia patients. *Gerontologist* 30:206–211.

Hamilton M (1989) Depressive disorders. In: Kaplan RI, Sadock BJ, eds. *Comprehensive Textbook of Psychiatry.* 5th ed., Vol. 1. Baltimore: Williams & Wilkins. pp. 892–912.

Hamilton M, White JM (1959) Clinical syndromes in depressive states. *J Ment Sci* 105:985–998.

Hamilton MS, Opler LA (1992) Akathisia, suicidality, and fluoxetine. *J Clin Psychiatry* 53:401–406.

Hamilton N (1967) Development of a rating scale for primary depressive illness. *Br J Social Clin Psychol* 6:278–296.

Hammer R, Giachetti A (1982) Muscarinic receptor subtypes: M1 and M2, bio-chemical and functional characterization. *Life Sci* 31:2991–2998.

Handwerker JV Jr, Palmer RF (1985) Clonidine in the treatment of "restless leg" syndrome. *N Engl J Med* 313:1228–1229.

Harriman DG, Taverner D, Woolf AL (1970) Ekbom's syndrome and burning paraesthesiae: a biopsy study by vital staining and electron microscopy of the intramuscular innervation with a note on age changes in motor nerve endings in distal muscles. *Brain* 93:393–406.

Harris JC, Tune LE, Allen M, et al (1981) Management of akathisia in a severely retarded adolescent male with help of an anticholinergic drug assay. *Lancet* 2:414.

Haskovec L (1902) Akathisie. *Arch Bohemes Med Clin* 17:704–708.

Haymaker W (1970) Kinnier Wilson. In: Haymaker K, Schiller F, eds. *The Founders of Neurology*. Springfield, IL: Thomas. pp. 535–542.

Heiman EM, Christie M (1986) Lithium-aggravated nocturnal myoclonus and restless legs syndrome. *Am J Psychiatry* 143:1191–1192.

Heinze EG, Frame B, Fine G (1967) Restless legs and orthostatic hypotension in primary amyloidosis. *Arch Neurol* 16:497–500.

Helms PM (1985) Efficacy of antipsychotics in the treatment of the behavioral complications of dementia. *J Am Geriatr Soc* 33:206–209.

Henderson D, Gillespie RD (1956) *A Textbook of Psychiatry*, 8th ed. London: Oxford University Press.

Hening W, Walters A, Cote L, et al (1983) Opiate responsive myoclonus. *Ann Neurol* 14:112.

Hening WA, Walters A, Kavey N, et al (1986) Dyskinesias while awake and periodic movements in sleep in restless legs syndrome: treatment with opioids. *Neurology* 36:1363–1366.

Hening WA, Walters AS (1989) Successful long-term therapy of the restless legs syndrome with opioid medication. *Sleep* 18:241.

Henniger G, DiMascio A, Klerman GL (1965) Personality factors in variability of response to phenothiazines. *Am J Psychiatry* 121:1091–1094.

Henningfield JE, Goldberg SR (1983) Nicotine as a reinforcer in human subjects and laboratory animals. *Pharmacol Biochem Behav* 19:989–992.

Hermesh H, Aizenberg D, Friedberg G, et al (1992) Electroconvulsive therapy for persistent neuroleptic-induced akathisia and parkinsonism: a case report. *Biol Psychiatry* 31:407–411.

Hermesh H, Molcho A, Munitz H (1988) Successful propranolol therapy for neuroleptic-induced akathisia resistant to anticholinergic and benzodiazpine drugs. *Clin Neuropharmacol* 11:369–372.

Hershon HI, Kennedy PF, McGuire RJ (1972) Persistence of extrapyramidal disorders and psychiatric relapse after withdrawal of long-term phenothiazine therapy. *Br J Psychiatry* 117:152–153.

Heylen SLE, Gelders YG (1992) Risperidone: a new antipsychotic with serotonin 5-HT2 and dopamine D2 antagonistic properties. *Clin Neuropharmacol* 15:180A–181A.

Hill JM (1988) The distribution of iron in the brain. In: Youdim MBH, ed. *Brain Iron: Neurochemistry and Behavioral Aspects*. London: Taylor & Francis. pp. 1–24.

Hill JM, Ruff MR, Weber RJ, et al (1985) Transferrin receptors in rat brain: neuropeptide-like pattern and the relationship to iron distribution. *Proc Natl Acad Sci USA* 82(3):4553–4557.

Hinsey JC, Ranson SW, McNattin RF (1930) The role of the hypothalamus and mesencephalon in locomotion. *Arch Neurol Psychiat* 23:1–43.

Hirsch SR (1982) Depression "revealed" in schizophrenia. *Br J Psychiatry* 140:421–424.

Hirsch SR (1983) The causality of depression in schizophrenia. *Br J Psychiatry* 142:624–625.

Hodge JR (1959) Akathisia: the syndrome of motor restlessness. *Am J Psychiatry* 116:337–338.

Hoeck A, Demmel U, Schicha H (1975) Trace element concentration in human brain: activation analysis of cobalt, iron, selenium, zinc, chromium, silver, cesium, antimony and scandium. *Brain* 98:49–64.

Hoffmeister F (1975) Negative reinforcing properties of some psychotropic drugs in drug-naive rhesus monkeys. *J Pharmacol Exp Ther* 192:468–477.

Hoffmeister F (1977) Reinforcing properties of perphenazine, haloperidol and amitriptyline in rhesus monkeys. *J Pharmacol Exp Ther* 200:516–522.

Hogarty GE, Schooler NR, Ulrich R, et al (1979) Fluphenazine and social therapy in the aftercare of schizophrenic patients: relapse analyses of a two-year study of fluphenazine decanoate and fluphenazine hydrochloride. *Arch Gen Psychiatry* 36:1283–1294.

Hollister LE (1957) Medical progress: complications from the use of tranquilizing drugs. *N Engl J Med* 257:170–177.

Hollister LE (1961) Current concepts in therapy: complications from psychotherapeutic drugs. *N Engl J Med* 264:291–293.

Hollister LE (1992) Neuroleptic dysphoria: So what's new? *Biol Psychiatry* 31: 531–537.

Hollister LE, Eikenberry DJ, Raffel S (1960) Chlorpromazine in nonpsychotic patients with pulmonary tuberculosis. *Ann Rev Resp Dis* 81:562–566.

Holman RB, Seagraves E, Elliott GR, et al (1976) Stereotyped hyperactivity in rats treated with tranylcypromine and specific inhibitors of 5-HT reuptake. *Behavioral Biology* 16:507–514.

Hordern A (1965) *Depressive States: A Pharmacotherapeutic Study.* Springfield, IL: Thomas.

Horiguchi J (1991) Low serum iron in patients with neuroleptic-induced akathisia and dystonia under antipsychotic drug treatment. *Acta Psychiatr Scand* 84:301–303.

Horiguchi J, Inami Y, Sasaki A, et al (1992) Periodic leg movements in sleep with restless legs syndrome: effect of clonazepam treatment. *Jpn J Psychiatry Neurol* 46:727–732.

Horiguchi J, Nishimatsu O (1992) Usefulness of antiparkinsonian drugs during neuroleptic treatment and the effect of clonazepam on akathisia and parkinsonism occurred after antiparkinsonian drug withdrawal: a double-blind study. *Jpn J Psychiatry Neurol* 46:733–739.

Hornykiewicz O (1966) Dopamine (3-hydroxytyramine) and brain functions. *Pharmacol Rev* 18:925–964.

Hsiao JK, Bartko JJ, Potter ZZ (1989) Diagnosing diagnoses: receiver operating characteristic methods and psychiatry. *Arch Gen Psychiatry* 46:664–667.

Hudson AJ, Brown WF, Gilbert JJ (1978) The muscular pain-fasciculation syndrome. *Neurology* 28:1105–1109.

Hughes JR, Hatsukami D (1986) Signs and symptoms of tobacco withdrawal. *Arch Gen Psychiatry* 43:289–294.

Huizinga J (1957) Hereditary acromelalgia. *Acta Gen* 7:121–123.

Hullett FJ, Levy AB (1983) Amoxapine-induced akathisia. *Am J Psychiatry* 140:820.

Hunter R, Earl CJ, Thornicroff S (1964) An apparently irreversible syndrome of abnormal movements following phenothiazine medication. *Proc R Soc Med* 57:758–762.

Hwang E, Van Woert M (1980) Acute versus chronic effects of serotonin uptake blockers on potentiation of the serotonin syndrome. *Commun Psychopharmacol* 4:161–176.

Hyman SE, Arana GW (1987) *Handbook of Psychiatric Drug Therapy.* Boston: Little, Brown. pp. 115–123.

Iager A-C, Kirch DG, Wyatt RJ (1985) A negative symptom rating scale. *Psychiatry Res* 16:27–36.

Inada T, Ichikawa T, Kato Y, et al (1988) A case of tardive akathisia. *Japan J Psychiatric Treat* 3:772–774.

Inada T, Yagi G, Kaijima K, et al (1991) Clinical variants of tardive dyskinesia in Japan. *Japan J Psychiatry Neurol* 45:67–71.

Ioannou C (1992) Media coverage versus fluoxetine as the cause of suicidal ideation [letter]. *Am J Psychiatry* 149:572.

Ireland WW (1877) *On Idiocy and Imbecility.* London: Churchill.

Irwin M, Sullivan G, Van Putten T (1988) Propranolol as a primary treatment of neuroleptic-induced akathisia. *Hillside J Clin Psychiatry* 10:244–250.

Iversen SD, Wilkinson S, Simpson B (1971) Enhanced amphetamine responses after frontal cortex lesions in the rat. *Eur J Pharmacol* 13:387–390.

Jablensky A (1978) *Psychological Impairments Rating Schedule.* Geneva: World Health Organization.

Jacobs BL, Wise WD, Taylor KM (1974) Differential behavioral and neurochemical effects following lesions of the doral or median raphe nuclei in rats. *Brain Res* 79:353–361.

Jacobs MB (1983) Diltiazem and akathisia. *Ann Intern Med* 99:794–795.

Jacobsen JH, Rosenberg RS, Huttenlocker PR, et al (1986) Familial nocturnal cramping. *Sleep* 9:54–60.

Jaffe JH (1989) Drug dependence: opioids, nonnarcotics, nicotine (tobacco), and caffeine. In: Kaplan RI, Sadock BJ, eds. *Comprehensive Textbook of Psychiatry.* 5th ed. Baltimore: Williams & Wilkins. pp. 642–686.

Jann MW, Saklad SR, Ereshefsky L, et al (1985) Effects of smoking on fluphenazine clearance in psychiatric inpatients. *Biol Psychiatry* 20:329–352.

Janssen PAJ, Niemegeers CJE, Awouters F, et al (1988) Pharmacology of risperidone (R 64 766): A new antipsychotic with serotonin-S2 and dopamine-D2 antagonistic properties. *J Pharmacol Exp Ther* 244:685–693.

Janssen Research Foundation (1992) Risperidone in the treatment of chronic schizophrenic patients: an international multicentre double-blind parallel-group comparative study versus haloperidol. *Clin Res Rep* RIS-INT-2. Beerse, Belgium: Janssen Research Foundation. pp. 1–27.

Jaspers K (1963) *General Psychopathology.* Hoenig J, Hamilton MW, trans. Chicago: University of Chicago Press.

Javoy-Agid F, Agid Y (1980) Is the mesocortical dopaminergic system involved in Parkinson disease? *Neurology* 30:1326–1330.

Jelliffe SC (1932) *Psychopathology of Forced Movements and the Oculogyric Crises of Lethargic Encephalitis.* Washington, DC: Nervous & Mental Disease Publishing.

Jeste DV, Caligiuri MP (1993) Tardive dyskinesia. *Schizophr Bull* 19(2):303–315.

Jeste DV, Wyatt RJ (1982) *Understanding and Treating Tardive Dyskinesia.* New York: Guilford.

Johnson DAW (1981) Studies of depressive symptoms in schizophrenia. *Br J Psychiatry* 139:89–101.

Johnson J (1969) Depressive changes after fluphenazine treatment. *Br Med J* 3:718.

Jolivet B (1953) *Paresthésies agitantes nocturnes des membres inférieurs, impatiences.* These de Paris (unpublished).

Jones MR (1943a) Studies in 'nervous' movements. I. The effect of mental arithmetic on the frequency and patterning of movements. *J Gen Psychol* 29:47–62.

Jones MR (1943b) Studies in 'nervous' movements. II. The effect of inhibition of micturition on the frequency and patterning of movements. *J Gen Psychol* 29:303–312.

Judah LN, Josephs ZM, Murphree OD (1961) Results of simultaneous abrupt withdrawal of ataraxics in 500 chronic psychotic patients. *Am J Psychiatry* 118:156–158.

Jungmann E, Schoffling K (1982) Akathisia and metoclopramide. *Lancet* 2:221.

Jus A, Pineau R, Lachance R, et al (1976) Epidemiology of tardive dyskinesia. II. *Dis Nerv Syst* 37(5):257–261.

Kabes J, Sikora J, Pisvecj J, et al (1982) Effect of piracetam on extrapyramidal side effects induced by neuroleptic drugs. *Int Pharmacopsychiatry* 17:185–192.

Kachanoff R, Leveille R, McLelland JP, et al (1973) Schedule induced behavior in humans. *Physiol Behav* 11:395–398.

Kalinowsky LB (1958) Appraisal of the 'tranquilizers' and their influence on other somatic treatments in psychiatry. *Am J Psychiatry* 115:294–300.

Kameyama T, Suzuki M, Nameshima T (1980) Effects of 5-hydroxytryptamine on defecation in open-field behavior in rats. *Pharmacol Biochem Behav* 12(6): 875–882.

Kane J, Honigfeld G, Singer J, et al (1988) Clozapine for the treatment-resistant schizophrenic: a double-blind comparison with chlorpromazine. *Arch Gen Psychiatry* 45:789–796.

Kane J, Woerner M, Borenstein M (1986) Integrating incidence and prevalence of tardive dyskinesia. *Psychopharmacol Bull* 22:254–258.

Kane JM (1990) Treatment programme and long-term outcome in chronic schizophrenia. *Acta Psychiatr Scand* 358:151–157.

Karn WN Jr, Kasper S (1959) Pharmacologically induced Parkinson-like signs as index of therapeutic potential. *Dis Nerv Syst* 20:284–293.

Kastin AJ, Kullender S, Borglin NE, et al (1968) Extrapigmentary effects of melanocyte-stimulating hormone in amenorrhoeic women. *Lancet* 1:1107–1110.

Kavey N, Walters AS, Hening W, et al (1988) Opioid treatment of periodic leg movements in sleep in patients without restless legs. *Neuropeptides* 11:181–184.

Kavey NB, Whyte J, Gidro-Frank S, et al (1987) Treatment of restless legs syndrome and periodic movements in sleep with propoxyphene. *Sleep Res* 16:367. Abstract.

Kazic I (1973) Norepinephrine synthesis and turnover in the brain: acceleration by physostigmine. In: Usdin E, Snyder SH, eds. *Frontiers in Catecholamine Research*. Oxford: Pergamon. pp. 897–899.

Kebabian JW, Caine DB (1979) Multiple receptors for dopamine. *Nature* 277:93–96.

Keckich WA (1978) Neuroleptics: violence as a manifestation of akathisia. *JAMA* 240:2185.

Keepers GA, Clappison VJ, Casey DE (1983) Initial anticholinergic prophylaxis for neuroleptic-induced extrapyramidal syndromes. *Arch Gen Psychiatry* 40:1113–1117.

Keidar S, Binenboim C, Palant A (1982) Muscle cramps during treatment with nifedipine. *Br Med J* 285:1241–1242.

Kendler KS (1976) A medical student's experience with akathisia. *Am J Psychiatry* 133:4.

Kennedy PF (1969) Chorea and phenothiazines. *Br J Psychiatry* 115:103–104.

Kennedy PF, Hershon HI, McCruire RJ (1971) Extrapyramidal disorders after prolonged phenothiazine therapy. *Br J Psychiatry* 118:509–518.

Kent T, Wilber R (1982) Reserpine withdrawal psychosis. *J Nerv Ment Dis* 170:502–504.

Keskiner A (1973) A long-term follow up of fluphenazine enanthate treatment. *Curr Ther Res* 15:305–313.

Khot V, Egan MF, Hyde TM, et al (1992) Neuroleptics and classic tardive dyskinesia. In: Lang A, Weiner WJ, eds. *Drug-induced Movement Disorders.* New York: Futura. pp. 121–166.

Kidger T, Barnes TRE, Trauer T, et al (1980) Sub-syndromes of tardive dyskinesia. *Psychol Med* 10:513–520.

Kiloh LG (1961) Pseudodementia. *Acta Psychiatr Scand* 37:336–351.

Kiloh LG, Garside RF (1963) The independence of neurotic depression and endogenous depression. *Br J Psychiatry* 109:451–463.

Kim A, Adler L, Angrist B, et al (1989) Efficacy of low-dose metoprolol in neuroleptic-induced akathisia. *J Clin Psychopharmacol* 9:294–296.

Kirch DG, Gerhardt GA, Shelton RC, et al (1987) Effect of chronic nicotine administration on monoamine and monoamine metabolite concentration in brain iron. *Clin Neuropharmacol* 10:376–383.

Klawans HL (1973) The pharmacology of tardive dyskinesia. *Am J Psychiatry* 130:82–86.

Klawans HL, Curvey PM, Tanner CM, et al (1986) Drug-induced myoclonus. *Adv Neurol* 43:251–264.

Klawans HL, Rubovits R (1974) Effects of cholinergic and anticholinergic agents on tardive dyskinesia. *J Neurol Neurosurg Psychiatry* 27:941–947.

Klawans HL Jr, Bergen D, Bruyn GW (1973) Prolonged drug-induced parkinsonism. *Confinia Neurol* 35:368–377.

Klee B, Kronig MH (1993) Case report of probable sertraline-induce akathisia [letter]. *Am J Psychiatry* 150:986–987.

Klein DF, Gittelman R, Quitkin F (1980) *Diagnosis and Drug Treatment of Psychiatric Disorders: Adults and Children.* 2nd ed. Baltimore: Williams & Wilkins.

Klerman GL, DiMascio A, Greenblatt M, et al (1959) The influence of specific personality tic patterns on the reactions of phrenotropic agents. In: Masserman J, ed. *Biological Psychiatry.* New York: Grune & Stratton. pp. 224–242.

Klett CJ, Caffey E (1972) Evaluating the long-term need for antiparkinson drugs by chronic schizophrenics. *Arch Gen Psychiatry* 26:374–379.

Knights A, Hirsch SR (1981) Revealed depression and drug treatment for schizophrenia. *Arch Gen Psychiatry* 38:806–811.

Koch HL (1935) An analysis of some measures of the behavior of preschool children. *J Genet Psychol* 46:139–169.

Koller WC (1984) Sensory symptoms in Parkinson's disease. *Neurology* 34:957–959.

Kornetsky C, Humphries O (1957) Relationship between effects of a number of centrally acting drugs and personality. *AMA Arch Neurol & Psychiat* 77:325.

Kostowski W, Giacalone E, Garattini S et al (1968) Studies on behavioural and biochemical changes in rats after lesion of midbrain raphe. *Eur J Pharmacol* 4:567–574.

Kraepelin E (1911) *Dementia Praecox and Paraphrenia.* Edinburgh: Livingstone.

Kraepelin E (1921) *Manic-depressive Insanity and Paranoia.* Edinburgh: Livingstone.

Kral VA (1962) Stress and mental disorders of the senium. *Med Serv J Can* 18:363–370.

Kramer MS, DiJohnson C, Davis P, et al (1990) L-Tryptophan in neuroleptic-induced akathisia. *Biol Psychiatry* 27:671–672.

Kramer MS, Gorkin R, DiJohnson C (1989) Treatment of neuroleptic-induced akathisia with propranolol: a controlled replication study. *Hillside J Clin Psychiatry* 11:107–119.

Kramer MS, Gorkin RA, DiJohnson C, et al (1988) Propranolol in the treatment of neuroleptic-induced akathisia (NIA) in schizophrenics: a double-blind, placebo-controlled study. *Biol Psychiatry* 24:823–827.

Krauthamer GM (1979) Sensory functions of the neostriatum. In: Divac I, Oberg RGE, eds. *The Neostriatum.* Oxford: Pergamon.

Krishnan KR, France RD, Ellinwood EH, Jr (1984) Tricyclic-induced akathisia in patients taking conjugated estrogens. *Am J Psychiatry* 141:696–697.

Krout MH (1954a) An experimental attempt to determine the significance of unconscious manual symbolic movements. *J Gen Psychol* 51:121–152.

Krout MH (1954b) An experimental attempt to produce unconscious manual symbolic movements. *J Gen Psychol* 51:93–120.

Kruse W (1960a) Persistent muscular restlessness after phenothiazine treatment: report of three cases. *Am J Psychiatry* 117:152–153.

Kruse W (1960b) Treatment of drug-induced extrapyramidal symptoms. *Dis Nerv Syst* 21:79–81.

Kucharski LT, Wagner RL, Friedman JH (1987) An investigation of the coexistence of abnormal involuntary movements, parkinsonism, and akathisia in chronic psychiatric inpatients. *Psychopharmacol Bull* 23:215–217.

Kumar BB (1979) An unusual case of akathisia. *Am J Psychiatry* 136:1088.

Kuniyoshi M, Arikawa K, Miura C, et al (1991) Effect of clonazepam on tardive akathisia. *Human Psychopharmacol* 6:39–42.

Kurlan R, Lichter D, Hewitt D (1989) Sensory tics in Tourette's syndrome. *Neurology* 39:731–734.

Kutcher SP, MacKenzie S, Galarraga W, et al (1987) Clonazepam treatment of adolescents with neuroleptic-induced akathisia. *Am J Psychiatry* 144:823–824.

Kuzuhara S, Kohara N, Ohkawa Y, et al (1989) [Parkinsonism, depression and akathisia induced by flunarizine, a calcium entry blockade: report of 31 cases]. *Rinsho Shinkeigaku* 29:681–686.

LaBan MM, Viola SL, Femminineo AF, et al (1990) Restless legs syndrome associated with diminished cardiopulmonary compliance and lumbar spinal stenosis: a motor concomitant of 'Vesper's curse.' *Arch Phys Med Rehabil* 71:384–388.

Lai H, Carino MA, Horito A (1978) Effects of ethanol on central dopamine functions. *Life Sci* 27:19–28.

Lambert NM, Sandoval J, Sassone D (1978) Prevalence of hyperactivity in elementary school children as a function of social system definers. *Am J Orthopsychiatry* 48:446–463.

Lang AE (1987) Restless legs syndrome and Parkinson's disease: insights into pathophysiology. *Clin Neuropharmacol* 10:476–478.

Lang AE (1991) Patient perception of tics and other movement disorders. *Neurology* 41:223–228.

Lang AE (1992) Akathisia and restless legs syndrome. In: Jankovic J, Tolosa E, eds. *Parkinson's Disease and Movement Disorders.* Munich: Urban Schwarzenberg. pp. 399–418.

Lang AE (1994) Withdrawal akathisia: case reports and a proposed classification of chronic akathisia. *Mov Disord* 9(2):188–192.

Lang AE, Johnson K (1987) Akathisia in idiopathic Parkinson's disease. *Neurology* 37:477–481.

Lang AW, Moore RA (1961) Acute toxic psychosis concurrent with phenothiazine therapy. *Am J Psychiatry* April:939–940.

Langer SZ (1980) Presynaptic receptors and the modulation of neurotransmission: pharmacological implications and therapeutic relevance. *Trends Neurosci* 3:110–112.

Layne OL, Jr, Yudofsky SC (1971) Postoperative psychosis in cardiotomy patients: the role of organic and psychiatric factors. *N Engl J Med* 284:518–520.

Le Moal M, Cardo B, Stinus L (1969) Influence of ventral mesencephalic lesions on various spontaneous and conditional behaviours in the rat. *Physiol Behav* 4:567–574.

Le Moal M, Galey D, Cardo B (1975) Behavioral effects of local injection of 6-hydroxydopamine in the medial ventral tegmentum in the rat: possible role of the mesolimbic dopaminergic system. *Brain Res* 88:190–194.

Le Moal M, Simon H (1991) Mesocorticolimbic dopaminergic network: functional and regulatory roles. *Physiol Res* 71:155–234.

Le Moal M, Stinus L, Galey D (1976) Radiofrequency lesion of the ventral mesencephalic tegmentum: neurological and behavioural considerations. *Exp Neurol* 50:521–535.

Lee RG (1989) Quantitation of cerebellar dysmetria using a three-dimensional motion analysis system. *Mov Disord* 4:97–98. Abstract.

Lee T, Tang SW (1984) Loxapine and clozapine decrease serotonin (S2) but do not elevate dopamine (D2) receptor numbers in the rat brain. *Psychiatry Res* 12:277–285.

Lees AJ (1990) Movement disorders in psychiatry. *Curr Opin Neurol Neurosurg* 3:342–345.

Leibovici A, Tariot PN (1988) Agitation associated with dementia: a systematic approach to treatment. *Psychopharmacol Bull* 24:49–53.

Leonard DP, Kidson MA, Thompson PJ, et al (1974) Double-blind trial of lithium carbonate and haloperidol in Huntington's chorea. *Lancet* 2:1208–1209.

Lepola U, Koskinen T, Rimon R, et al (1989) Sulpiride and perphenazine in schizophrenia: a double-blind clinical trial. *Acta Psychiatr Scand* 80:92–96.

Levin H, Chengappa KN, Kambhampati RK, et al (1992) Should chronic treatment-refractory akathisia be an indication for the use of clozapine in schizophrenic patients? *J Clin Psychiatry* 53:248–251.

Levin HS, Grossman RG (1978) Behavioral sequelae of closed head injury: a quantitative study. *Arch Neurol* 35:720–727.

Levin JD, Lane SR, Gordon NC, et al (1982) A spinal opioid synapse mediates the interaction of spinal and brainstem sites in morphine analgesia. *Brain Res* 236:85–91.

Levinson DF, Simpson GM, Singh H, et al (1990) Fluphenazine dose, clinical response, and extrapyramidal symptoms during acute treatment. *Arch Gen Psychiatry* 47:761–768.

Lewis A (1934) Melancholia: a clinical survey of depressive states. *J Ment Sci* 8:277–378.

Leysen JE, Gommeren W, van Compel P, et al (1985) Receptor binding properties in vitro and in vivo of ritanserin: a very potent and long-acting serotonin-S2 antagonist. *Mol Pharmacol* 27:600–611.

Lidz CW, Meisel A, Osterweis M, et al (1983) Barriers to informed consent. *Ann Intern Med* 99:539–543.

Lieberman J, Johns C, Cooper T, et al (1989) Clozapine pharmacology and tardive dyskinesia. *Psychopharmacology* 99:554–559.

Liljequist S (1978) Changes in the sensitivity of dopamine receptors in the nucleus accumbens and in the striatum induced by chronic ethanol administration. *Acta Pharmacol Toxicol (Copenhagen)* 43:19–28.

Linazasoro G, Marti Masso JF, Suarez JA (1993) Nocturnal akathisia in Parkinson's disease: treatment with clozapine. *Mov Disord* 8(2):171–174.

Lindstrom LH, Wieselgren IM, Struwe G, et al (1990) A double-blind comparative multicentre study of remoxipride and haloperidol in schizophrenia. *Acta Psychiatr Scand* 358(suppl):130–135.

Lindvall O, Bjorklund A, Skajerberg G (1983) Dopamine-containing neurons in the spinal cord: anatomy and some functional aspects. *Ann Neurol* 14:255–260.

Linet LS (1985) Tourette syndrome, pimozide, and school phobia: the neuroleptic separation anxiety syndrome. *Am J Psychiatry* 142:613–615.

Lipinski JF, Hudson JI, Cunningham SL, et al (1991) Polysomnographic characteristics of neuroleptic-induced akathisia. *Clin Neuropharmacol* 14:413–419.

Lipinski JF, Mallya G, Zimmerman P, et al (1990) Akathisia and fluoxetine: reply [letter]. *J Clin Psychiatry* 51:211–212.

Lipinski JF, Zubenko GS, Barreira P, et al (1983) Propranolol in the treatment of neuroleptic-induced akathisia. *Lancet* 2:685–686.

Lipinski JF Jr, Keck PE Jr, McElroy SL (1988) Beta-adrenergic antagonists in psychosis: is improvement due to treatment of neuroleptic-induced akathisia? *J Clin Psychopharmacol* 8:409–416.

Lipinski JF Jr, Mallya G, Zimmerman P, et al (1989) Fluoxetine-induced akathisia: clinical and theoretical implications [see comments]. *J Clin Psychiatry* 50:339–342.

Lipinski JF Jr, Zubenko GS, Cohen BM, et al (1984) Propranolol in the treatment of neuroleptic-induced akathisia. *Am J Psychiatry* 141:412–415.

Lipowski ZJ (1990) *Delirium: Acute Confusional States.* New York: Oxford University Press.

Little JT, Jankovic J (1987) Tardive myoclonus. *Mov Disord* 2:307–312.

Lorens SA, Guldberg FC, Hole K, et al (1976) Activity, avoidance learning and regional 5-hydroxytryptamine following intra-brain stem 517-hydroxytryptamine and electrolytic midbrain raphe lesion in the rat. *Brain Res* 108:97–113.

Luft R, Muller R (1947) 'Crampi' och 'restless legs' vid akut poliomyelit. *Nord Med* 33:748.

Lugaresi E, Cirignotta F, Coccagna G, et al (1986) Nocturnal myoclonus and restless legs syndrome. *Adv Neurol* 43:295–307.

Lugaresi E, Coccagna G, Berti Ceroni G, et al (1968) Restless legs syndrome and nocturnal myoclonus. In: Gastaug H, Berti Ceroni G, Coccagna G, eds. *The Abnormalities of Sleep in Man.* Bologna: Gaggi. pp. 285–294.

Lugaresi E, Coccagna G, Mantovani M, et al (1972) Some periodic phenomena arising during drowsiness and sleep in man. *Electroencephalogr Clin Neurophysiol* 32:701–705.

Lugaresi E, Tassarini CA, Coccagna C, et al (1965) Particularites cliniques et polygraphiques du syndrome d'impatience des membres inferieurs. *Rev Neurol (Paris)* 113:545–555.

Lund CE, Mortimer AM, Rogers D, et al (1991) Motor, volitional and behavioural disorders in schizophrenia. I: Assessment using the Modified Rogers Scale. *Br J Psychiatry* 158:323–327.

Lund Lauersen A, Gerlach J (1986) Antipsychotic effect of remoxipride: a new substituted benzamide with selective antidopaminergic activity. *Acta Psychiatr Scand* 73:17–21.

Lundvall O, Abom PE, Holm R (1983) Carbamazepine in restless legs: a controlled pilot study. *Eur J Clin Pharmacol* 25:323–324.

Lutz EG (1976) Neuroleptic-induced akathisia and dystonia triggered by alcohol. *JAMA* 236:2422–2423.

Lutz EG (1978) Restless legs, anxiety and caffeinism. *J Clin Psychiatry* 39:693–698.

Maany I, Dhopesh V (1990) Akathisia and fluoxetine [letter; comment]. *J Clin Psychiatry* 51:210–212.

Mackler B, Finch C (1982) Iron in central nervous system oxidative metabolism. In: Pollitt E, Leibel RL, eds. *Iron Deficiency: Brain Biochemistry and Behavior*. New York: Raven. pp. 31–38.

MacMillan JC, Snell RG, Tyler A, et al (1993) Molecular analysis and clinical correlations of the Huntington's disease mutation. *Lancet* 342(8877):954–958.

Magliozzi JR, Gillespie H, Lombrozo L, et al (1985) Mood alteration following oral and intravenous haloperidol and relationship to drug concentration in normal subjects. *J Clin Pharmacol* 25:285–290.

Magnussen I, Braengaard H (1982) *p,p'*-DDT induced myoclonus in mice: the role of serotonin. *Acta Neurol Scand* 65(suppl 90):66.

Maltbie AL, Cavenar JO Jr (1977) Akathisia diagnosis: an objective test. *Psychosomatics* 18:36–39.

Mann K, Bartels M, Bauer H, et al (1984) Amisulpride: an open clinical study of a new benzamide in schizophrenic patients. *Pharmacopsychiatry* 17:111–115.

Mano T, Schiozawa Z, Sobue I (1982) Extrapyramidal involuntary movements during sleep. *Electroencephalogr Clin Neurophysiol* (suppl 35):431–442.

Manos N, Gkiouzepas J, Logothetis J (1981) The need for continuous use of antiparkinsonian medication with chronic schizophrenic patients receiving long-term neuroleptic therapy. *Am J Psychiatry* 138(2):184–188.

Manschreck TC (1986) Motor abnormalities in schizophrenic disorders. In: Nasrallah HA, Weinberger DR, eds. *Handbook of Schizophrenia, Vol. 1: The Neurology of Schizophrenia*. Amsterdam: Elsevier. pp. 65–96.

Marder SR, Van Putten T (1988) Who should receive clozapine? *Arch Gen Psychiatry* 45:865–867.

Marjot DH (1969) Depression following fluphenazine treatment. *Br Med J* 3:780.

Marley E, Wozniak K (1984) Interactions of a nonselective monoamine oxidase inhibitor, phenelzine, with inhibitors of 5-hydroxytryptamine copamine or noradrenoline re-uptake. *Psychiat Res* 18:173–180.

Marsden CD (1980) The physiology of myoclonus and its relation to epilepsy. *Res Clin Forums* 2:31–45.

Marsden CD, Hallett M, Fahn S (1982) The nosology and pathophysiology of myoclonus. In: Marsden CD, Fahn S, eds. *Neurology, II: Movement Disorders*. London: Butterworth Scientific. pp. 196–248.

Marsden CD, Jenner P (1980) The pathophysiology of extrapyramidal side-effects of neuroleptic drugs. *Psychol Med* 10:55–72.

Marsden CD, Meadows JC, Large GW, et al (1969) Variations in human physiological finger tremor, with particular reference to changes in age. *Electroencephalogr Clin Neurophysiol* 27:169–178.

Marsden CD, Tarsy D, Baldessarini RJ (1975) Spontaneous and drug-induced movement disorders in psychotic patients. In: Benson DF, Blumer D, eds. *Psychiatric Aspects of Neurologic Disease*. New York: Grune & Stratton. pp. 219–266.

Martensson B, Nyberg S, Toresson G, et al (1989) Fluoxetine treatment of depression. *Acta Psychiatr Scand* 79:586–596.

Martinelli P, Coccagna G, Lugaresi E (1987) Nocturnal myoclonus, restless legs syndrome, and abnormal electrophysiological findings [letter]. *Ann Neurol* 21:515.

Masland RL (1947) Myokymia – cause of 'restless legs.' *JAMA* 134:1298.

Mathews E (1923) A study of emotional stability in children. *Journal of Delinquency* 3:1–40.

Mattes JA (1985) Metoprolol for intermittent explosive disorder. *Am J Psychiatry* 142:1108–1109.

Matthews WB (1979) Treatment of the restless legs syndrome with clonazepam [letter]. *Br Med J* 1:751.

Matthysse S (1986) Animal models in psychiatric research. *Prog Brain Res* 65:259–270.

May PRA, Lee MA, Bacon RC (1983) Quantitative assessment of neuroleptic-induced extrapyramidal symptoms: clinical and non-clinical approaches. *Clin Neuropharmacol* 6(suppl):S35–S52.

Mayer-Gross W (1920) Uber die Stellungsnahme auf abgelaufenen akuten Psychose. *Z Gesante Neurol Psychiatr* 60:160–212.

McClelland HA, Farquarson RG, Leyburn P, et al (1976) Very high dose fluphenazine decanoate: a controlled trial in chronic schizophrenia. *Arch Gen Psychiatry* 33:1435–1439.

McCreadie RG, Robertson LJ, Wiles DH (1992) The Nithsdale Schizophrenia Surveys. IX: akathisia, parkinsonism, tardive dyskinesia and plasma neuroleptic levels. *Br J Psychiatry* 160:793–799.

McCreadie RG, Todd N, Livingstone M, et al (1988) A double blind comparative study of remoxipride and thioridazine in the acute phase of schizophrenia. *Acta Psychiatr Scand* 78:49–56.

McDonald CS, Zepelin H, Zammit GK (1981) Age and sex patterns in auditory awakening thresholds. *Sleep Res* 19:115.

McGlashan T, Carpenter WT (1976) Postpsychotic depression in schizophrenia. *Arch Gen Psychiatry* 33:231–241.

McGrae JD, Winkelmann RE (1963) Generalised essential telangiectasia. *JAMA* 185:909–913.

Medinar C, Kramer MD, Kurland AA (1962) Biperidin in the treatment of phenothiazine-induced extrapyramidal reactions. *JAMA* 182:1127–1128.

Mehrabian A, Friedman SL (1986) An analysis of fidgeting and associated individual differences. *J Pers* 54:406–429.

Mehrabian A, Williams M (1969) Nonverbal concomitants of perceived and intended persuasiveness. *Journal of Personal and Social Psychology* 13:37–58.

Meltzer H, Young M, Metz J, et al (1979) Extrapyramidal side effects and increased serum prolactin following fluoxetine, a new antidepressant. *J Neural Transm* 45:165–175.

Meltzer HY (1991) The mechanism of action of novel antipsychotic drugs. *Schizophr Bull* 17:263–287.

Meltzer HY, Matsubara S, Lee JC (1989) Classification of typical and atypical antipsychotic drugs on the basis of dopamine D-1, D-2 and serotonin2 pKi values. *J Pharmacol Exp Ther* 251:238–246.

Mendels J, Cochrane C (1968) The nosology of depression: the endogenous-reactive concept. *Am J Psychiatry* 124(suppl):1–11.

Menza MA, Grossman N, Van Horn M, et al (1991) Smoking and movement disorders in psychiatric patients. *Biol Psychiatry* 30:109–115.

Merriam AE, Aronson MK, Gaston P, et al (1988) The psychiatric symptoms of Alzheimer's disease. *J Am Geriatr Soc* 36:7–12.

Metcalfe RA, MacDermott N, Chalmers RJ (1986) Restless red legs: an association of the restless legs syndrome with arborizing telangiectasia of the lower limbs. *J Neurol Neurosurg Psychiatry* 49:820–823.

396   *References*

Meyboom RH, Ferrari MD, Dieleman BP (1986) Parkinsonism, tardive dyskinesia, akathisia, and depression induced by flunarizine. *Lancet* 2:292.

Meyers M (1951) *Lang's German–English Medical Dictionary.* 4th ed. Philadelphia: Blakiston.

Micheli F, Pardal MF, Gatto M, et al (1987) Flunarizine- and cinnarizine-induced extrapyramidal reactions. *Neurology* 37:881–884.

Mikkelsen EJ, Detlor J, Cohen DJ (1981) School avoidance and social phobia triggered by haloperidol in patients with Tourette's disorder. *Am J Psychiatry* 138:1572–1576.

Miller CH, Fleischhacker WW, Ehrmann H, et al (1990) Treatment of neuroleptic induced akathisia with the 5-HT2 antagonist ritanserin. *Psychopharmacol Bull* 26:373–376.

Miller CH, Hummer M, Pycha R, et al (1992) The effect of ritanserin on treatment-resistant neuroleptic induced akathisia: case reports. *Prog Neuropsychopharmacol Biol Psychiatry* 16:247–251.

Miller LG, Jankovic J (1988) Variable expression of neuroleptic-induced movement disorders: a study of 125 patients. Presented at the Symposium on Drug Induced Movement Disorders, Philadelphia.

Miller LG, Jankovic J (1989) Metoclopramide-induced movement disorders: clinical findings with a review of the literature. *Arch Intern Med* 149:2486–2492.

Miller LG, Jankovic J (1990) Neurologic approach to drug-induced movement disorders: a study of 125 patients. *South Med J* 83:525–532.

Miller RJ, Hiley CR (1974) Antimuscarinic properties of neuroleptics and drug-induced parkinsonism. *Nature* 248:596–597.

Mills R, Hening W, Walters A, et al (1993) Successful use of actigraphy to quantify motor symptoms in the restless legs syndrome. Presented at the Annual Meeting of the American Academy of Neurology, New York City, April. *Neurology* 43:A387 (Abstract).

Milne IK (1992) Akathisia associated with carbamazepine therapy. *N Z Med J* 105:182.

Missak SS (1987) Does the human body produce a substance similar to caffeine? *Med Hypotheses* 24:161–165.

Misu Y, Goshima Y, Ueda H, et al (1985) Presynaptic inhibitory dopamine receptors on noradrenergic nerve terminals: analysis of biphasic actions of dopamine and apomorphine on the release of endogenous norepinephrine in rat hypothalamic slices. *J Pharmacol Exp Ther* 235:771–777.

Mitler MM, Browman CP, Menn SJ, et al (1986) Nocturnal myoclonus: treatment efficacy of clonazepam and temazepam. *Sleep* 9:385–392.

Moldofsky H, Tullis C, Quance G, et al (1986) Nitrazepam for periodic movements in sleep (sleep-related myoclonus). *Can J Neurol Sci* 13:52–54.

Moller HJ, Kissling W, Dietzfelbinger T, et al (1989) Efficacy and tolerability of a new antipsychotic compound (Savoxepine): results of a pilot study. *Pharmacopsychiatry* 22:38–41.

Montagna P, Coccagna G, Cirignotta F, et al (1983) Familial restless legs syndrome: long-term follow-up. In: Guilleminault C, Lugaresi E, eds. *Sleep/Wake Disorders: Natural History, Epidemiology and Long-term Evolution.* New York: Raven. pp. 231–235.

Montagna P, Sassoli de Bianchi L, Zucconi M, et al (1984) Clonazepam and vibration in restless legs syndrome. *Acta Neurol Scand* 69:428–430.

Montplaisir J, Godbout R, Boghen D, et al (1985) Familial restless legs with periodic movements in sleep: electrophysiologic, biochemical, and pharmacologic study. *Neurology* 35:130–134.

Montplaisir J, Godbout R, Poirier G, et al (1986) Restless legs syndrome and periodic movements in sleep: physiopathology and treatment with L-dopa. *Clin Neuropharmacol* 9:456–463.

Montplaisir J, Lorrain D, Godbout R (1991) Restless legs syndrome and periodic leg movements in sleep: the primary role of dopaminergic mechanism. *Eur Neurol* 31(1):41–43.

Moorthy SS, Dierdorf SF (1990) Restless legs during recovery from spinal anesthesia. *Anesth Analg* 70:337.

Morgan LK (1967) Restless limbs: a commonly overlooked symptom controlled by 'Valium.' *Med J Aust* 2:589–594.

Morgenstern H, Glazer WM (1993) Identifying risk factors for tardive dyskinesia among long-term outpatients maintained with neuroleptic medications. Results of the Yale Tardive Dyskinesia Study. *Arch Gen Psychiatry* 50(a):723–733.

Morosini C (1967) Osservasioni sui fenomeni neurodislettici da haloperidol. Presented at the Symposium Internazionale Sull Haloperidol e Triperidol, Institute Luso Farmaxo d'Italia, Milan, Italy.

Mosko SS, Nudleman KL (1986) Somatosensory and brainstem auditory evoked responses in sleep-related periodic leg movements. *Sleep* 9:399–404.

Mukherjee S (1984) Tardive dysmentia: a reappraisal. *Schizophr Bull* 10:151–152.

Mukherjee S, Wisniewski A, Bider R, et al (1985) Possible association between tardive dyskinesia and altered carbohydrate metabolism [letter]. *Arch Gen Psychiatry* 42(2):205.

Munetz MR (1980) Oculogyric crisis and tardive dyskinesia [letter]. *Am J Psychiatry* 137:1628.

Munetz MR (1986) Akathisia variants and tardive dyskinesia [letter]. *Arch Gen Psychiatry* 43:1015.

Munetz MR, Benjamin S (1990) Who should perform the AIMS examination? *Hosp Community Psychiatry* 41:912–915.

Munetz MR, Cornes CL (1982) Akathisia, pseudoakathisia and tardive dyskinesia: clinical examples. *Compr Psychiatry* 23:345–352.

Munk-Anderson E, Behnke K, Heltberg J, et al (1989) Sulpiride versus haloperidol – a clinical trial in schizophrenia: a preliminary report. *Acta Psychiatr Scand* 311(suppl):31–41.

Murphy G (1959) Acroparestesias agitantes nocturnas. *Rev Neurol (Buenos Aires)* 7:201–205.

Murray TJ, Kelly P, Campbell L, et al (1977) Haloperidol in the treatment of stuttering. *Br J Psychiatry* 130:370–373.

Mussio Fournier JC, Rawak F (1940) Agitation paresthesique des extremites. *Rev Neurol (Paris)* 79:337–341.

Myslobodsky MS (1986) Anosognosia in tardive dyskinesia. *Schizophr Bull* 12:1–6.

Myslobodsky MS (1993) Central determinants of attention and mood disorder in tardive dyskinesia ('tardive dysmentia'). *Brain Cogn* 23:88–101.

Nace GS, Wood AJ (1987) Pharmacokinetics of long acting propranolol: implications for therapeutic use. *Clin Pharmacokinet* 13:51–64.

Nakama M, Ochia T, Kowa Y (1972) Effects of psychotropic drugs in emotional behavior: exploratory behavior of naive rats in holed open-field. *Jpn J Pharmacol* 22:767–775.

Nasrallah HA, Pappas NJ, Crowe BR (1980) Oculogyric dystonia in tardive dyskinesia. *Am J Psychiatry* 137:850–851.

Nath A, Jankovic J, Pettigrew LC (1987) Movement disorders and AIDS. *Neurology* 37:37–41.

Nathan PW (1978) Painful legs and moving toes: evidence on the site of the lesion. *J Neurol Neurosurg Psychiatry* 41:934–939.

National Institute of Mental Health (1976) Abnormal Involuntary Movement Scale. In: Guy W, ed. *Early Clinical Drug Evaluation Unit Assessment Manual.* Rockville, MD: US Dept of Health and Human Sciences. pp. 534–537.

National Institute of Mental Health. (1985) Clinical global impressions. *Psychopharmacol Bull* 21:839–843.

Nauta WJ, Domesick VB (1978) Cross roads of limbic and striatal circuitry: hypothalamo–nigral connections. In: Livingston KE, Hornykiewicz O, ed. *Limbic Mechanisms.* New York: Plenum. pp. 75–93.

Nauta WJH, Smith GP, Faull RLM, et al (1978) Efferent connections and the nigral afferents of the nucleus accumbens septi in the rat. *Neuroscience* 3:385–401.

Needleman HL, Gunnoe C, Leviton A, et al (1979) Deficits in psychologic and classroom performance of children with elevated dentine lead levels. *N Engl J Med* 300:689–695.

Nelson JC, Charney DS (1981) The symptoms of major depressive illness. *Am J Psychiatry* 138:1–13.

Nemes Z, Volavka J, Bitter I, et al (1990) Rhythmic movements of chronic akathisia. *Biol Psychiatry* 27:465–466.

Nemes ZC, Rotrosen J, Angrist B, et al (1991) Serum iron levels and akathisia. *Biol Psychiatry* 29:411–413.

Neppe VM (1982) Carbamazepine in the psychiatric patient [letter]. *Lancet* 2:334.

Newhouse PA, Sunderland T, Tariot PN, et al (1988) The effects of acute scopolamine in geriatric depression. *Arch Gen Psychiatry* 45:906–912.

Niederehe G (1988) TRIMS Behavioral Problem Checklist (BPC). *Psychopharmacol Bull* 24:771–778.

Nishikawa T, Kuwahara H, Tsuda A, et al (1992) Distinguishing acute and tardive akathisia by monitoring microvibration: a pilot study. *Jpn J Psychiatry Neurol* 46:665–672.

Nishimatsu O, Horiguchi J, Inami Y, et al (1992) Nocturnal myoclonus observed in a patient with neuroleptic-induced akathisia. *Jpn J Psychiatry Neurol* 46:121–126.

Nordic Dyskinesia Study Group. (1986) Effect of different neuroleptics in tardive dyskinesia and parkinsonism: a video-controlled multicenter study with chlorprothixene, perphenazine, haloperidol and haloperidol + biperiden. *Psychopharmacology* 90:423–429.

Nordlander NB (1953) Therapy in restless legs. *Acta Med Scand* 143:453–457.

Nordlander NB (1954) Restless legs. *Br J Phys Med* 17:160.

Nordstrom AL, Farde L, Halldin C (1992) Time course of D_2-dopamine receptor occupancy examined by PET after single oral doses of haloperidol. *Psychopharmacology* 106:433–438.

Nutt JG (1992) Dyskinesia induced by levodopa and dopamine agonists in patients with Parkinson's disease. In: Lang AE, Weiner WJ, eds. *Drug-induced Movement Disorders.* Mt. Kisco: Futura. pp. 281–314.

Nutt JG, Carter JH (1984) Sensory symptoms in parkinsonism related to central dopaminergic function. *Lancet* 2:456–457.

Ohanna N, Peled R, Rubin AE, et al (1985) Periodic leg movements in sleep: effect of clonazepam treatment. *Neurology* 35:408–411.

Ollerenshaw DP (1973) The classification of the functional psychoses. *Br J Psychiatry* 122:517–530.

O'Loughlin V, Dickie AC, Ebmeier KP (1991) Serum iron and transferrin in acute neuroleptic induced akathisia. *J Neurol Neurosurg Psychiatry* 54:363–364.

Olson WC (1929) *The Measurement of Nervous Habits in Normal Children.* Minneapolis: University of Minnesota Press.

Opler LA (1991) Akathisia and suicide [letter]. *Am J Psychiatry* 148:1259.

Oppenheim H (1923) *Lehbuch der Nervenkrankheiten.* 7th ed. Berlin: S. Karger.

Oreland L (1971) Purification and properties of pig liver mitochondrial monoamine oxidase. *Arch Biochem Biophys* 146:410–421.

Orlovsky GN (1969) Spontaneous and induced locomotion in the thalamic cat. *Biophysics* 14:1154–1162.

Oshtory MA, Vijayan N (1980) Clonazepam treatment of insomnia due to sleep myoclonus. *Arch Neurol* 37:119–120.

Oster J (1972) Growing pains: a symptom and its significance. *Dan Med Bull* 19:72–79.

Oswald I (1959) Sudden bodily jerks on falling asleep. *Brain* 82:82–103.

Ouagazzal A, Nieoillon A, Amalric M (1993) Effects of dopamine D1 and D2 receptor blockade on MK-801-induced hyperlocomotion in rats. *Psychopharmacology* 111:427–434.

Overall JE, Gorham DR (1962) The brief psychiatric rating scale. *Psychol Rep* 10:799–812.

Paik IH, Lee C, Choi BM, et al (1989) Mianserin-induced restless legs syndrome [see comments]. *Br J Psychiatry* 155:415–417.

Parker G, Brotchie H (1992) Psychomotor change as a feature of depressive disorders: an historical overview. *Aust N Z J Psychiatry* 26:146–155.

Parker G, Hadzi-Pavlovic D, Boyce P, et al (1990) Classifying depression by mental stage signs. *Br J Psychiatry* 157:55–65.

Parker G, Hadzi-Pavlovic D, Brodaty H, et al (1993) Psychomotor disturbance in depression: defining the constructs. *J Affect Disord* 27:255–265.

Parkes JD, Calver DM, Zilkha KJ (1970) Controlled trial of amantadine hydrochloride in Parkinson's disease. *Lancet* 1:259–263.

Passouant P, Cadillac J, Baldy-Moulinier M, et al (1970) Etude de sommeil chez des uremiques chroniques soumis a une epuration extrarenale. *Electroencephalogr Clin Neurophysiol* 29:441–449.

Patterson JF (1986) Pseudoakathisia associated with atenolol [letter]. *J Clin Psychopharmacol* 6:390.

Patterson JF (1988) Akathisia associated with buspirone. *J Clin Psychopharmacol* 8:296–297.

Peled R, Lavie P (1987) Double-blind evaluation of clonazepam on periodic leg movements in sleep. *J Neurol Neurosurg Psychiatry* 50:1679–1681.

Pelletier G, Lorrain D, Montplaisir J (1992) Sensory and motor components of the restless legs syndrome. *Neurology* 42:1663–1666.

Penfield W, Welch K (1951) The supplementary motor area of the cerebral cortex. *Arch Neurol Psychiatry* 66:289–317.

Perenyi A, Kuncz E, Bagdy G (1985) Early relapse after sudden withdrawal or dose reduction of clozapine. *Psychopharmacology* 86:244.

Peroutka SJ (1988) 5-Hydroxytryptamine receptor subtypes. *Annu Rev Neurosci* 11:45–60.

Peroutka SJ, Snyder SH (1980) Relationship of neuroleptic drug effects at brain dopamine, serotonin, alpha-adrenergic, and histamine receptors to clinical potency. *Am J Psychiatry* 137:1518–1522.

Perry KW, Fuller RW (1992) Effect of fluoxetine on serotonin and dopamine concentration in microdialysis fluid from rat striatum. *Life Sci* 50:1683–1690.

Petrie WM, Ban TA (1981) Propranolol in organic agitation. *Lancet* 1:324.

Pfeiffer E (1975) A short portable mental status questionnaire for the assessment of organic brain deficit in elderly patients. *J Am Geriatr Soc* 23:433–441.

Pijnenburg AJJ, Honig WMM, Van der Heyden JAM, et al (1975) Effects of chemical stimulation of the mesolimbic dopamine system upon locomotor activity. *Eur J Pharmacol* 41:87–95.

Pineau R, Lachance R, Pelchat G, et al (1976) Epidemiology of tardive dyskinesia. *Dis Nerv Syst* 37 (4 pt. 1):210–214.

Pohl R, Yeragani VK, Balon R, et al (1988) The jitteriness syndrome in panic disorder patients with antidepressants. *J Clin Psychiatry* 49:100–104.

Pohl R, Yeragani VK, Ortiz A (1986) Response of tricyclic-induced jitteriness to a phenothiazine in two patients. *J Clin Psychiatry* 47:427.

Polizos P, Engelhardt DM (1978) Dyskinetic phenomena in children treated with psychotropic medications. *Psychopharmacol Bull* 145:621–624.

Pollitt E, Leibel RL (1982) *Iron Deficiency: Brain Biochemistry and Behaviour.* New York: Raven Press.

Pradhan N, Arunasmitha S (1991) Correlations of motility, defecatory behavior and striatal dopaminergic activity in rats. *Physiol Behav* 50:135–138.

Price WA, Zimmer B (1987) Lithium-induced akathisia. *J Clin Psychiatry* 48:81.

Prien RF, Klet J, Calley EM (1976) Polypharmacy in the psychiatric treatment of elderly hospitalized patients: a survey of 12 veterans administration hospitals. *Disord Nerv Syst* 37:333–336.

Pryce IG, Edwards H (1966) Persistent oral dyskinesia in female mental hospital patients. *Br J Psychiatry* 112:983–987.

Purdon-Martin J (1946) Acroparesthesia in the lower limbs: unexplained pains in the legs at night. *Br Med J* 1:307.

Rall TW (1990) Hypnotics and sedatives; ethanol. In: Gilman AG, Rall TW, Nies AS, et al, eds. *The Pharmacological Basics of Therapeutics.* New York: Pergamon Press. pp. 345–382.

Randrup A, Munkvad I (1966) Role of catecholamines in the amphetamine excitation response. *Nature* 211:540.

Rao JM, Cowie VA, Mathew B (1987) Tardive dyskinesia in neuroleptic medicated mentally handicapped subjects. *Acta Psychiatr Scand* 76:507–513.

Rao JM, Cowie VA, Mathew B (1989) Neuroleptic-induced parkinsonian side effects in the mentally handicapped. *J Ment Def Res* 33:81–86.

Rapoport A (1989) Unilateral akathisia [letter]. *Neurology* 39:1648.

Raskin A, Crook T (1988) Mood scales: elderly. *Psychopharmacol Bull* 24:727–732.

Raskin DE (1985) Antipsychotic medication and the elderly. *J Clin Psychiatry* 46:36–40.

Ratey JJ, Mikkelsen EJ, Bushnell-Smith G, et al (1986) Beta blockers in the severely and profoundly mentally retarded. *J Clin Psychopharmacol* 6:103–107.

Ratey JJ, Sorgi P, Polakoff S (1985) Nadolol as a treatment for akathisia. *Am J Psychiatry* 142:640–642.

Ray I (1972) Amotivational syndrome. *Can Med Assoc J* 107–279.

Ray WA, Federspiel CF, Schaffner W (1980) A study of antipsychotic use in nursing homes: epidemiologic evidence suggesting misuse. *Am J Public Health* 70:485–491.

Read DJ, Feest TG, Nassim MA (1981) Clonazepam: effective treatment for restless legs syndrome in uraemia. *Br Med J* 283:885–886.

Reisberg B, Borenstein J, Salob SP, et al (1987) Behavioural symptoms in Alzheimer's disease: phenomenology and treatment. *J Clin Psychiatry* 48(suppl 5):9–15.

Reitan RM, Davison LA (1974) *Clinical Neuropsychology: Current Status and Applications.* New York: Hemisphere.

Reiter S, Adler L, Angrist B, et al (1987a) Atenolol and propranolol in neuroleptic-induced akathisia. *J Clin Psychopharmacol* 7:279–280.

Reiter S, Adler L, Erle S, et al (1987b) Neuroleptic-induced akathisia treated with pindolol. *Am J Psychiatry* 144:383–384.

Remington G, Fornazzari L, Sethna R (1993) Placebo response in refractory tardive akathisia. *Can J Psychiatry* 38:248–250.

Resek G, Haines J, Sainsbury P (1981) An ultrasound technique for the measurement of tardive dyskinesia. *Br J Psychiatry* 138:474–478.

Reyes RL, Bhattacharya AK, Heller D (1981) Traumatic head injury: restlessness and agitation as prognosticators of physical and psychologic improvements in patients. *Arch Phys Med Rehabil* 62:20–23.

Reynolds G, Blake DR, Pall HS, Williams A (1986) Restless legs syndrome and rheumatoid arthritis. *Br Med J* 292:659–660.

Richards PD, Flaum MA, Bateman M, et al (1986) The anti-emetic efficacy of secobarbital and chlorpromazine compared to metoclopramide, diphenhydramine and dexamethasone. *Cancer* 58:959–962.

Richardson MA, Craig TJ (1982) The co-existence of parkinsonism-like symptoms and tardive dyskinesia. *Am J Psychiatry* 139(3):341–343.

Richardson MA, Craig TJ, Branchey MH (1982) Intra-patient variability in the measurement of tardive dyskinesia. *Psychopharmacology* 76:269–272.

Richardson MA, Haugland G, Craig TJ (1991) Neuroleptic use, parkinsonian symptoms, tardive dyskinesia, and associated factors in child and adolescent psychiatric patients. *Am J Psychiatry* 148:1322–1328.

Richelson E (1984) Neuroleptic affinities for human brain receptors and their use in predicting adverse effects. *J Clin Psychiatry* 45:331–336.

Richelson E (1985) Pharmacology of neuroleptics in use in the United States. *J Clin Psychiatry* 46(8 pt. 2):8–14.

Richelson E, Nelson A (1984) Antagonism by neuroleptics of neurotransmitter receptors of normal human brain in vitro. *Eur J Pharmacol* 103:197–204.

Rifkin A, Doddi S, Karajgi B, et al (1991) Dosage of haloperidol for schizophrenia. *Arch Gen Psychiatry* 48:166–170.

Rifkin A, Quitkin F, Klein DF (1975) Akinesia. *Arch Gen Psychiatry* 32:672–674.

Risse C, Barnes R (1986) Pharmacologic treatment of agitation associated with dementia. *J Am Geriat Soc* 34:368–376.

Ritchie EC, Bridenbaugh RH, Jabbari B (1988) Acute generalized myoclonus following buspirone administration. *J Clin Psychiatry* 49:242–243.

Robertson MM, Schneiden V, Lees WJ (1990) Management of Gilles de la Tourette syndrome using sulpiride. *Clin Neuropharmacol* 13(3):229–235.

Roger SD, Harris DCH, Stewart JH (1991) Possible relation between restless legs and anaemia in renal dialysis patients. *Lancet* 337:1551.

Rogers D (1985) The motor disorders of severe psychiatric illness: a conflict of paradigms. *Br J Psychiatry* 147:221–232.

Rogers D (1992) Neuropsychiatry of movement disorders. *Curr Opin Psychiatry* 5:84–87.

Rosenthal SH, Gudeman JE (1967) The endogenous depressive pattern: an empirical investigation. *Br J Psychiatry* 16:241–249.

Rosenthal SH, Klerman GL (1966) Content and consistency in the endogenous depressive pattern. *Br J Psychiatry* 112:471–484.

Ross DR, Walker JI, Peterson J (1983) Akathisia induced by amoxapine. *Am J Psychiatry* 140:115–116.

Rothstein C, Zelterman I, White HR (1962) Discontinuation of maintenance dosages of ataractic drugs on a psychiatric continued treatment ward. *J Nerv Ment Dis* 134:555–560.

Rozovsky F (1990) *Consent to Treatment: A Practical Guide.* 2nd ed. Boston: Little, Brown.

Russell KH, Hagenmeyer-Houser SH, Sanberg PR (1987a) Haloperidol-induced emotional defecation: a possible model for neuroleptic anxiety syndrome. *Psychopharmacology (Berlin)* 91:45–49.

Russell KH, Hagenmeyer-Houser SH, Sanberg PR (1987b) Haloperidol produces increased defecation in rats habituated to environments. *Bull Psychonomic Soc* 25:13–16.

Rutter M (1967) A children's behaviour questionnaire for completion by teachers: preliminary findings. *J Child Psychol Psychiat* 8:8–11.

Rutter M, Cox A, Tupling C, et al (1975) Attainment and adjustment in two geographical areas. I. The prevalence of psychiatric disorder. *Am J Psychiatry* 126:493–509.

Rutter M, Greenfield D, Lockyer L (1967) A five to fifteen-year follow-up study of infantilie psychosis. *Br J Psychiatry* 113:1183–1199.

Rutter M, Tizard J, Whitmore K (1970) *Education, Health and Behaviour.* London: Longmans.

Sachdev P (1986) Lithium potentiation of neuroleptic-induced EPSE (case report). *Am J Psychiatry* 143:942.

Sachdev P (1991) Psychoactive drug use in an institution for intellectually handicapped persons. *Med J Aust* 155:75–79.

Sachdev P (1992) Drug-induced movement disorders in institutionalised adults with mental retardation: clinical characteristics and risk factors. *Aust N Z J Psychiatry* 26:242–248.

Sachdev P (1993a) The neuropsychiatry of brain iron. *J Neuropsychiatry Clin Neurosci* 5:18–29.

Sachdev P (1993b) Clinical characteristics of 15 patients with tardive dystonia. *Am J Psychiatry* 150:498–500.

Sachdev P (1994a) Research diagnostic criteria for drug-induced akathisia: conceptualization, rationale and proposal. *Psychopharmacology* 114(1):181–186.

Sachdev P (1994b) Tardive akathisia, tardive dyskinesia and serum iron status. *J Clin Psychopharmacol* 14:147–149.

Sachdev P (1994c) A rating scale for drug-induced akathisia: development, reliability and validity. *Biol Psychiatry* 35(4):263–271.

Sachdev P, Chee KY (1990) Pharmacological characterization of tardive akathisia. *Biol Psychiatry* 28:809–818.

Sachdev P, Kiloh LG (1994) The nondepressive pseudodementias. In: Emery VOB, Oxman TE, eds. *Dementia: Presentations, Differential Diagnosis, and Nosology.* Baltimore: Johns Hopkins University Press. pp. 277–297.

Sachdev P, Kruk J (1994) Clinical characteristics and risk factors for acute neuroleptic-induced akathisia. *Arch Gen Psychiatry* 51:963–974.

Sachdev P, Loneragan C (1991a) The present status of akathisia. *J Nerv Ment Dis* 179:381–391.

Sachdev P, Loneragan C (1991b) Acute drug-induced akathisia is not associated with low serum iron status. *Psychopharmacology* 103:138–139.

Sachdev P, Loneragan C (1993a) Intravenous challenges of benztropine and propranolol in tardive akathisia. *Psychopharmacology* 116:324–331.

Sachdev P, Loneragan C (1993b) Intravenous challenges of benztropine and propranolol in acute neuroleptic-induced akathisia. *Clin Neuropharmacol* 16:324–331.

Sachdev P, Loneragan C (1993c) Low-dose apomorphine challenge in tardive akathisia. *Neurology* 43:544–547.

Sachdev P, Loneragan C, Westbrook F (1993) Neuroleptic-induced defecation in rats as a model for neuroleptic dysphoria. *Psychiatry Res* 47:37–45.

Sachdev P, Smith JS, Angus-Leppan H, et al (1990) Pseudodementia twelve months on. *J Neurol Neurosurg Psychiatry* 53:254–259.

Sacks O (1983) *Awakenings*. New York: Dutton.

Safferman AZ, Lieberman JA, Pollack S, et al (1992) Clozapine and akathisia. *Biol Psychiatry* 31:753–754.

Safferman AZ, Lieberman JA, Pollack S, et al (1993) Akathisia and clozapine treatment. *J Clin Psychopharmacol* 13:286–287.

Salamone JD (1992) Complex motor and sensorimotor functions of striatal and accumbens dopamine: involvements in instrumental behavior processes. *Psychopharmacology* 107:160–174.

Sale I, Kristall H (1978) Schizophrenia following withdrawal from chronic phenothiazine administration: a case report. *Aust N Z J Psychiatry* 12:73–75.

Saller CF, Chiodo LA (1980) Glucose suppresses basal firing and haloperidol-induced increase in firing rate of central dopaminergic neurons. *Science* 210:1269–1271.

Saller R, Hellenbrecht D (1985) Comparison of the antiemetic efficacy of two high-dose benzamides, metoclopramide and alizapride, against cisplatin-induced emesis. *Can Treat Rep* 69:1301–1303.

Saltz BL, Woerner MG, Kane JM, et al (1991) Prospective study of tardive dyskinesia incidence in the elderly. *JAMA* 266:2402–2406.

Salvi F, Montagna P, Plasmati R, et al (1990) Restless legs syndrome and nocturnal myoclonus: initial clinical manifestation of familial amyloid polyneuropathy. *J Neurol Neurosurg Psychiatry* 53:522–525.

Salzman C, van der Kolk BA (1979) Psychotropic drugs and polypharmacy in elderly patients in a general hospital. *J Ger Res* 12:167–176.

Salzman SC (1987) Treatment of the elderly agitated patient. *J Clin Psychiatry* 48(5 suppl):19–21.

Sanberg PR (1989) Neuroleptic-induced emotional defecation: effects of pimozide and apomorphine. *Physiol Behav* 46:199–202.

Sanberg PR, Pisa M, Faulks IJ, et al (1980) Experiential influences on catalepsy. *Psychopharmacology* 69:225–226.

Sanberg PR, Russell KH, Hagenhauser-Houser SH, et al (1989) Neuroleptic-induced emotional defecation effects of scopolamine and haloperidol. *Psychopharmacology* 99:60–63.

Sandoz Pharmaceutical Corporation. (1991) *Hospital Pharmacist's Guide to the Clozaril Patient Management System*. East Rutherford, NJ: Sandoz.

Sandyk R (1985a) The endogenous opioid system in neurological disorders of the basal ganglia. *Life Sci* 37:1655–1663.

Sandyk R (1985b) Propranolol-induced tardive dyskinesia in a patient with akathisia [letter]. *Ann Neurol* 18:370.

Sandyk R (1986) L-Tryptophan in the treatment of restless legs syndrome. *Am J Psychiatry* 143:554–555.

Sandyk R (1989) Melanocyte stimulating hormone (MSH) in the restless-legs syndrome. *Int J Neurosci* 46:197–199.

Sandyk R, Bernick C, Lee SM, et al (1987) L-Dopa in uremic patients with the restless legs syndrome. *Int J Neurosci* 35:233–235.

Sandyk R, Iacono RP, Bamford CR (1988) Spinal cord mechanisms in amitriptyline responsive restless legs syndrome in Parkinson's disease. *Int J Neurosci* 38:121–124.

Sandyk R, Kay SR (1990a) Sulcal size and neuroleptic-induced akathisia. *Biol Psychiatry* 27:466–467.

Sandyk R, Kay SR (1990b) Relationship of neuroleptic-induced akathisia to drug-induced parkinsonism. *Ital J Neurol Sci* 11:439–442.

Sandyk R, Kay SR, Awerbuch GI, et al (1991) Risk factors for neuroleptic-induced movement disorders. *Int J Neurosci* 61:149–188.

Sarwer-Foner GJ (1960a) The role of neuroleptic medication in psychotherapeutic interaction. *Compr Psychiatry* 1:291–300.

Sarwer-Foner GJ (1960b) Recognition and management of drug-induced extrapyramidal reactions and 'paradoxical' behavioural reactions in psychiatry. *Can Med Assoc J* 83:312–318.

Sarwer-Foner GJ (1961) Comments on the psychodynamic aspects of the extrapyramidal reactions. *Rev Can Biol* 20:527–533.

Sarwer-Foner GJ (1963) On the mechanisms of action in neuroleptic drugs: a theoretical psychodynamic explanation. *Recent Adv Biol Psychiatry* 20:527–533.

Sarwer-Foner GJ, Ogle W (1956) Psychosis and enhanced anxiety produced by reserpine and chlorpromazine. *Can Med Assoc J* 74:526–532.

Saskin P, Moldofsky H, Lue FA (1985) Periodic movements in sleep and sleep-wake complaint. *Sleep* 8:319–324.

Scatton B, Rouguier L, Javoy-Agid F, et al (1982) Dopamine deficiency in cerebral cortex in Parkinson's disease. *Neurology* 32:1039–1040.

Schachar R, Rutter M, Smith A (1981) The characteristics of situationally and pervasively hyperactive children: implications for syndrome definition. *J Child Psychol Psychiat* 22:375–392.

Schmidt WR, Jarcho LW (1966) Persistent dyskinesia following phenothiazine therapy. *Arch Neurol* 14:369–373.

Schoenen J, Gonce M, Delwaide PJ (1984) Painful legs and moving toes: a syndrome with different physiopathic mechanisms. *Neurology* 34:1108–1113.

Schonecker M (1957) Ein eigentumliches syndrome in oralen Bereich bein Magaphen Applikation. *Nervenarzt* 28:35.

Schooler N, Kane J (1982) Research diagnoses for tardive dyskinesias. *Arch Gen Psychiatry* 39:486–487.

Schooler N, Severe J, Levine J, et al (1982) Der abruck der neuroleptischen behandlung bei schizophrenen patienten und dessen einfluss auf ruckfalle und auf symptome der spatdyskinesi. In: Kryspin-Exner K, Hinterhuber H, Schubert H, eds. *Ergebnisse der Psychiatrischen Therapieforschung.* Stuttgart: FK Schattauer Verlag.

Schott GD (1981) Painful legs and moving toes: the role of trauma. *J Neurol Neurosurg Psychiatry* 44:344–346.

Schreiber G, Avissar S, Umansky R, et al (1988) Implications of muscarinic receptor heterogeneity for research on tardive dyskinesia. In: Wolf ME, Mosnaim AD, eds. *Tardive Dyskinesia.* Washington, DC: American Psychiatric Press.

Schuckit MA, Petrich J, Chiles J (1978) Hyperactivity: diagnostic confusion. *J Nerv Ment Dis* 166(2):279–299.

Schulte JR (1985) Homicide and suicide associated with akathisia and haloperidol. *Am J Foren Psychiatry* 6:3–7.

Schwarcz G, Gosenfeld L, Gilderman A, et al (1986) Akathisia associated with carbamazepine therapy. *Am J Psychiatry* 143:1190–1191.

Schwartz GE (1983) Development and validation of the Geriatric Evaluation by Relatives Rating Instrument (GERRI). *Psychol Rep* 53:479–458.

Seeman P (1977) Anti-schizophrenic drugs: membrane receptor sites of action. *Biochem Pharmacol* 26:1741–1748.

Seeman P, Lee T, Chau-Wong M, et al (1976) Antipsychotic drug doses and neuroleptic/dopamine receptors. *Nature* 261:717–719.

Seham M, Boardman DV (1934) A study of motor automatisms. *Arch Neurol Psychiatry* 32:154–173.

Seifert R, Jamieson J, Gardner R (1983) Use of anticholinergics in the nursing home: an empirical study and review. *Drug Intell Clin Pharm* 17:470–473.

Seligman MEP (1972) Preface. In: Seligman MEP, Hager IL, eds. *Biological Boundaries in Learning.* New York: Appleton-Century-Crofts. pp. 8–9.

Settle EC (1993) Akathisia and sertraline [letter]. *J Clin Psychiatry* 54:321.

Severson JA, Marcusson J, Winbald B, et al (1982) Age-correlated loss of dopaminergic binding sites in human basal ganglia. *J Neurochem* 39:1623–1631.

Shapiro AK, Shapiro ES (1993) Neuroleptic drugs. In: Kurlan R, ed. *Handbook of Tourette's Syndrome and Related Tic and Behavioral Disorders.* New York: Marcel Dekker. pp. 347–376.

Shapiro AK, Shapiro ES, Young JG, Feinberg TE (1988) *Gilles de la Tourette Syndrome.* 2nd ed. New York: Raven Press.

Shaw ED, Mann JJ, Weiden PJ, et al (1986) A case of suicidal and homicidal ideation and akathisia in a double-blind neuroleptic crossover study. *J Clin Psychopharmacol* 6:196–197.

Shear MK, Frances A, Weiden P (1983) Suicide associated wih akathisia and depot fluphenazine treatment. *J Clin Psychopharmacol* 3:235–236.

Sheard MH (1969) The effect of *p*-chlorophenylanine on behaviour in rats: relation to brain serotonin and 5-hydroxyindoleacetic acid. *Brain Res* 15:524–528.

Shearer RM, Brownes IT, Curran P (1984) Tardive akathisia and agitated depression during metoclopramide therapy. *Acta Psychiatr Scand* 70:428–431.

Shen WW (1981) Akathisia: an overlooked, distressing, but treatable condition. *J Nerv Ment Dis* 169:599–600.

Shen WW (1983) The management of amoxapine-induced akathisia. *Am J Psychiatry* 140:1102–1103.

Shen WW (1984) Alcohol, amoxapine, and akathisia. *Biol Psychiatry* 19:929–930.

Sher NS (1962) Hallucinations and chlorpromazine in an otosclerotic. *Am J Psychiatry* February: 746–747.

Sicard JA (1923) Akathisie and tasikinesie. *Presse Med* 31:265–266.

Sieker HO, Heyman A, Birchfield RI (1960) The effects of natural sleep and hypnosomnolent states on respiratory function. *Ann Intern Med* 53:500–516.

Sigwald J, Grossiord A, Duriel P, et al (1947) Le traitement de la maladie de Parkinson et des manifestations extrapyramidalles par le diethylaminoethyl *n*-thiophyenylamine (2987 RP): resultants d'une anee d'application. *Rev Neurol* 79:683–687.

Sigwald J, Solignac J (1960) Manifestations douloureuses de lad maladie de Parkinson et paresthesies provoquees par les neuroleptiques. *Sem Hop Paris* 44:2222–2225.

Silver JM, Yudofsky SC, Kogan M, et al (1986) Elevation of thioridazine plasma levels by propranolol. *Am J Psychiatry* 143:1290–1292.

Simpson GM (1977) Neurotoxicology of major tranquilizers In: Roizen L, Shiraki H, Grcevic H, eds. *Neurotoxicology.* New York: Raven Press. pp. 1–7.

Simpson GM, Amuso D, Blair JH, et al (1964) Phenothiazine-produced extra-pyramidal system disturbance. *Arch Gen Psychiatry* 10:199–208.

Simpson GM, Angus JWS (1970) A rating scale for extrapyramidal side-effects. *Acta Psychiatr Scand* 213:11–19.

Simpson GM, Voitachevsky A, Young MA, et al (1977) Deanol in the treatment of tardive dyskinesia. *Psychopharmacology* 52:257–261.

Singh MM, Kay SR (1979) Dysphoria response to neuroleptic treatment in schizophrenia: its relationship to autonomic arousal and prognosis. *Biol Psychiatry* 14:277–294.

Sinha D, Zelman FP, Nelson S, et al (1992) A new scale for assessing behavioral agitation in dementia. *Psychiatry Res* 41:73–88.

Siris SG (1985) Three cases of akathisia and 'acting out.' *J Clin Psychiatry* 46:395–397.

Skarsfeldt T, Perregaard J (1990) Sertindole, a new neuroleptic with extreme selectivity on A10 versus A9 dopamine neurons in the rat. *Eur J Pharmacol* 182:613–614.

Slawson P (1989) Psychiatric malpractice: ten years' loss experience. *Medicine Law* 8:415–427.

Smith A (1973) *Symbol Digits Modalities Test.* Los Angeles: Western Psychological Services.

Smith RC (1985) Relationship of periodic movements in sleep (nocturnal myoclonus) and the Babinski sign. *Sleep* 8:239–243.

Smith RC (1988) Is the dopaminergic supersensitivity theory of tardive dyskinesia valid? In: Wolf ME, Mosnaim AD, eds. *Tardive Dyskinesia: Biological Mechanisms and Clinical Aspects.* Washington, DC: American Psychiatric Press. pp. 1–22.

Snider SR, Fahn S, Isgreen WP, et al (1976) Primary sensory symptoms in parkinsonism. *Neurology* 26:423–429.

Sokoloff P, Giros B, Martres MP, et al (1990) Molecular cloning and characterization of a novel dopamine receptor (D3) as target for neuroleptics. *Nature* 347:146–151.

Sovner R, DiMascio A (1978) Extrapyramidal syndromes and other neurological side-effects of psychotropic drugs. In: Lipton MA, DiMascio A, Killam KF, eds. *Psychopharmacology: A Generation of Progress.* New York: Raven Press. pp. 1021–1032.

Spielberger CD, Gorsuch RL, Lushenc RE (1967) *State-Trait Anxiety Inventory.* Tallahassee: Florida State University Press.

Spillane JD (1970) Restless legs syndrome in chronic pulmonary disease. *Br Med J* 4:796–798.

Spillane JD, Nathan PW, Kelly RE, et al (1971) Painful legs and moving toes. *Brain* 94:541–556.

Stahl SM (1985) Akathisia and tardive dyskinesia: changing concepts. *Arch Gen Psychiatry* 42:915–917.

Stahl SM, Faull KF, Barchas JD, et al (1985) CSF monoamine metabolites in movement disorders and normal aging. *Arch Neurol* 42:166–169.

Steck H (1954) [The extrapyramidal syndrome in the course of treatment with largactil and serpasil] Le syndrome extrapyramidal et d'encephalique au cours des traitements au largactil et au serpasil. *Ann Med Psychol* 112:737–743.

Stefano GB (1982) Comparative aspects of opioid–dopamine interaction. *Cell Mol Neurobiol* 2:167–178.

Stein JA, Tschudy DP (1970) Acute intermittent porphyria: A clinical and biochemical study of 46 patients. *Medicine* 49:1–16.

Stein MB, Pohlman ER (1987) Tardive akathisia associated with low-dose haloperidol use. *J Clin Psychopharmacol* 7:202–203.

Steinberg HR, Green R, Durell J (1967) Depression occurring during the course of recovery from schizophrenic symptoms. *Am J Psychiatry* 124:699–702.

Steiner JC (1987) Clonidine in restless legs syndrome. *Neurology* 37(1 suppl):278. Abstract.

Stern MJ, Pillsbury JA, Sonnenberg SM (1972) Postpsychotic depression in schizo-phrenics. *Compr Psychiatry* 13:519–598.

Stewart JT (1989) Akathisia following traumatic brain injury: treatment with bromocriptine. *J Neurol Neurosurg Psychiatry* 52:1200–1201.

Stewart MA, Cumming C, Singer S, et al (1981) The overlap between hyperactive and unsocialized aggressive children. *J Child Psychol Psychiat* 22:35–45.

Stewart MA, Pitts FN, Craig HG, et al (1966) The hyperactive child syndrome. *Am J Orthopsychiatry* 36:861–867.

Stone RK, Alvarez WF, Ellman G (1989) Lifetime antipsychotic-drug exposure, dyskinesia and related movement disorders in the developmentally disabled. *Pharmacol Biochem Behav* 34:759–763.

Stone RK, May JE, Alvarez WF, et al (1989) Prevalence of dyskinesia and related movement disorders in a developmentally disabled population. *J Ment Defic Res* 33:41–53.

Strang PR (1967) The symptom of restless legs. *Med J Aust* 1:1211–1213.

Strange PG (1990) Subtypes of the D2 dopamine receptor [letter]. *Trends Pharmacol Sci* 11:357.

Strange PG (1992) *Brain Biochemistry and Brain Disorders.* Oxford University Press.

Sunderland T, Alterman IS, Yount D, et al (1988) A new scale for the assessment of depressed mood in demented patients. *Am J Psychiatry* 145:955–959.

Sunderland T, Cohen BM (1987) Blood to brain distribution of neuroleptics. *Psychiatry Res* 20:299–305.

Symposium (1989) Abstracts of the Symposium on High Technology in the Quantitation of Movement Disorders. *Mov Disord* 4:97–104.

Swedberg B (1952) Anemi och sideropeni simulerande hjartsjukdom. *Svenska Lakartidn* 49:2591.

Symonds CP (1953) Nocturnal myoclonus. *J Neurol Neurosurg Psychiatry* 16:166–171.

Tariot PN, Cohen RM, Sunderland T, et al (1987) L-Deprenyl in Alzheimer's dis-ease: preliminary evidence for behavioral change with monoamine oxidase B inhibition. *Arch Gen Psychiatry* 44:427–433.

Tassin JP, Stinus L, Simon M, et al (1978) Relationship between the locomotor hy-peractivity induced by A10 lesions and the destruction of the fronto-cortical dopaminergic innervation in the rat. *Brain Res* 141:267–281.

Taylor MA (1990) Catatonia: a review of a behavioral neurologic syndrome. *Neuropsychiat Neuropsychol Behav Neurol* 3:48–72.

Teicher MH, Glod C, Cole JO (1990) Emergence of intense suicidal preoccupation during fluoxetine treatment. *Am J Psychiatry* 147:207–210.

Telstad W, Sorensen O, Larsen S, et al (1984) Treatment of the restless legs syn-drome with carbamazepine: a double blind study. *Br Med J (Clin Res Ed)* 288:444–446.

Terao T, Terao M, Yoshimura T, et al (1991) Restless legs syndrome induced by lithium. *Biol Psychiatry* 30:1167–1170.

Teri L, Borson S, Kiyak HA, et al (1989) Behavioral disturbance, cognitive dys-function, and functional skill: prevalence and relationship in Alzheimer's dis-ease. *J Am Geriatr Soc* 37:109–116.

Teri L, Larson EB, Reifler B (1988) Behavioral disturbance in dementia of the Alzheimer type. *J Am Geriatr Soc* 36:1–6.

Thierry AM, Stinus L, Blanc G, et al (1973) Some evidence for the existence of dopaminergic neurons in the rat cortex. *Brain Res* 50:230–234.

Thorley G (1984) Review of follow-up and follow-back studies of childhood hy-peractivity. *Psychol Bull* 96:116–132.

TiPS Receptor Nomenclature Supplement. (1992) *Trends Pharmacol Sci* (special suppl 20).

Tominaga H, Fukuzako H, Izumi K, et al (1987) Tardive myoclonus [letter]. *Lancet* 1:322.

Tryon WW, Pologe B (1987) Accelerometric assessment of tardive dyskinesia. *Am J Psychiatry* 144:1584–1587.

Trzepacz PT, Violette EJ, Sateia MJ (1984) Response to opioids in three patients with restless legs syndrome. *Am J Psychiatry* 141:993–995.

Tune L, Coyle JT (1981) Acute extrapyramidal side effects: serum levels of neuroleptics and anticholinergics. *Psychopharmacology* 75:9–15.

Tuvo F (1949) Contributo clinico alla conoscenza della sindrome cosiddetta 'irritables legs.' *Minerva Med* 40:741–743.

Tyron AF (1968) Thumb-sucking and manifest anxiety: a note. *Child Dev* 39: 1158–1163.

Ugedo L, Grenhoff J, Svensson TH (1989) Ritanserin, a 5-HT2 receptor antagonist, activates midbrain dopamine neurons by blocking serotonergic inhibition. *Psychopharmacology* 98:45–50.

Uhrbrand L, Faurbye A (1960) Reversible and irreversible dyskinesia after treatment with perphenazine, chlorpromazine, reserpine, and electroconvulsive therapy. *Psychopharmacologia* 1:408–418.

Van Putten T (1974) Why do schizophrenic patients refuse to take their drugs? *Arch Gen Psychiatry* 31:67–72.

Van Putten T (1975) The many faces of akathisia. *Compr Psychiatry* 16:43–47.

Van Putten T, Crumpton E, Yale C (1976) Drug refusal in schizophrenia and the wish to be crazy. *Arch Gen Psychiatry* 33:1443–1446.

Van Putten T, Marder SR (1986) Toward a more reliable diagnosis of akathisia. *Arch Gen Psychiatry* 43:1015–1016.

Van Putten T, Marder SR (1987) Behavioral toxicity of antipsychotic drugs. *J Clin Psychiatry* 48(suppl):13–19.

Van Putten T, Marder SR, Mintz J (1990) A controlled dose comparison of haloperidol in newly admitted schizophrenic patients. *Arch Gen Psychiatry* 47:754–758.

Van Putten T, Marder SR, Wirshing WC, et al (1991) Neuroleptic plasma levels. *Schizophr Bull* 17:197–216.

Van Putten T, May PR, Marder SR (1984a) Response to antipsychotic medication: the doctor's and the consumer's view. *Am J Psychiatry* 141:16–19.

Van Putten T, May PR, Marder SR (1984b) Akathisia with haloperidol and thiothixene. *Psychopharmacol Bull* 20:114–117.

Van Putten T, May PR, Marder SR (1984c) Akathisia with haloperidol and thiothixene. *Arch Gen Psychiatry* 41:1036–1039.

Van Putten T, May PRA (1978a) Subjective response as a predictor of outcome in pharmacotherapy. *Arch Gen Psychiatry* 35:477–480.

Van Putten T, May PRA (1978b) 'Akinetic depression' in schizophrenia. *Arch Gen Psychiatry* 35:1101–1107.

Van Putten T, May PRA, Jenden DJ, et al (1980) Plasma and saliva levels of chlorpromazine and subjective response. *Am J Psychiatry* 137:1241–1242.

Van Putten T, May PRA, Marder SR (1981) Subjective response to antipsychotic drugs. *Arch Gen Psychiatry* 38:187–190.

Van Putten T, Mutalipassi LR, Malkin MD (1974) Phenothiazine induced decompensation. *Arch Gen Psychiatry* 30:13–19.

Van Tol HH, Bunzow JR, Guan HC, et al (1991) Cloning of the gene for a human dopamine D4 receptor with high affinity for the antipsychotic clozapine. *Nature* 350:610–614.

Vernallis FF (1955) Teeth-grinding: some relationships to anxiety, hostility, and hyperactivity. *J Clin Psychol* 11:389–391.

Vetulani J, Suster F (1975) Action of various antidepressant treatments reduces reactivity of noradrenergic cyclic AMP-generating system in limbic forebrain. *Nature* 257:495–496.

Viukari M, Linnoila M (1977) Effect of fusaric acid on tardive dyskinesia and mental state in psychogeriatric patients: a pilot study. *Acta Psychiatr Scand* 56:57–61.

von Economo C (1931) *Encephalitis Lethargica: Its Sequelae and Treatment.* London: Oxford University Press.

von Scheele C (1986) Levodopa in restless legs. *Lancet* 2:426–427.

von Scheele C, Kempi V (1990) Long-term effect of dopaminergic drugs in restless legs: a 2-year follow-up. *Arch Neurol* 47:1223–1224.

Waddington JL (1989) Schizophrenia, affective psychoses, and other disorders treated with neuroleptic drugs: the enigma of tardive dyskinesia, its neurobiological determinants, and the conflict of paradigms. *Int Rev Neurobiol* 31:297–353.

Waddington JL, Youssef HA, Dolphin C, et al (1987) Cognitive dysfunction, negative symptoms, and tardive dyskinesia in schizophrenia: their association in relation to topography of involuntary movements and criterion of their abnormality. *Arch Gen Psychiatry* 44:907–912.

Waldmeier PC, Delini-Stula AA (1979) Serotonin-dopamine interactions in the nigrostriatal system. *Eur J Pharmacol* 55:363–373.

Walker BA, Ziskind E (1977) Relationship of nail-biting to sociopathy. *J Nerv Ment Dis* 164:64–65.

Wallace M, Singer G (1975) Adjunctive behavior in humans during game playing. *Physiol Behav* 14:651–654.

Wallace M, Singer G (1976) Adjunctive behavior and smoking induced by a maze solving schedule in humans. *Physiol Behav* 17:849–852.

Walters A, Hening W, Chokroverty S, et al (1985) Opioid responsiveness of neuroleptic-induced akathisia [letter]. *Ann Neurol* 18:137.

Walters A, Hening W, Chokroverty S, et al (1986) Opioid responsiveness in patients with neuroleptic-induced akathisia. *Mov Disord* 1:119–127.

Walters AS, Hening A (1989) Opioids, a better treatment for acute than tardive akathisia: possible role for the endogenous opiate system in neuroleptic-induced akathisia. *Med Hypotheses* 28:1–2.

Walters AS, Hening W (1987) Review of the clinical presentation and neuropharmacology of restless legs syndrome. *Clin Neuropharmacol* 10:225–237.

Walters AS, Hening W, Chokroverty S, et al (1989) Restlessness of the arms as the principal manifestation of neuroleptic-induced akathisia. [letter]. *J Neurol* 236:435.

Walters AS, Hening W, Rubinstein M, et al (1991) A clinical and polysomnographic comparison of neuroleptic-induced akathisia and the idiopathic restless legs syndrome. *Sleep* 14:339–345.

Walters AS, Hening WA, Chokroverty S (1988a) Frequent occurrence of myoclonus while awake and at rest, body rocking and marching in place in a subpopulation of patients with restless legs syndrome. *Acta Neurol Scand* 77:418–421.

Walters AS, Hening WA, Kavey N, et al (1988b) A double-blind randomized crossover trial of bromocriptine and placebo in restless legs syndrome. *Ann Neurol* 24:455–458.

Walters AS, Picchietti D, Hening W, et al (1990) Variable expressivity in familial restless legs syndrome. *Arch Neurol* 47:1219–1220.

Warnes H (1968) Suicide in schizophrenics. *Dis Nerv Syst* 11:312–321.

Watson R, Hollander C (1987) Familial nocturnal myoclonus. *Sleep Res* 16:309–319.

Webb TE, Oski FA (1974) Behavioural status of young adolescents with iron deficiency anemia. *J Spec Educ* 8:153–156.

Webster DD (1966) Rigidity in extrapyramidal disease. *J Neurosurg* 24:299.

Wechsler LR, Stakes JW, Shahani BT, et al (1986) Periodic leg movements of sleep (nocturnal myoclonus): an electrophysiological study. *Ann Neurol* 19:168–173.

Weddington WW Jr, Banner A (1986) Organic affective syndrome associated with metoclopramide: case report. *J Clin Psychiatry* 47:208–209.

Weiden P, Bruun R (1987) Worsening of Tourette's disorder due to neuroleptic-induced akathisia. *Am J Psychiatry* 144:504–505.

Weiden PJ, Mann JJ, Dixon L, et al (1989) Is neuroleptic dysphoria a healthy response? *Compr Psychiatry* 33:546–552.

Weil A (1970) Hermann Oppenheim. In: Haymaker W, Schiller F, eds. *The Founders of Neurology*. Springfield, IL: Thomas. pp. 492–495.

Weinberg J, Dallman PR, Levine S (1980) Iron deficiency during early development in the rat: behavioural and physiological consequences. *Pharmacol Biochem Behav* 12:493–502.

Weinberger DR, Berman KF, Suddath R, et al (1992) Evidence of a dysfunction of a prefronto-limbic network in schizophrenia: a magnetic resonance imaging and regional cerebral blood flow study of discordant monozygotic twins. *Am J Psychiatry* 149:890–987.

Weinberger DR, Bigelow LB, Klein ST, et al (1981) Drug withdrawal in chronic schizophrenic patients: in search of neuroleptic-induced supersensitivity psychosis. *J Clin Psychopharmacol* 1:120–123.

Weiner HL, Lajtha A, Sershen H (1989) Dopamine D1 receptor and dopamine D2 receptor binding activity changes during chronic administration of nicotine in a 1-methyl-4-phenyl-1,2,3,6-tetra-hydropyridine-treated mice. *Neuropharmacology* 28:535–537.

Weiner WJ, Goetz CG, Nausieda PA, et al (1978) Respiratory dyskinesias: extrapyramidal dysfunction and dyspnea. *Ann Intern Med* 88:327–331.

Weiner WJ, Luby ED (1983) Persistent akathisia following neuroleptic withdrawal. *Ann Neurol* 13:466–467.

Weiss B, Hechtman L (1979) The hyperactive child syndrome. *Science* 205:1348–1354.

Weiss B, Hechtman LT (1986) *Hyperactive Children Grown Up: Empirical Findings and Theoretical Considerations*. New York: Guilford Press.

Wells BG, Cold JA, Marken PA, et al (1991) A placebo-controlled trial of nadolol in the treatment of neuroleptic-induced akathisia. *J Clin Psychiatry* 52:255–260.

Wersall J (1952) Restless legs. *Svenska Lakartidn* 49:2032–2035.

West R, Hajek P, Belcher M (1989) Time course of cigarette withdrawal symptoms while using nicotine gum. *Psychopharmacology* 99:143–153.

Wetzel H, Wiedemann K, Holsboer F, et al (1991) Savoxepine: invalidation of an 'atypical' neuroleptic response pattern predicted by animal models in an open clinical trial with schizophrenic patients. *Psychopharmacology* 103:280–283.

Whittacker CB, Hoy RM (1963) Withdrawal of perphenazine in chronic schizophrenia. *Br J Psychiatry* 109:422–427.

Whittier JR, Mettler FA (1949) Studies on the subthalamus of the rhesus monkey. *J Comp Neurol* 90:319–372.

Wiesel FA (1976) Effects of high dose propranolol treatment on dopamine and norepinephrine metabolism in regions of rat brain. *Neurosci Lett* 2:35–38.

Wilbur R, Kulik AV (1983) Propranolol for akathisia. *Lancet* 2:917.

Wilbur R, Kulik FA, Kulik AV (1988) Noradrenergic effects in tardive dyskinesia, akathisia and pseudoparkinsonism via the limbic system and basal ganglia. *Prog Neuropsychopharmacol Biol Psychiatry* 12:849–864.

Williams DG (1973) So-called 'nervous habits'. *J Psychol* 83:103–109.

Williams K, Goldstein G (1979) Cognitive and affective response to lithium in patients with organic brain syndrome. *Am J Psychiatry* 136:800–803.

Willis T (1685) *The London Practice of Physick.* London: Thomas Bassett & William Crooke.

Wilson IC, Garbutt JC, Lanier CF, et al (1983) Is there a tardive dysmentia? *Schizophr Bull* 9:187–192.

Wilson SAK (1940) *Neurology.* Vols I and II. Baltimore: Williams & Williams.

Wilson SAK (1952) Disorders of motility and of muscle tone, with special reference to the corpus striatum. *Lancet* 2:1–10.

Wilson SAK (1955) *Neurology.* 2nd ed. London: Butterworths.

Winkleman NW (1961) The inter-relationship between the physiological and psychological etiologies of akathisia. In: Bordeleau JM, ed. *Extrapyramidal Systems and Neuroleptics.* Montreal: Editions Psychiatriques. pp. 563–568.

Wirsching WC, Cummings JL, Dencker SJ (1991) Electromechanical characteristics of tardive dyskinesia. *J Neuropsychiatry Clin Neurosci* 3:10–17.

Wirshing WC, Phelan CK, Van Putten T, et al (1990) Effects of clozapine on treatment-resistant akathisia and concomitant tardive dyskinesia. *J Clin Psychopharmacol* 10:371–373.

Wirshing WC, Van Putten T, Rosenberg J, et al (1992) Fluoxetine, akathisia, and suicidality: is there a causal connection? *Arch Gen Psychiatry* 49:580–581.

Witschy J, Malone G, Holden L (1984) Neuroleptic withdrawal psychosis in a manic depressive patient. *Am J Psychiatry* 141:105–106.

Wittig R, Zorick F, Piccione P, et al (1983) Narcolepsy and disturbed nocturnal sleep. *Clin Electroencephalogr* 14:130–134.

Wittmaack T (1861) *Pathologic und Therapie der Sensibilitat-Neurosen.* Leipzig: E. Schafer.

Woolf NJ, Butcher LL (1989) Cholinergic systems: synopsis of anatomy and overview of physiology and pathology. In: Scheibel AB, Wechsler AF, ed. *The Biological Substrates of Alzheimer's Disease.* New York: Academic Press. pp. 73–86.

Wykes T, Sturt E (1986) The measurement of social behaviour in psychiatric patients: an assessment of the reliability and validity of the SBS schedule. *Br J Psychiatry* 148:1–11.

Yassa R, Bloom D (1990) Lorazepam and anticholinergics in tardive akathisia. *Biol Psychiatry* 27:463–464.

Yassa R, Groulx B (1989) Lorazepam in the treatment of lithium-induced akathisia. *J Clin Psychopharmacol* 9:70–71.

Yassa R, Iskandar H, Nastase C (1988) Propranolol in the treatment of tardive akathisia: a report of two cases. *J Clin Psychopharmacol* 8:283–285.

Yassa R, Lal S (1986) Respiratory irregularity and tardive dyskinesia. *Acta Psychiatr Scand* 73:506–510.

Yassa R, Lal S, Korpassy A, et al (1987) Nicotine exposure and tardive dyskinesia. *Biol Psychiatry* 22:67–72.

Yeragani VK, Pohl R, Balon R, et al (1992) Imipramine-induced jitteriness and decreased serum iron levels. *Neuropsychobiology* 25:8–10.

Youdim MBH, Ashkenazi R, Ben-Shachar D, et al (1983) Modulation of brain receptor in striatum by iron: behavioral and biochemical correlates. *Adv Neurol* 40:159–173.

Youdim MBH, Ben-Shachar D, Yehuda S (1989) Putative biological mechanisms of the effect of iron deficiency on brain biochemistry and behavior. *Am J Clin Nutr* 50:607–617.

Young RR (1992) Tremor: an overview. In: Joseph AB, Young RR, eds. *Movement Disorders in Neurology and Neuropsychiatry.* Boston: Blackwell Scientific. pp. 565–568.

Youssef HA, Waddington JL (1987) Morbidity and mortality in tardive dyskinesia: associations in chronic schizophrenia. *Acta Psychiatr Scand* 75:74–77.

Yudosfky SC, Silver JM, Schneider SE (1987) Pharmacologic treatment of aggression. *Psychiatr Ann* 17:397–404.

Yudofsky SC, Stevens L, Silver J, et al (1984) Propranolol in the treatment of rage and violent behavior associated with Korsakoff's psychosis. *Am J Psychiatry* 141:114–115.

Zarit SH, Reever KE, Bach-Peterson J (1980) Relatives of the impaired elderly: correlates of feelings of burden. *Gerontologist* 29(6):649–655.

Zelman S (1978) Terbutaline and muscular symptoms. *JAMA* 239:930.

Zitrin CM, Klein DF, Woerner MG (1978) Behavior therapy, supportive psychotherapy, imipramine and phobias. *Arch Gen Psychiatry* 35:307–316.

Zitrin CM, Klein DF, Woerner MG (1980) Treatment of agoraphobia with group exposure in vivo and imipramine. *Arch Gen Psychiatry* 37:63–72.

Zorick F, Roth T, Salis P, et al (1978) Insomnia and excessive day-time sleepiness as presenting symptoms in nocturnal myoclonus. *Sleep Res* 7:256.

Zubenko GS, Barreira P, Lipinski JF Jr (1984a) Development of tolerance to the therapeutic effect of amantadine on akathisia. *J Clin Psychopharmacol* 4:218–220.

Zubenko GS, Cohen BM, Lipinski JF Jr, et al (1984b) Use of clonidine in treating neuroleptic-induced akathisia. *Psychiatry Res* 13:253–259.

Zubenko GS, Cohen BM, Lipinski JFJ (1987) Antidepressant-related akathisia. *J Clin Psychopharmacol* 7:254–257.

Zubenko GS, Lipinski JF, Cohen BM, et al (1984c) Comparison of metoprolol and propranolol in the treatment of akathisia. *Psychiatry Res* 11;143–149.

Zucconi M, Coccagna G, Petronelli R, et al (1989) Nocturnal myoclonus in restless legs syndrome effect of carbamazepine treatment. *Funct Neurol* 4:263–271.

Zuckerman M, Lubin B (1965) *Manual for the Multiple Affect Check List.* San Diego: Educational and Industrial Testing Service.

Zung WWK (1965) A self-rating depression scale. *Arch Gen Psychiatry* 12:63–70.

Index